Challenging Concepts in Paediatric Critical Care

Published and forthcoming titles in the
Challenging Concepts in series

Anaesthesia (Edited by Dr Phoebe Syme, Dr Robert Jackson,
and Dr Timothy Cook)

Cardiovascular Medicine (Edited by Dr Aung Myat, Dr Shouvik
Haldar, and Professor Simon Redwood)

Critical Care (Edited by Dr Christopher Gough, Dr Justine Barnett,
Professor Tim Cook, and Professor Jerry Nolan)

Emergency Medicine (Edited by Dr Sam Thenabadu, Dr Fleur Cantle,
and Dr Chris Lacy)

Infectious Diseases and Clinical Microbiology
(Edited by Dr Amber Arnold and Professor George E. Griffin)

Interventional Radiology (Edited by Dr Irfan Ahmed,
Dr Miltiadis Krokidis, and Dr Tarun Sabharwal)

Neurology (Edited by Dr Krishna Chinthapalli, Dr Nadia Magdalinou,
and Professor Nicholas Wood)

Neurosurgery (Edited by Mr Robin Bhatia and Mr Ian Sabin)

Obstetrics and Gynaecology (Edited by Dr Natasha Hezelgrave,
Dr Danielle Abbott, and Professor Andrew Shennan)

Oncology (Edited by Dr Madhumita Bhattacharyya, Dr Sarah Payne,
and Professor Iain McNeish)

Oral and Maxillofacial Surgery (Edited by Mr Matthew Idle and
Group Captain Andrew Monaghan)

Respiratory Medicine (Edited by Dr Lucy Schomberg,
Dr Elizabeth Sage, and Dr Nick Hart)

Challenging Concepts in Paediatric Critical Care
Cases with Expert Commentary

Edited by

Dr Hari Krishnan

Consultant Paediatric Intensivist, Birmingham Children's Hospital, Birmingham, UK

Dr Miriam R. Fine-Goulden

Consultant, Paediatric Intensive Care and South Thames Retrieval Service,
Evelina London Children's Hospital, Guy's & St Thomas' NHS Foundation Trust, London, UK

Dr Sainath Raman

Senior Medical Officer, Paediatric Intensive Care, Queensland Children's Hospital, Brisbane,
QLD, Australia

Dr Akash Deep

Director, Paediatric Intensive Care Unit, King's College Hospital, London, UK

Series editors

Dr Aung Myat

NIHR Academic Clinical Lecturer in Interventional Cardiology, Brighton and Sussex Medical School,
Brighton, UK

Dr Shouvik Haldar

Consultant Cardiologist and Electrophysiologist, Heart Rhythm Centre,
Royal Brompton and Harefield NHS Foundation Trust, Honorary Clinical Senior Lecturer, Imperial College London, London, UK

Professor Simon Redwood

Professor of Interventional Cardiology and Honorary Consultant Cardiologist, King's College London and St Thomas' Hospital, London, UK

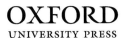

OXFORD
UNIVERSITY PRESS

UNIVERSITY PRESS

Great Clarendon Street, Oxford, OX2 6DP,
United Kingdom

Oxford University Press is a department of the University of Oxford.
It furthers the University's objective of excellence in research, scholarship,
and education by publishing worldwide. Oxford is a registered trade mark of
Oxford University Press in the UK and in certain other countries

Published in the United States of America by Oxford University Press
198 Madison Avenue, New York, NY 10016, United States of America

British Library Cataloguing in Publication Data

Data available

Library of Congress Control Number: 2020938759

ISBN 978-0-19-879459-2

Printed and bound by
CPI Group (UK) Ltd, Croydon, CR0 4YY

Despite stressful circumstances, critically ill children and families place their faith in the paediatric critical care team to provide expert clinical care. Paediatric critical care clinicians dedicate their life's work to the cause of alleviating pain and suffering in children. It is to those children, families, and healthcare professionals that we wish to dedicate this book.

FOREWORD BY JOSEPH CARCILLO

This is a really fun book to learn from which approaches critical illness in children using a series of venues devoted to the most challenging of clinical problems. Though one may or may not agree on all points made by the experts whom illustrate each case, the reader will surely come away with an enriched view of the things to think about when approaching critically ill children. I think this case method of teaching and learning is sadly slipping away in modern medical education, but happily not gone yet! Students of the art of medicine, including those of us with many years' experience, are presently left reading consensus statements and evidence evidence-based documents that in the end are not really very helpful. The structure of Dr Krishnan's book focuses on being helpful. The student is given the opportunity to think about a case as it progresses, consider what one would might do to help the theoretical child along the progression of presentation and admission to the PICU, observe what the experts would do at each point in time, and then review what rationale and logic the experts have used to come to their considered course of action(s). This is followed by a review of literature pertaining to each treatment decision with final teaching points summarizing where the field is going in this regard.

We all learn differently. Dr Krishnan and colleagues' case method approach is delightful because it reads like a short novel, is experienced by the reader as though one is at the child's bedside, and is illustrative of all those concepts that textbooks, guidelines, and evidence-based documents want to teach in a way that is engaging and rewarding.

J. A. Carcillo
Professor of Critical Care Medicine and Pediatrics
University of Pittsburgh School of Medicine

FOREWORD BY KEVIN MORRIS

We live in an era of easy-to-access information on our smartphones and computers. As a result, it can be a challenge for a book to provide added value over and above a plethora of electronic information, as well as providing something different to the range of book texts that exist. Despite this challenge, I am impressed that Krishnan and colleagues have been able to produce a book 'with a difference', which for me does provide added value and something different.

Using a series of chapters, each built around a clinical case, they have developed a book that encompasses a clever blend of aspects of bedside care, including 'clinical tips', background epidemiology and science, 'evidence base' highlights, 'learning points', and 'expert comments'. A focused list of around 20–25 references is provided at the end of each chapter for further reading. The experts who have provided their personal slants on the topics being discussed are all well-known senior clinicians in the field of paediatric critical care, and many of their unique insights would be difficult to find in any other published material. I particularly liked the last section of each chapter entitled 'A final word from the expert'.

At times the nature of the book, with the different angles described above, does result in a style that is less flowing and more a collection of pocket-sized *pearls of wisdom* around the topic under discussion, but I suspect that this style will prove popular with the new generation of intensive care doctors, nurses, and allied health professionals who have more adaptable minds than my generation! I see the book as having a particular appeal for those in training, as they build their knowledge around the common clinical presentations that they will encounter, though there is much in this book for more senior colleagues to enjoy and to learn from.

Professor Kevin Morris

PREFACE

This textbook, *Challenging Concepts in Paediatric Critical Care*, has been designed to cater to the needs of paediatric intensivists, and current and future clinicians in training. Similar to its predecessors in the 'Challenging concepts' series, this book aims to educate clinicians by describing scenarios in paediatric intensive care medicine that range from common, such as bronchiolitis and sepsis, to those that are more complex, such as mechanical circulatory support and end-of-life decision-making.

As Sir William Osler stated: 'Medicine is a science of uncertainty and an art of probability'.

With the novel approach, based on typical cases rather than the more standard textbook system-based structure, we have endeavoured to focus on both the science and the art of paediatric critical care. Every chapter has 'expert commentary' written by an international expert, providing practical advice on their approach to each clinical scenario. Many chapters include results and imaging to enhance the fidelity and narrative style of text. These encourage the reader to understand the patient journey and feel part of the decision-making process. The textbook is not meant to be an exhaustive theoretical treatise; it is designed to help facilitate the practical application of the theoretical aspects of paediatric intensive care medicine on a day-to-day basis. The clinical topics in this book are aligned with curricula of the UK Royal College of Paediatrics and Child Health's paediatric intensive care medicine, the Paediatric Basic Assessment and Support in Intensive Care (BASIC) course, and the relevant domains of the "European Paediatric / Neonatal Intensive Care Diploma™ (EPIC)". However, we anticipate that the contents of and concepts within this book will be of great value to paediatric critical care clinicians worldwide.

Science and medicine are ever-changing, with newer breakthroughs rendering earlier beliefs, concepts, and medicines less relevant, if not obsolete. While we have strived to ensure that the information contained is as up to date as possible, clinicians should keep abreast of developments in evidence base and practice, and be aware of any local guidelines and protocols. We hope that this practical case-based book helps raise the standards of care for critically ill children worldwide.

Hari Krishnan
Miriam R. Fine-Goulden
Sainath Raman
Akash Deep

ACKNOWLEDGEMENTS

This textbook would not have been possible without the efforts of a large team of people. Our families endured not only the long clinical hours to support our professional careers, but also the additional time we spent editing to publish this book in its current, high-quality format. Among the many who we owe, the editors wish to thank the following people, in particular:

• all the contributors and the experts for providing high-quality content;

• Geraldine Jeffers, Fiona Sutherland, and the team at Oxford University Press;

• Ahila, Abhinav, and Arnav Krishnan(s);

• the late Mrs Ramesh Rani—a tribute to his mum by Akash Deep and his dad, Faqir Singh, 'who always supported his career'.

• All of the Fines, the Gouldens and the Fine Gouldens.

CONTENTS

EXPERTS

Rachel Agbeko, Consultant in Paediatric Intensive Care, Department of Paediatric Intensive Care, Great North Children's Hospital, The Newcastle upon Tyne Hospitals NHS Foundation Trust, Newcastle upon Tyne, UK; Associate Clinical Lecturer, Translational and Clinical Research Institute, Newcastle University, Newcastle upon Tyne, UK

Gail Annich, Director of Quality and Safety and Emergency Preparedness, Department of Critical Care Medicine, Director of CCRT/Code Blue and Resuscitation Oversight, Medical Lead for Mass Casualty, The Hospital for Sick Children, Professor, Department of Paediatrics, University of Toronto, Toronto, ON, Canada

Joe Brierley, Consultant in Paediatric and Neonatal Intensive Care and Director of Bioethics, Great Ormond Street Hospital, London, UK

Timothy E. Bunchman, Professor and Director, Pediatric Nephrology and Transplantation, Children's Hospital of Richmond at Virginia Commonwealth University, Richmond, VA, USA

Mike Champion, Consultant in Paediatric Inherited Metabolic Disease and Clinical Lead, Evelina Children's Hospital, London, UK

Akash Deep, Director, Paediatric Intensive Care Unit, King's College Hospital, London, UK

Andrew Durward, Attending Physician, Paediatric Intensive Care, Sidra Medicine, Doha, Qatar

Roxanne Kirsch, Cardiac Critical Care Staff Physician, Critical Care Bioethics Associate, Assistant Professor of Pediatrics, The Hospital for Sick Children, University of Toronto, Toronto, ON, Canada

Hari Krishnan, Consultant Paediatric Intensivist, Birmingham Children's Hospital, Birmingham, UK

Nilesh M. Mehta, Professor of Anaesthesia, Harvard Medical School, Boston, MA, USA; Chair, Critical Care Nutrition and Metabolism, Department of Anesthesiology, Critical Care and Pain Medicine, Boston Children's Hospital, Boston, MA, USA

Vinay M. Nadkarni, Endowed Chair, Professor, Department of Anesthesiology and Critical Care Medicine, Children's Hospital of Philadelphia, Philadelphia, PA, USA; Medical Director, CHOP Center for Simulation, Advanced Education, and Innovation, The Children's Hospital of Philadelphia, Philadelphia, PA, USA; Associate Director, University of Pennsylvania Center for Resuscitation Science, Department of Emergency Medicine, Philadelphia, PA, USA

Mark J. Peters, Professor of Paediatric Intensive Care, Great Ormond Street Hospital, London, UK

Adrian Plunkett, Consultant, Paediatric Intensive Care, Birmingham Children's Hospital, Birmingham, UK

Padmanabhan Ramnarayan, PICU and Retrieval Consultant, Great Ormond Street Hospital and St Mary's Hospital, Children's Acute Transport Service, London, UK

Fiona Reynolds, Consultant in Paediatric Intensive Care, Birmingham Children's Hospital, Birmingham, UK

Peter C. Rimensberger, Director, Service of Neonatology and Paediatric Intensive Care, Department of Paediatrics, University Hospital of Geneva, Geneva, Switzerland

Robert C. Tasker, Professor of Anaesthesia (Pediatrics), Department of Anesthesia, Critical Care and Pain Medicine, and Department of Neurology, Boston Children's Hospital, Harvard Medical School, Boston, MA, USA

Kentigern Thorburn, Clinical Director of Critical Care and Consultant in Paediatric Intensive Care, Alder Hey Children's Hospital, Liverpool, UK; Honorary Lecturer, Department of Clinical Infection, Microbiology and Immunology, The University of Liverpool, Liverpool, UK

Shane Tibby, Clinical Lead for Paediatric Intensive Care and South Thames Retrieval Service, Evelina London Children's Hospital, Guy's & St Thomas' NHS Foundation Trust, London, UK

CONTRIBUTORS

Ben D. Albert, Associate Program Director, Critical Care Medicine Fellowship Program, Boston Children's Hospital, Boston, MA, USA; Instructor of Anaesthesia, Harvard Medical School, Boston, MA, USA

Katelyn Ariagno, Pediatric Clinical Nutrition Specialist III, Center for Nutrition, Boston Children's Hospital, Boston, MA, USA; Medical/Surgical Intensive Care Unit, Division of Critical Care Medicine, Department of Anesthesiology, Critical Care and Pain Medicine, Boston Children's Hospital, Boston, MA, USA

Omer Aziz, Paediatric Intensive Care Consultant, Bristol Royal Hospital for Children, Bristol, UK

Ryan P. Barbaro, Assistant Professor of Pediatrics, Division of Critical Care Medicine, University of Michigan Medical School, Ann Arbor, MI, USA

Reshma Bholah, Assistant Professor of Pediatrics, Weill Cornell Medicine—Qatar, Doha, Qatar

Thomas Breen, Consultant Paediatric Anaesthetist, St George's Hospital, London, UK

Lisa A. DelSignore, Attending Physician, Division of Pediatric Critical Care, Department of Pediatrics, Floating Hospital for Children at Tufts Medical Center, Boston, MA, USA; Assistant Professor, Tufts University School of Medicine, Boston, MA, USA

Christiane S. Eberhardt, Deputy Chief, Centre for Vaccinology, University of Geneva, Switzerland; Department of Pediatrics, University Hospitals of Geneva, Switzerland

Miriam R. Fine-Goulden, Consultant, Paediatric Intensive Care and South Thames Retrieval Service, Evelina London Children's Hospital, Guy's & St Thomas' NHS Foundation Trust, London, UK

Crawford Fulton, PICU Trainee, Alder Hey Children's Hospital, Liverpool, UK

Arun Ghose, Consultant Paediatric Intensivist PICU, KIDS Retrieval Service, Birmingham Children's Hospital, Birmingham, UK

Thomas D. Jerrom, Consultant in Paediatric Intensive Care, Paediatric Intensive Care Unit, Directorate of Children's Services, Bristol Royal Hospital for Children, Bristol, UK

Andrew Jones, Consultant, GOSH, King's College Hospital, London, UK

Andrew J. Lautz, Department of Anesthesiology and Critical Care Medicine, Children's Hospital of Philadelphia, PA, USA; Physician, Division of Critical Care Medicine, Department of Pediatrics, Cincinnati Children's Hospital Medical Center, Cincinnati, OH, USA

Jon Lillie, Consultant, Paediatric Intensive Care and South Thames Retrieval Service, Evelina London Children's Hospital, Guy's & St Thomas' NHS Foundation Trust, London, UK

Ryan W. Morgan, Assistant Professor of Anesthesia, Critical Care Medicine, and Pediatrics, Department of Anesthesiology and Critical Care Medicine, Children's Hospital of Philadelphia, Philadelphia, PA, USA

Andrew Nyman, Consultant, Paediatric Intensive Care and South Thames Retrieval Service, Evelina London Children's Hospital, Guy's & St Thomas' NHS Foundation Trust, London, UK

Elizabeth O'Donohoe, Consultant Paediatric Anaesthetist, St George's Hospital, London, UK

Sainath Raman, Senior Medical Officer, Paediatric Intensive Care, Queensland Children's Hospital, Brisbane, QLD, Australia

Samiran Ray, Paediatric Intensive Care Consultant, Great Ormond Street Hospital, London, UK

Dilanee Sangaran, Consultant, Paediatric Intensive Care, St George's Hospital, London, UK

Justin Q.Y. Wang, Consultant and Senior Lecturer, Department of Paediatrics, University of Malaya, Kuala Lumpur, Malaysia

ABBREVIATIONS

ABG	arterial blood gas
ACCM	American Critical Care Medicine
ACT	activated clotting time
ADEM	acute disseminated encephalomyelitis
ADRENAL	Adjunctive Corticosteroid Treatment in Critically Ill Patients with Septic Shock
A&E	Accident and Emergency
AED	antiepileptic drug
aEEG	amplitude integrated electroencephalogram
AKI	acute kidney injury
AKIN	Acute Kidney Injury Network
ALF	acute liver failure
ALL	acute lymphoblastic leukaemia
ALP	alkaline phosphatase
AMA	American Medical Association
AoMRC	Academy of Medical Royal Colleges
APAGBI	Association of Paediatric Anaesthetists of Great Britain and Ireland
APLS	Advanced Paediatric Life Support
ARDS	acute respiratory distress syndrome
ARDSNet	Acute Respiratory Distress Syndrome Clinical Network
ARISE	Australasian Resuscitation in Sepsis Evaluation
AS	aortic stenosis
ASD	atrial septal defect
ASPEN	American Society for Parenteral and Enteral Nutrition
ATP	adenosine triphosphate
AV	atrioventricular
$\beta2M$	beta-2 microglobulin
BBB	blood–brain barrier
BE	base excess
BESS	Bronchiolitis Endotracheal Surfactant Study
BIDS	Bronchiolitis of Infancy Discharge Study
BMI	body mass index
BMP	basic metabolic panel
BP	blood pressure
BPF	bronchopleural fistula
bpm	beats per minute
BTS	British Thoracic Society
BUN	blood urea nitrogen
BVM	bag valve mask
CBC	complete blood count
CBF	cerebral blood flow
CBV	cerebral venous blood volume
CDC	Centers for Disease Control
cDSA	colour density spectral array
cEEG	continuous electroencephalogram
CESAR	Conventional ventilatory support versus Extracorporeal membrane oxygenation for Severe Adult Respiratory failure
CFAM	cerebral function analysing monitoring
CFM	cerebral function monitoring
CI	cardiac index
CICV	cannot intubate, cannot ventilate
CKD	chronic kidney disease
$CMRO_2$	cerebral metabolic rate for oxygen
CMV	cytomegalovirus
CO	cardiac output
ConSEPT	Convulsive Status Epilepticus Paediatric Trial
COPP	coronary perfusion pressure
CPAP	continuous positive airway pressure
CPB	cardiopulmonary bypass
CPP	cerebral perfusion pressure
CPR	cardiopulmonary resuscitation
CRRT	continuous renal replacement therapy
CSC	Children's Social Care
CSF	cerebrospinal fluid
CT	computed tomography
CVP	central venous pressure
CVVH	continuous veno-venous haemofiltration
CVVHD	continuous veno-venous haemodiafiltration
CysC	cystatin C
CXR	chest X-ray
DAS	Difficult Airway Society
DBP	diastolic blood pressure
DCD	donation after circulatory death
DEFG	don't ever forget glucose
DGH	district general hospital
DNC	death by neurological criteria
ECG	electrocardiogram
echo	echocardiogram

EcLiPSE	Emergency treatment with Levetiracetam or Phenytoin in convulsive Status Epilepticus in children	HSV	herpes simplex virus
		HVP	high-volume plasma exchange
		IBW	ideal body weight
ECLS	extracorporeal life support	IC	indirect calorimetry
ECMO	extracorporeal membrane oxygenation	ICH	intracranial haemorrhage
ECP	extracorporeal photophoresis	ICP	intracranial pressure
E-CPR	extracorporeal cardiopulmonary resuscitation	ICU	Intensive Care Unit
		IGFBP	insulin-like growth factor binding protein
ED	Emergency Department	IHCA	in-hospital cardiac arrest
Edi	electrical activity of the diaphragm	IJ	internal jugular
EDTA	ethylenediaminetetraacetic acid	IL	interleukin
EEG	electroencephalogram	IMD	inherited metabolic disorder
EGDT	early goal-directed therapy	iNO	inhaled nitrous oxide
Ela-2	elastase 2	INR	international normalized ratio
ELSO	Extracorporeal Life Support Organization	IO	intra-osseous
EN	enteral nutrition	IPS	idiopathic pulmonary syndrome
ENT	ear, nose, and throat	IV	intravenous
ESETT	Established Status Epilepticus Treatment Trial	IVA	isovaleric acidaemia
		JET	junctional ectopic tachycardia
ESPNIC	European Society of Paediatric and Neonatal Intensive Care	JVP	jugular venous pressure
		kcal	kilocalories
etCO$_2$	end-tidal carbon dioxide	KDIGO	Kidney Disease Improving Global Outcomes
ETT	endotracheal tube		
EVD	external ventricular drain	KIM-1	kidney injury molecule 1
FDA	US Food and Drugs Administration	LA	left atrial
FEAST	Fluid Expansion as Supportive Therapy	LAP	left atrial pressure
FFP	fresh frozen plasma	LCOS	low cardiac output state
FGM	female genital mutilation	LMA	laryngeal mask airway
FII	fabricated or induced illness	LP	lumbar puncture
FiO$_2$	fraction of inspired oxygen	LV	left ventricle/left ventricular
FIRES	febrile infection-related epilepsy syndrome	MAP	mean arterial pressure
GABA	γ-aminobutyric acid	MCADD	medium-chain acyl-CoA dehydrogenase deficiency
GBS	group B streptococcus		
GMC	General Medical Council	MCS	mechanical circulatory support
GP	general practitioner	MMIF	macrophage migration inhibition factor
GVHD	graft-versus-host disease	MMP	matrix metalloproteinase
GWTG-R	Get With The Guidelines–Resuscitation	mPaw	mean airway pressure
HSCT	haematopoietic stem cell transplant	MRI	magnetic resonance imaging
HD	haemodialysis	MRSA	methicillin-resistant *Staphylococcus aureus*
HE	hepatic encephalopathy	MSUD	maple syrup urine disease
HES	hydroxyethyl starch	MUAC	mid-upper arm circumference
HFNC	high-flow nasal cannula	NABI	non-accidental brain injury
HFOV	high-frequency oscillatory ventilator	NAI	non-accidental injury
HLA	human leukocyte antigen	NAVA	neutrally adjusted ventilatory assist
HLH	hypoplastic left heart	NGAL	neutrophil gelatinase-associated lipocalin
HLHS	hypoplastic left heart syndrome	NGT	nasogastric tube
hMPV	human metopneumovirus	NIBP	non-invasive blood pressure
HR	heart rate	NIPPV	non-invasive positive pressure ventilation

NIV	non-invasive ventilation	RIFLE	Risk for renal dysfunction, Injury to the kidney, Failure of kidney function, Loss of kidney function and End-stage renal disease
NMDA	N-methyl-D-aspartate		
OA	organic acidaemia		
OHCA	out-of-hospital cardiac arrest		
OI	oxygenation index	RNA	ribonucleic acid
paCO₂	partial pressure of carbon dioxide	ROSC	return of spontaneous resuscitation
PALF	paediatric acute liver failure	RR	respiratory rate
PALICC	Paediatric Acute Lung Injury consensus conference	RRT	renal replacement therapy
		RSE	refractory status epilepticus
PaO₂	partial pressure of oxygen	RSI	rapid sequence induction
PARDS	paediatric acute respiratory distress syndrome	RSV	respiratory syncytial virus
		RV	right ventricle
pO₂	partial pressure of oxygen	SAKI	sepsis-induced acute kidney injury
PCR	polymerase chain reaction	SALT-ED	Saline against Lactated Ringer's or Plasma-Lyte in the Emergency Department
PD	peritoneal dialysis		
PDE	phosphodiesterase	SaO₂	oxygen saturation
PEA	pulseless electrical activity	SBS	shaken baby syndrome
PEEP	positive end expiratory pressure	SCCM	Society of Critical Care Medicine
PEG	percutaneous endoscopic gastrostomy	SD	standard deviation
PELOD2	Paediatric Organ Dysfunction 2	SDH	subdural haemorrhage
PI	pulsatility index	SE	status epilepticus
PIC	Paediatric Intensive Care	SIRS	systemic inflammatory response syndrome
PICS	Paediatric Intensive Care Society	SjvO₂	jugular venous oxygen saturation
PICU	Paediatric Intensive Care Unit	SLED	slow low-efficiency dialysis
p-IHCA	paediatric in-hospital cardiac arrest	SMART	Isotonic Solutions and Major Adverse Renal Events Trial
PIP	peak inspiratory pressure		
PN	parenteral nutrition	SNOD	Specialist Nurse for Organ Donation
ppm	parts per million	SOFA	Sequential Organ Failure Assessment
PPV	positive pressure ventilation	SPLIT	0.9% Saline vs Plasma-Lyte 148 (PL-148) for ICU Fluid Therapy
pRIFLE	paediatric-modified Risk for renal dysfunction, Injury to the kidney, Failure of kidney function, Loss of kidney function and End-stage renal disease		
		SpO₂	peripheral capillary oxygen saturation
		SPROUT	Sepsis, Prevalence, Outcome and Therapies
ProCESS	Protocolized Care for Early Septic Shock	SSC	Surviving Sepsis Campaign
ProMISe	Protocolised Management in Sepsis	SRSE	super-refractory status epilepticus
PRS	Pierre Robin sequence	STC	stem cell transplant
PT	prothrombin time	SVR	systemic vascular resistance
PVR	pulmonary vascular resistance	SVT	supraventricular tachycardia
qEEG	quantitative electroencephalogram	T3	tri-iodothyronine
QoL	quality of life	TAPVD	total anomalous pulmonary venous discharge
qSOFA	quick Sequential Organ Failure Assessment		
RAI	renal angina index	TA-TMA	transplant-associated thrombotic microangiopathy
RCPCH	Royal College of Paediatrics and Child Health		
		TBI	traumatic brain injury
RCT	randomized controlled trial	TCD	transcranial Doppler
REE	resting energy expenditure	TGA	transposition of the great arteries
RH	retinal haemorrhage	THAN	transient hyperammonaemia of the newborn

THAPCA	Therapeutic Hypothermia after Pediatric Cardiac Arrest		VCO_2	breath-to-breath carbon dioxide
			VF	ventricular fibrillation
TIMP	tissue inhibitor of metalloproteinase		VO_2	breath-to-breath oxygen
TMS	tandem mass spectrometry		VOD	veno-occlusive disease
TPA	tissue plasminogen activator		VSD	ventricular septal defect
TSF	triceps skinfold		VT	ventricular tachycardia
UCD	urea cycle defect		Vt	tidal volume
UNICEF	United Nations Children's Fund		VV	veno-venous
VA	veno-arterial		WBC	white blood cell
$VACO_2$	venous:arterial carbon dioxide difference		WD	Wilson's disease
VAD	ventricular assist device		WHO	World Health Organization
VAV	veno-arterio-venous			

Septic shock in children

Sainath Raman

🕐 **Expert commentary** by Mark J. Peters

Case history

A 12-year old girl, weighing 50 kg, presented to the Emergency Department (ED) with a 2-day history of fever and lethargy. She was admitted to the paediatric ward. Her vital signs on arrival were: pulse oximetry saturations 95%, respiratory rate (RR) 25 breaths per minute, and heart rate (HR) 100 beats per minute (bpm). She deteriorated over the next 24 hours with hypotension (88/38; mean 50mmHg) and lactic acidosis (5 mmol/L on a venous blood gas). A provisional diagnosis of sepsis was made. However, the focus of infection was unclear. The local team initiated resuscitation. She received 2 litres of normal saline as fluid boluses. Her blood pressure remained low. She was started on dopamine infusion at 5 µg/kg/min through a peripheral venous cannula. Her perfusion and blood pressure improved briefly. She received ceftriaxone, clindamycin, and gentamicin as empirical antibiotics. Dopamine was titrated up to 10 µg/kg/min—to target a mean blood pressure of 55 mmHg—while retrieval to a Paediatric Intensive Care Unit (PICU) was organized. In the next few hours, she was transferred to the PICU.

⊗ **Learning point** Definition of sepsis

Paediatric systemic inflammatory response syndrome (SIRS) has been defined as the clinical state wherein either an abnormal temperature or abnormal leukocyte count is present. Either an abnormal HR (>2 standard deviations (SDs) above normal for age or <10th percentile for age) or an abnormal RR (>2 SDs above normal for age) should also be documented. Sepsis has been defined as SIRS caused by an infection while septic shock is sepsis with cardiovascular organ dysfunction (see Figure 1.1).[1]

These definitions are neither sensitive nor specific. Similar problems with adult definitions prompted the Sepsis-3 initiative, which discarded the term SIRS and defined sepsis as 'a life-threatening organ dysfunction caused by a dysregulated response to infection'.[2] In this new system 'septic shock' is a subset of sepsis that involves significant circulatory, metabolic, and cell abnormalities associated with an increased risk of death. Importantly, these definitions achieve something new: sepsis can now be distinguished from uncomplicated infection. This has important implications for early recognition of a patient with sepsis. The key feature of sepsis in this system is an increase in the Sequential Organ Failure Assessment (SOFA) score by more than 2 points from baseline in the context of suspected infection.

The quick SOFA (qSOFA) is a pragmatic alternative. It has been validated in adult patients admitted to hospital with an infection. It incorporates the Glasgow Coma Scale, systolic blood pressure, and RR. In the Intensive Care Unit (ICU) patient, the SOFA score has a better predictive value, but qSOFA remains a valid measure for the patient in the ED. Work is underway to establish an international collaboration to create a paediatric sepsis registry that will enable creation of a similar definition to Sepsis 3.0.

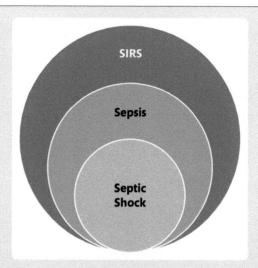

Figure 1.1 Septic shock is a subset of sepsis. Sepsis, in turn, is a subset of systemic inflammatory response syndrome (SIRS).

Refractory septic shock in children has been defined as high blood lactate with high-dose vasoactive drugs in the presence of myocardial dysfunction. Any future paediatric sepsis definition needs an organ failure score analogous to SOFA score. The Paediatric Organ Dysfunction 2 score (PELOD2) might be suitable for this purpose.

⊘ **Evidence base** Sepsis definition

Although the sepsis definitions mentioned above are current, there is much debate about their utility. For instance, in a point prevalence study in hospitalized children with a fever, nearly 75% met SIRS criteria. Furthermore, the prevalence of SIRS in patients admitted to the PICU has been reported to be in excess of 70%. Scott et al.[3] noted that the majority of medical paediatric patients with SIRS were discharged from the ED. Interestingly, the Sepsis, Prevalence, Outcome and Therapies study (SPROUT) demonstrated only a moderate agreement between physician diagnosis and consensus criteria, questioning the applicability of these criteria at the bedside.

Case history (continued)

Her vital signs were abnormal on admission to the PICU. Pulse oximeter saturations were 92% in 5 L/minute face mask oxygen. Mean blood pressure remained low at 50 mmHg. HR rose again to 120 bpm following a brief drop after the initial fluid resuscitation. One litre of 4.5% albumin was administered for further resuscitation.

➕ **Clinical tip** History and clinical examination

A structured and focused clinical examination along with a detailed history will ensure prompt recognition of a seriously ill child. The examination should follow the ABCD approach.

● Airway and breathing—this usually includes abnormal RR, abnormal breathing pattern (includes grunting), and inefficient breathing efforts.

- Circulation—deranged HR, delayed capillary refill time (may not be present in warm shock), abnormal skin colour (erythema, purpuric rash, mottling, pallor, or cyanosis), cool peripheries, reduced pulse volume, and low blood pressure (terminal sign).
- Disability—abnormal consciousness level, posturing, and pupils (size and reaction to light).

Shock should be diagnosed by clinical examination before the onset of hypotension. Abnormal temperature (hypo- or hyperthermia), altered mental status, and vasodilation or deranged capillary refill time are the prime signs commonly employed to diagnose shock. Community-acquired septic shock may present more often as cold shock, while shock associated with central venous line infection often exhibits as warm shock.[4]

> **Learning point** Epidemiology of paediatric sepsis
>
> The proportion of children admitted with sepsis, using the international paediatric sepsis consensus criteria, to the PICU varies from 7.7% to 27.3%.[5] It is on the rise. Mortality estimates range from 14% to 25%. The SPROUT study in children aged <18 years with severe sepsis showed a prevalence of 8.2% and a mortality of 25%.
>
> More than half of deaths as a result of sepsis occur within 24 hours of referral to the PICU.[6] Interestingly, a recent retrospective study observed that a lower proportion (one-quarter) died in the first day. Refractory shock and multiple organ dysfunction syndrome after shock recovery were the top two causes of death in this group. This may reflect a failure of early recognition or suboptimal resuscitation.

> **Expert comment** Echocardiography
>
> 'Cold shock' and 'warm shock' cannot reliably be distinguished clinically. Extended monitoring, including echocardiography, may be useful in this scenario, to determine the haemodynamic pattern of shock. Echocardiography may quantify cardiac function. However, with no dynamic measure of systemic vascular resistance (i.e. loading conditions), this assessment of cardiac function should be interpreted with caution.

Case history (continued)

A decision was made to intubate her due to her worsening clinical state. A peripheral adrenaline infusion was started at 0.1 μg/kg/min prior to intubation to optimize her haemodynamic state. She had already been starved for the last 6 hours. Fentanyl, ketamine, and vecuronium were used as induction agents. A senior trainee was the first intubator. She tolerated the procedure well. An endotracheal tube was placed on first pass. End-tidal carbon dioxide trace, auscultation, and chest X-ray confirmed ideal tube tip position. She was established on mechanical ventilatory support.

A central venous line and arterial line were placed. She received a total of 5 L of resuscitation fluid in the first 12 hours since deterioration on the ward. This comprised of normal saline and albumin solutions. She was started on adrenaline through the central venous line. This had to be increased to 0.3 μg/kg/min. Her admission arterial blood lactate was 12 mmol/L and central venous saturation (right internal jugular $ScvO_2$) was 50%. After her haemodynamic status stabilized, $ScvO_2$ improved to 60%. She had significant peripheral oedema and was difficult to ventilate, requiring high airway pressures. At this point, a vascath was inserted. She was started on continuous veno-venous haemofiltration with the aim of improving acid–base and fluid balance.

> **Clinical tip** Lactate
>
> Lactate >2 mmol/L is associated with increased mortality in adults with severe sepsis. In addition, lactate clearance (normalization) within 6 hours of presentation to the ED may be associated with decreased mortality. This, however, is being challenged (discussed later). Scott et al.[7] observed that a high lactate level on admission had a significant association with the development of organ dysfunction within 24 hours in children with sepsis. Admission lactate may be a better predictor of outcome in sepsis than base excess.

> **Clinical tip** Early inotropes
>
> In our practice, we start adrenaline peripherally while central venous access is achieved. Typically, adrenaline is started early in resuscitation (usually, but not necessarily always, after administration of 40 mL/kg crystalloid). The escalation of vasoactive drugs is determined by the physiological state. If the child presents in a 'cold shock' state, adrenaline is preferred. We describe 'cold shock' as hypotension with a narrow pulse pressure. However, in a 'warm shock' state (hypotension, wide pulse pressure, and low central venous saturations), noradrenaline and/or vasopressin are chosen. Excessive doses of catecholamines (>0.2–0.3 μg/kg/min) can induce acidosis and also cause endocardial necrosis. In sepsis, however, this may not be the case. Nonetheless, when reaching doses in the higher range other options should be considered.

⭐ **Learning point**   Choice of fluids

A systematic review of paediatric septic shock patients demonstrated no mortality benefit from the use of colloids. The recommendation was to use blood as a volume expander if the haemoglobin was <10 g/dL and $ScvO_2$ <70% during acute resuscitation.[6] This was in line with the guidance in septic shock in adults at the time. Since then, the guidance in adults has been modified to reflect a lower haemoglobin target (7 g/dL) for transfusion. In most other situations, crystalloids remain the preferred fluid of choice in the first instance.

✅ **Evidence base**   Fluid resuscitation

Fluid resuscitation and prompt administration of antibiotics are the two cornerstones of management of septic shock.

Type of resuscitation solution

Colloids that have been investigated are albumin (4.5%), hydroxyethyl starch (HES), modified gelatin, and dextran. A recent Cochrane review showed no benefit in their use compared to crystalloids in critically ill adult patients. Moreover, HES was observed to cause more renal impairment.

The most commonly used crystalloid solution is normal saline. In fact, most ED clinicians in Australia use saline as their first-choice resuscitation fluid. This practice is probably similar worldwide, owing to the ease of availability, low cost, and perceived safety. Saline administration is, however, associated with hyperchloraemic acidosis. Healthy volunteers have demonstrated worse renal blood flow velocity after receiving saline versus balanced crystalloid solution such as Plasma-Lyte 148™.

✅ **Evidence base**   Balanced crystalloids

Despite clear theoretical and observational evidence of superiority of balanced crystalloids over normal saline solution, the evidence from clinical trials is inconclusive.

The SPLIT trial compared the use of saline versus Plasma-Lyte 148™ for resuscitation in approximately 1000 patients admitted to adult ICUs. They reported no difference in the primary outcome measure—incidence of acute kidney injury. The SMART trial recruited approximately 15,000 critically ill adults in ICUs. They observed a statistically significant but marginal benefit, i.e. 1% reduction in the composite outcome of death from any cause, new renal replacement therapy, or persistent renal dysfunction, from balanced crystalloids compared with saline. The SALT-ED trial demonstrated no benefit in hospital-free days from the use of balanced solutions in non-critically ill adults. They did note a decrease in the incidence of major adverse kidney events within 30 days. With nearly equivocal evidence, the choice between balanced solutions and saline remains with the individual clinician.

ℹ️ **Expert comment**
Resuscitation endpoints

Resuscitation endpoints are complex but may include mixed venous oxygen saturations and lactate clearance. The value of fluid resuscitation and the utility of these endpoints depends on the standard of care available in a healthcare system and the baseline mortality rate. The mandated hour-1 bundle of care, which includes blood cultures, administration of antibiotics, and fluid resuscitation, has been shown to reduce mortality in paediatric sepsis.[12]

✅ **Evidence base**   Early goal-directed therapy

Carcillo et al. reported on a small retrospective analysis of fluid volumes and outcomes in children. They found a linear relationship between fluid volume received in the first 6 hours and survival. Almost a decade later, Rivers et al. published their landmark study. They demonstrated a significant reduction in mortality in septic adult patients who were managed according to an early goal-directed therapy (EGDT) protocol. They focused on early resuscitation aimed at clinical targets such as central venous pressure between 8 and 12 mmHg, mean arterial pressure ≥ 65 mmHg, central venous saturations ≥ 70%, and urine output ≥ 0.5 mL/kg/h. This protocol has been mirrored in numerous settings. The Surviving Sepsis Campaign (SSC) draws on this protocol. We will discuss the SSC later.[8,9]

Oliveira et al. conducted the first randomized control trial assessing the benefit of EGDT in paediatric septic shock (n = 102). The intervention group had target superior vena cava oxygenation saturations >70% and had a significantly lower 28-day mortality (11.8% vs 39.2%; p = 0.002). These children received more crystalloids, blood transfusion, and inotropic support in the first 6 hours than those where $ScvO_2$ was not targeted.[10]

More recent studies (ARISE, ProCESS, and ProMISe) indicate that EGDT now offers no advantage over usual resuscitation.[11] This may well reflect significant improvements in routine care that mean that EGDT is no longer meaningfully different. The current standard of practice is aggressive fluid resuscitation in the initial hours after presentation, with careful attention paid to the possibility of fluid overload. This has been reinforced in the hour-1 bundle in the 2018 update to the SSC. There have been criticisms to this approach, as it does not titrate care to individual patients.

The time course of multiorgan failure differs between adults and children. Organ failure scores peak on day 3–4 of ICU admission in adults versus an earlier rise in children (<3 days). This difference suggests that aggressive fluid resuscitation might be more important in children. However, the FEAST trial demonstrated that children with infections in sub-Saharan Africa, with a high prevalence of malaria and anaemia, had higher mortality when fluid boluses were administered (saline or albumin) than a no resuscitation fluid arm. The SQUEEZE trial is investigating the fluid resuscitation regime in septic shock in children.

Case history (continued)

The haemofiltration strategy for the first 24 hours was to accomplish acid–base homeo-stasis and electrolyte balance. By the first 4 hours in PICU, she was noted to be anuric, with blood chemistry suggestive of acute kidney injury. The blood flow rate was set at 150 mL/min with an ultrafiltrate of 2.2 L/h. Neutral balance was targeted. Lactate clearance was achieved by 12 h. She was in a considerable positive fluid state by day 2. Unsurprisingly, her mechanical ventilatory requirements increased. As her haemo-dynamic state was more stable, the filtration strategy was altered to achieve negative fluid balance for the next few days.

> ⊕ **Clinical tip** Fluid removal (de-resuscitation)
>
> Invariably, septic patients end up with a significant positive fluid balance after the initial phase of resuscitation. Positive fluid balance impedes gas exchange in the lung and oxygen delivery to the tissues.
>
> There are three main strategies to achieve negative balance on patients.
>
> 1. Fluid restriction—most intensive care patients are fluid restricted to two-thirds maintenance allowance. One might consider restricting this further, if unable to achieve the right balance, especially in the context of hyponatraemia.
> 2. Diuresis—the most common diuretic used is furosemide. It may be used either as intermittent bolus doses or as a continuous infusion. While there are proponents of both modes, in our experience, continuous infusion gives a better response profile and limits sudden dumps of urine output. Furosemide may be used in conjunction with a potassium-sparing diuretic to limit electrolyte imbalance.
> 3. Renal replacement therapy (RRT)—early initiation of RRT in sepsis is still debated but may be useful, especially in the presence of acute kidney injury or significant acid-base derangement.

> ⊘ **Evidence base** Fluid overload
>
> There is an association between positive fluid balance and mortality in adult septic shock patients. Similarly, positive fluid balance in paediatric septic shock was associated with impaired oxygenation and increased morbidity.[13] However, paediatric studies have not shown a direct causal link between fluid overload and mortality. A systematic review found an association between conservative fluid management and an increase in ventilator-free days and ICU length of stay. Notably, the study did not find a link to mortality.[14]
>
> An interesting risk stratification approach to children with septic shock has been reported recently. The authors stratified mortality risk on admission into low, moderate, and severe. Increased cumulative per cent positive fluid balance at 7 days was associated with mortality in the low-risk group but not the others.[15] This finding contradicts the current dogma supported by adult and paediatric studies that fluid overload is detrimental to outcome in all patients.

⊘ **Evidence base** Dopamine versus adrenaline

One hundred and twenty children, aged <15 years, with septic shock were randomized to either receive incremental doses of dopamine or adrenaline. A significant reduction in mortality was noted with the use of adrenaline compared with dopamine (7% vs 20.6%; p = 0.03).[18]

> ✪ **Learning point** Renal replacement therapy
>
> The most appropriate timing of initiation of RRT in sepsis is unclear. A small study (n = 29) in children with sepsis receiving continuous RRT (CRRT) within 48 hours showed improved oxygenation and haemodynamics, but not a mortality benefit. RRT has been shown to be associated with a reduction in macrophage migration inhibition factor (MMIF) in patients with septic shock. Higher levels of MMIF were associated with increased mortality and use of RRT was associated with survival.[16] However, randomized studies in adults show no benefit of a protocol of early RRT versus standard care.

Case history (continued)

This patient had received antibiotics soon after admission to the paediatric ward. The cover was broadened immediately following the deterioration. She received one dose of intravenous immunoglobulin for suspected toxic shock syndrome. On day 2, her blood culture was positive for *Staphylococcus aureus*. Gentamicin and clindamycin were stopped. She received a 2-week course of flucloxacillin.

> ✚ **Clinical tip** Antibiotics
>
> Early administration of antibiotics makes intuitive sense and is supported by the SSC recommendations. Association between delay in initiation of antibiotics and in-hospital mortality has been reported. In a paediatric study, a 3-hour delay in antibiotics versus immediate administration was associated with an increased odds ratio of death of 3.9.[17] Therefore, good sepsis care mandates early antibiotic delivery. Initiatives such as Paediatric Sepsis 6 may help operational delivery of early recognition and antibiotic administration targets.

Case history (continued)

As noted earlier, she was on peripheral dopamine infusion on arrival to PICU, which was changed to adrenaline. Subsequently, she required addition of both noradrenaline and vasopressin. These were titrated towards a target mean arterial blood pressure of > 55 mmHg. Her inotropic and vasopressor requirement peaked at adrenaline of 0.2 μg/kg/min, noradrenaline of 0.3 μg/kg/min, and vasopressin 0.02 units/kg/h during the first 24 hours of her PICU stay. The rationale for adrenaline was the documented association of cardiac dysfunction and severe sepsis. The vasopressors were necessary owing to the 'warm shock' physiology with a wide pulse pressure, warm peripheries, and low central venous saturations.

> ⊘ **Evidence base** Choice and place of inotropes
>
> Most of the clinical practice guidelines in paediatric intensive care draw evidence from extrapolation from adult studies. The use of inotropes and vasopressors are no different. The American College of Critical Care Medicine guidelines for haemodynamic support in pediatric and neonatal septic shock recommend the same inotrope and vasopressor use as the adult protocol, i.e. dopamine or adrenaline for cold shock, and noradrenaline for warm shock.

❝ **Expert comment** Choice of inotrope

The *choice* of inotrope may not be as important as the *appropriate* use for the clinical situation. However, data now suggest that adrenaline (epinephrine) may be superior to dopamine.

Case history (continued)

When the inotrope and vasopressor requirements were rapidly increasing on day 1, a decision was made to administer 6-hourly sepsis dose steroids (hydrocortisone 2 mg/kg). This helped wean vasoactive infusions. She received steroids for 48 hours.

⊘ Evidence base Steroids

In a multicentre, double-blind trial, 1241 critically ill adults with septic shock were randomized to either hydrocortisone–fludrocortisone combination or placebo. This trial demonstrated a marginal reduction in all-cause 90-day mortality in the hydrocortisone–fludrocortisone group.[19] In contrast, the ADRENAL trial, in which 3800 adults were randomized to receive either adjunctive hydrocortisone infusion or placebo, did not show a mortality benefit with the administration of hydrocortisone.[20] However, the hydrocortisone group did have faster resolution of shock and a lower rate of blood transfusion. Overall, the latest randomized controlled trials do not show an increased risk with the use of steroids in septic shock in adults.

In contrast, analysis of the SPROUT study[4] in children suggested that corticosteroids were associated with PICU mortality even after controlling for many confounders with an adjusted odds ratio of 1.58 (95% confidence interval 1.01–2.49). Similarly, a risk-stratified analysis (biomarker-based stratification tool—PERSEVERE) of paediatric septic shock observed more organ failure and worse outcome in the corticosteroid group than those who did not receive corticosteroids. Of note, this association was not apparent when individual risk strata were assessed.[21]

The answer might lie in better patient selection. Using a biomarker-based risk assessment model (PERSEVERE) and gene expression profile, Wong et al. reported a 10-fold reduction in the risk of persistent organ failure at 7 days or 28-day mortality in a particular subset (endotype B + intermediate-high risk on PERSEVERE) of the patient population.[21]

★ Learning point Steroids

Corticosteroids have been in use for severe infections for several decades. But the precise mechanism for the potential benefit is far from clear. The intuitive reasoning might be that steroids cause immunomodulation and control the host's pro-inflammatory state. However, the balance of pro- and anti-inflammatory pathways in septic shock is unclear and certainly vary between patients. These and other caveats have challenged the routine use of steroids.

⊘ Expert comment Steroids

The balance of risks may differ in children from adults. Children have lower overall mortality but a higher proportion of deaths in the context of failed shock resolution combined with a relatively short stay on intensive care. These factors can be interpreted as children having more to gain (earlier haemodynamic stability) and less to lose (increased daily risk of nosocomial infection) from steroids.

Therefore, our approach is to select the patient carefully. We believe that steroid supplementation should be a considered decision when shock fails to resolve with fluids and inotropes, rather than a default plan.

Case history (continued)

At the peak of fluid resuscitation, inotrope, vasopressor, and ventilator requirements and before established end organ dysfunction (specifically liver and renal), extracorporeal membrane oxygenation (ECMO) was considered. Fortunately, the patient improved and did not need escalation of therapy to ECMO.

✚ Clinical tip Extracorporeal membrane oxygenation

Outcomes following ECMO in septic shock patients are improving. Currently, despite variability in practice, review of the Extra Corporeal Life Support Organization registry suggests up to 60% survival in this group. ECMO may be considered for refractory respiratory failure as a veno-venous mode or, more likely, in the refractory shock scenario needing veno-arterial mode.

Case history (continued)

Our patient improved over the next few days. She came off vasoactive medications on day 3. She required CRRT for 2 weeks, while her kidney function improved gradually. She had a convalescence phase of several weeks. Eventually, however, she made a full recovery. The management of this child was based largely around the principles of the SSC.

> **ⓘ Expert comment** Care bundles
>
> 'Get organized'—this should be the overarching principle of management of paediatric sepsis. State- and hospital-wide systems, such as the New York Sepsis Mandate, that ensure bundles of care are observed have demonstrated better clinical outcomes. The New York initiative followed a paediatric death. The directive was for hospitals to complete an hour-1 bundle of care (blood culture, delivery of antibiotics, and fluid resuscitation) in all septic patients. Although the complete bundle was achieved in only 25% of the patients, there was a clear association between entire bundle completion and lower risk-adjusted odds of in-hospital mortality.[12] It is now agreed that hospitals should proactively dictate sepsis management by mandating adherence to care bundles.

Discussion

SSC

Sepsis is a medical emergency. The SSC guidelines recognize this fact and recommend an hour-1 bundle in adults. Key components of the hour-1 bundle are:

1. Monitor lactate; repeat if > 2 mmol/L.
2. Blood culture before administration of broad-spectrum antibiotics.
3. Aggressive fluid resuscitation with 30 mL/kg for hypotension.
4. Consider vasopressors if hypotension persists despite or during fluid resuscitation.[23,24]

The timeline in the American Critical Care Medicine (ACCM) paediatric sepsis algorithm is broadly in line with what has been described.[7]

Criticisms of the SSC

Several experts in critical care criticized the initial SSC, especially the EGDT component of the management based on the landmark study by Rivers et al.[9] There is a school of thought now that, perhaps, vasopressors should be initiated after resuscitation with 20–30 mL/kg of fluid. The proponents of 'early vasopressor use in septic shock' claim that excessive intravenous fluid administration only worsens the damage to the glycocalyx membrane (with some literature to back them) and causes tissue oedema.[25] Concerns about conflict of interest were expressed. Significant advances have been made with regard to transparency and disclosure in subsequent iterations of the SSC.

One of the targets of EGDT and SSC is lactate clearance. The rationale for aiming for lactate clearance is as follows: septic shock leads to tissue hypoxia, which triggers excess lactate production due to anaerobic metabolism. Although lactate per se is not toxic, lactate clearance might be used as a marker of improved oxygen delivery and consumption balance. Recent evidence suggests aerobic pathways may produce lactate as a result of stress-induced catecholamine release. Hence, some believe that aiming for lactate clearance may not be appropriate.[26] Despite these criticisms, the SSC has been associated with a dramatic impact on the mortality of sepsis.

Impact of the SSC

The current SSC guideline (fourth iteration) has arisen from robust supporting data. A long-term study of performance metrics and outcome data demonstrated lower mortality in high-compliance sites versus those with low compliance. Furthermore, there was a 0.7% reduction in mortality per site for every 3 months of participation. In addition, hospital and ICU length of stay dropped linearly with an increase in compliance with the resuscitation bundle.[28] No other medical intervention has been this consistent in its benefit.

The paediatric SSC guidelines were recently published.[29] The key recommendations to highlight are:

1. Fluid bolus therapy should depend on the setting, i.e. availability of intensive care in a health care system.
2. No clear difference between adrenaline and noradrenaline, but either of them is preferred to dopamine.
3. Reduced emphasis on the differentiation between 'cold' and 'warm' shock based solely on clinical examination.
4. Equipoise around the use of steroids in refractory catecholamine-resistant septic shock.
5. Time to antibiotic therapy—if a child presents in septic shock, they should receive antibiotics within 1 hour. However, if a child presents with sepsis but not in shock, the clinician has up to 3 hours to perform urgent diagnostics before starting empirical antibiotic therapy.

Protocolized care has been associated with a quicker resolution of organ dysfunction than non-protocolized care. Interestingly, evidence to the contrary can also be found. A retrospective cohort study of PICU admissions with paediatric sepsis from the ED comparing the subgroup whose management was consistent with the SSC bundle versus the usual care group, did not show better outcomes in the SSC cohort. However, as expected for paediatric sepsis, a low mortality rate was observed. More importantly, 75% of the study population had received the interventions within 3 hours, suggesting that the non-SSC compliant cohort were managed only slightly slower. This is in line with the observation of relatively prompt interventions (compared to historical data) in the control group in recent sepsis trials in adults, suggesting an overall improvement in sepsis care.

Role of sepsis bundles of care

Checklists foster efficient delivery of care. To provide well-organized care, the campaign created bundles. The bundle has two phases. The first (to be achieved within 3 hours of recognition of sepsis (1 hour in the latest guidance for adults)) includes measuring lactate level, obtaining a blood culture, administering antibiotics, and administering a fluid bolus if needed. The second phase (within 6 hours) requires providing goal-directed therapy.

The main issue in paediatric emergency sepsis care is that the bundle of care approach has not fully percolated to all hospitals. The prospective observational UK Paediatric Intensive Care Society sepsis audit confirmed this theory. Of the children admitted to UK PICUs, the ACCM Paediatric Advanced Life Support guideline for the management of severe sepsis was adhered to in only 38% of cases. Unfortunately, this problem is not unique to the UK. A prospective multicentre cohort study from the USA also reported significant variability in adherence to all metrics of paediatric sepsis bundle of care. This problem needs to be addressed.

This is remediable. Quality improvement projects have demonstrated that 100% bundle compliance can be achieved. Notably, the improvements were sustained over a 9-month period and led to a reduction in mortality. Therefore, paediatric severe sepsis management can be improved and sustained with ongoing education and training.

A final word from the expert

The early recognition of septic shock is paramount to achieve a positive outcome. It is prudent to titrate aggressive fluid resuscitation to the individual patient. Management using a bundle of care removes unwanted variability in the clinical process and improves outcomes. The future is likely to include improved recognition of different phenotypes of sepsis and more individualized treatments plans.

References

1. Goldstein B, Giroir B, Randolph A. International pediatric sepsis consensus conference: definitions for sepsis and organ dysfunction in pediatrics. *Pediatr. Crit. Care Med.* 2005;6:2–8.
2. Singer M, Deutschman CS, Seymour CW, et al. The Third International Consensus Definitions for Sepsis and Septic Shock (Sepsis-3). *JAMA* 2016;315:801.
3. Scott HF, Deakyne SJ, Woods JM, Bajaj L. The prevalence and diagnostic utility of systemic inflammatory response syndrome vital signs in a pediatric emergency department. *Acad. Emerg. Med.* 2015;22:381–9.
4. Brierley J, Peters MJ. Distinct hemodynamic patterns of septic shock at presentation to pediatric intensive care. *Pediatrics* 2008;122:752–9.
5. Souza DC de, Barreira ER, Faria LS. The epidemiology of sepsis in childhood. *Shock* 2016;47:2–5.
6. Cvetkovic M, Lutman D, Ramnarayan P, Pathan N, Inwald DP, Peters MJ. Timing of death in children referred for intensive care with severe sepsis: implications for interventional studies. *Pediatr. Crit. Care Med.* 2015;16:410–17.
7. Scott HF, Brou L, Deakyne SJ, Fairclough DL, Kempe A, Bajaj L. Lactate clearance and normalization and prolonged organ dysfunction in pediatric sepsis. *J. Pediatr.* 2016;170:149–55.
8. Davis AL, Carcillo JA, Aneja RK, et al. The American College of Critical Care Medicine Clinical Practice Parameters for Hemodynamic Support of Pediatric and Neonatal Septic Shock: executive summary. *Pediatr. Crit. Care Med.* 2017;18:884–890.
9. Carcillo JA, Davis AL, Zaritsky A. Role of early fluid resuscitation in pediatric septic shock. *JAMA* 1991;266:1242–5.
10. Rivers E, Nguyen B, Havstad S, et al. Early goal-directed therapy in the treatment of severe sepsis and septic shock. *N. Engl. J. Med.* 2001;345:1368–77.
11. Oliveira CF, Oliveira DSF, Gottschald AFC, et al. ACCM/PALS haemodynamic support guidelines for paediatric septic shock: an outcomes comparison with and without monitoring central venous oxygen saturation. *Intensive Care Med.* 2008;34:1065–75.
12. Angus DC, Barnato AE, Bell D, et al. A systematic review and meta-analysis of early goal-directed therapy for septic shock: the ARISE, ProCESS and ProMISe Investigators. *Intensive Care Med.* 2015;41:1549–60.
13. Evans IVR, Phillips GS, Alpern ER, et al. Association between the New York sepsis care mandate and in-hospital mortality for pediatric sepsis. *JAMA* 2018;320:358–67.
14. Arikan AA, Zappitelli M, Goldstein SL, Naipaul A, Jefferson LS, Loftis LL. Fluid overload is associated with impaired oxygenation and morbidity in critically ill children. *Pediatr. Crit. Care Med.* 2012;13:253–8.
15. Silversides JA, Major E, Ferguson AJ, et al. Conservative fluid management or deresuscitation for patients with sepsis or acute respiratory distress syndrome following the resuscitation phase of critical illness: a systematic review and meta-analysis. *Intensive Care Med.* 2017;43:155–70.
16. Abulebda K, Cvijanovich NZ, Thomas NJ, et al. Post-ICU admission fluid balance and pediatric septic shock outcomes. *Crit. Care Med.* 2014;42:397–403.

17. Pohl J, Papathanasiou M, Heisler M, et al. Renal replacement therapy neutralizes elevated MIF levels in septic shock. *J. Intensive Care* 2016;4:39.
18. Weiss SL, Fitzgerald JC, Balamuth F, et al. Delayed antimicrobial therapy increases mortality and organ dysfunction duration in pediatric sepsis. *Crit. Care Med.* 2014;42:2409–17.
19. Ventura AMC, Shieh HH, Bousso A, et al. Double-blind prospective randomized controlled trial of dopamine versus epinephrine as first-line vasoactive drugs in pediatric septic shock. *Crit. Care Med.* 2015;43:2292–302.
20. Annane D, Renault A, Brun-Buisson C, et al. Hydrocortisone plus fludrocortisone for adults with septic shock. *N. Engl. J. Med.* 2018;378:809–18.
21. Venkatesh B, Finfer S, Cohen J, et al. Adjunctive glucocorticoid therapy in patients with septic shock. *N. Engl. J. Med.* 2018;378:797–808.
22. Atkinson SJ, Cvijanovich NZ, Thomas NJ, et al. Corticosteroids and pediatric septic shock outcomes: a risk stratified analysis. *PLoS One* 2014;9:7–13.
23. Wong HR, Atkinson SJ, Cvijanovich NZ, et al. Combining prognostic and predictive enrichment strategies to identify children with septic shock responsive to corticosteroids. *Crit. Care Med.* 2016;44:e1000–3.
24. Rhodes A, Evans LE, Alhazzani W, et al. *Surviving Sepsis Campaign: International Guidelines for Management of Sepsis and Septic Shock: 2016.* Berlin Heidelberg: Springer; 2017.
25. Levy MM, Evans LE, Rhodes A. The Surviving Sepsis Campaign Bundle: 2018 update. *Intensive Care Med.* 2018;44:997–1000.
26. Chelazzi C, Villa G, Mancinelli P, De Gaudio AR, Adembri C. Glycocalyx and sepsis-induced alterations in vascular permeability. *Crit. Care* 2015;19:26.
27. Garcia-Alvarez M, Marik P, Bellomo R. Stress hyperlactataemia: present understanding and controversy. *Lancet Diabetes Endocrinol.* 2014;2:339–47.
28. Levy MM, Rhodes A, Phillips GS, et al. Surviving Sepsis Campaign: association between performance metrics and outcomes in a 7.5-year study. *Intensive Care Med.* 2014;40:1623–33.
29. Weiss SL, Peters MJ, Alhazzani W, et al. Surviving sepsis campaign international guidelines for the management of septic shock and sepsis-associated organ dysfunction in children. *Intensive Care Med.* 2020;46:10–67.

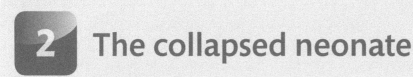

CASE

2 The collapsed neonate

Jon Lillie

Expert commentary by Shane Tibby

Case history

A 6-day-old boy presented to the Emergency Department (ED) with a 2-day history of poor feeding and a 1-day history of lethargy and increased work of breathing. There were no antenatal concerns and he was born at term, weighing 4 kg, and was discharged home after a normal routine examination by the paediatrician. The infant was fully breastfed.

On examination he was pale and mottled, with a temperature of 35°C. He had a respiratory rate of 70 breaths per minute, increased work of breathing, and was grunting. Oxygen saturations measured on the right hand were 93%. He was cold peripherally, central capillary refill time was 4 seconds, heart rate (HR) 200 beats per minute, and blood pressure (BP; taken with a cuff on the right arm) was 60/46 mmHg. Because he was so tachycardic, it was difficult to rule out a murmur on auscultation. He had hepatomegaly with liver edge extending 3 cm beyond the subcostal margin. He was drowsy and did not cry in response to the insertion of a peripheral intravenous cannula. His pupils were 3 mm wide, equal, and reactive to light. His anterior fontanelle was flat, abdomen soft, and peripheral genitalia were normal.

> **Learning point** Initial management of neonatal collapse
>
> The case history is a typical presentation of neonatal collapse, defined by respiratory and/or cardiovascular failure in a child aged up to 28 days. There are multiple causes of neonatal collapse; presenting symptoms are often similar and rarely identify the diagnosis. Signs and symptoms of respiratory distress can be due to respiratory or cardiac pathology, or may be a compensatory response to metabolic acidosis or anaemia. Similarly, signs and symptoms of cardiovascular shock may indicate a primary cardiac problem but could be secondary to sepsis, metabolic disease, bleeding, or abdominal pathology. Common symptoms such as drowsiness, poor feeding, and vomiting are all non-specific.
>
> Delineating the underlying cause of collapse is often difficult, so immediate life-saving management is usually initiated before making a definitive diagnosis. Resuscitation following the Advanced Paediatric Life Support (APLS) algorithm is useful, but certain key points need to be emphasized.[1]

> **Learning point** Airway and breathing
>
> High-flow oxygen should be given to all neonates in resuscitation, even if there are concerns that the collapse is due to congenital heart disease (see Expert commentary 'Oxygen therapy in congenital cardiac disease'). Intubation and ventilation is often necessary and the patient's cardiovascular status should be optimized prior to giving induction agents.

✪ **Learning point** Circulation, neurology, fluids, and antibiotics

Circulation

Intravascular access is often difficult to obtain, but potential sites that are often underutilized in the shocked neonate are scalp, external jugular, and umbilical vein. The intra-osseous (IO) route is often necessary, with APLS recommending that this should be used after three attempts at venous cannulation, or immediately if the child is peri-arrest.

In the shocked patient, 20 mL/kg crystalloid fluid should be delivered unless there are signs of heart failure (gallop, cardiomegaly, and hepatomegaly). Signs of heart failure may develop with fluid administration, so the patient's response should continue to be reassessed. If signs of heart failure develop then further fluid is unlikely to be beneficial and inotropes should be initiated.

There is no clear evidence to indicate which inotrope is most beneficial in neonates. Adrenaline, milrinone, and dopamine can be administered peripherally in dilute concentrations, and all inotropes can be given intra-osseously.[2] Surviving Sepsis Campaign guidelines recommend that inotropes are started after 40–60 mL/kg fluid;[3] however, if there are signs of cardiac failure or cardiac dysfunction, inotropes can be initiated earlier than this, especially if induction agents are to be given for intubation, which may cause further cardiovascular compromise.

A prostaglandin infusion should be started if there are any concerns that the child could have a duct-dependent lesion (see cardiac section in 'Causes of neonatal collapse' for more information on prostaglandin use and dosing).

Neurology

Seizures should be treated aggressively with anticonvulsants, but biochemical causes of seizures must be excluded immediately by blood gas analysis: hypoglycaemia, hyponatraemia, and hypocalcaemia are all causes of neonatal seizures. If the child has abnormal neurological signs, an urgent computed tomography (CT) scan of the brain is indicated to exclude intracranial pathology. If there are signs of respiratory failure or shock then the child should be intubated and ventilated prior to this scan. Signs of raised intracranial pressure (bradycardia and hypertension, bulging fontanelle, unequal or unresponsive pupils) need immediate treatment with a hyperosmotic agent such as hypertonic sodium chloride.

Fluids, temperature, and bleeding

All neonates are at risk of hypothermia and hypoglycaemia so both should be monitored closely and corrected if necessary. An overhead heater works well to facilitate access for procedures while keeping the patient warm. Maintenance fluid containing dextrose should be started in all neonates. Abnormal bleeding may be due to congenital causes, perinatal insults, trauma, or sepsis. The scalp, fontanelle, skin, and abdomen should be examined for signs of bleeding and if present the patient should be given vitamin K and clotting products. If haemoglobin is <70 g/L or the baby has bleeding and shock then packed red blood cells should be given. If bleeding is extensive, clotting products such as fresh frozen plasma should be administered without delay, before coagulation results are available from the laboratory.

Antimicrobials

Sepsis is the most common cause of neonatal collapse, and even when other pathologies such as cardiac disease are suspected, antimicrobials should be given immediately as infection is impossible to exclude at the time of presentation. Broad-spectrum antibiotics such as cefotaxime and amoxicillin or as per local guidelines should be given, and aciclovir should be added if herpes is suspected (see infection section in 'Causes of neonatal collapse').

⚫ **Expert comment** Oxygen therapy in congenital cardiac disease

Traditional teaching was that oxygen should be avoided in congenital cardiac disease, with concerns that an increased blood PaO_2 might stimulate the ductus arteriosus to close early. This, however, does not rule out the use of oxygen in the resuscitation of the collapsed neonate for several reasons:

- The cause for collapse in congenital heart disease is most likely to be due to the duct closing; these patients will be hypoxic and/or shocked so delivery of oxygen to the tissues must be optimized;
- Any baby with suspected cardiac disease will have prostaglandin commenced (see 'Clinical tip: prostaglandin dosing'), which prevents duct closure;
- If the duct is open in a baby with cyanotic congenital cardiac disease, the oxygenated blood from the pulmonary veins will mix with desaturated blood before it reaches the ductus arteriosus, which may reduce the risk of duct closure.

Oxygen use may be detrimental in a minority of congenital cardiac patients owing to its role as a pulmonary vasodilator. The reduction in pulmonary pressures increases pulmonary blood flow, and in cardiac lesions in which blood shunts freely between pulmonary and systemic circulations, this can lead to reduced systemic blood flow and exacerbate shock. In the neonatal period this is confined to lesions of obstructed outflow on the left, particularly hypoplastic left heart syndrome (HLHS) and critical aortic stenosis (AS) in which systemic blood flow is dependent on blood flowing right to left across the duct. Giving oxygen or lowering carbon dioxide in these cases can reduce the pulmonary pressures so that blood flows preferentially to the lungs rather than to the systemic circulation. In these specific examples, therefore, withholding oxygen may be beneficial. However, when presented initially with a collapsed neonate, it is almost impossible to identify this situation clinically and withholding oxygen in all other shocked patients would be detrimental. Use of oxygen is therefore recommended *even in known congenital heart disease* when a patient is collapsed.[4]

➕ **Clinical tip** Oxygen therapy

Providing high-flow oxygen is also of use diagnostically: if the saturations remain low despite oxygen, this makes cyanotic heart disease more likely, especially if there is no explanation for a respiratory cause for hypoxia on clinical assessment or chest X-ray.

A paediatric emergency call was placed. The anaesthetist delivered PEEP with 100% oxygen via an anaesthetic T-piece. Saturations improved and the patient stopped grunting, although he continued to have signs of respiratory distress. His oxygen saturations improved to 100% and there was no difference between preductal and postductal oxygen saturation measurements.

✪ **Learning point** Causes of neonatal collapse

While life-saving resuscitation is initiated and continued, careful examination and prioritization of specific investigations are necessary to make the diagnosis. It is important that treatment covering a range of possible pathologies continues until the diagnosis has been narrowed to one specific area. In broad terms, the following need consideration:

- cardiac causes;
- sepsis—infective causes;
- bleeding and trauma—including non-accidental injury
- metabolic, endocrine, and seizures

✪ **Learning point** Cardiac causes

Although congenital cardiac disease is has an incidence of 6–8 in 1000 births, only 2 in 1000 require intervention in infancy.[5,6] Cases may be diagnosed antenatally, on the routine postnatal check or outside of the neonatal period.

Congenital cardiac conditions that present as neonatal collapse are almost all duct-dependent, although there are exceptions. The duct tends to close at 5–14 days of age. Presence of a narrow pulse pressure, gallop, and hepatomegaly are signs of heart failure. The absence of a murmur or cyanosis does not exclude a cardiac diagnosis. Congenital, cardiac lesions can be divided into cyanotic and acyanotic.

➕ **Clinical tip** Cardiac investigations

Investigations such as pre- and postductal saturations, chest X-ray, four-limb BP, and electrocardiogram (ECG) are essential in any collapsed neonate, although a 12-lead ECG is rarely a priority in the resuscitation phase of treatment unless an arrhythmia is suspected.

✪ **Learning point** Acyanotic cardiac disease

Acyanotic cardiac disease that presents with neonatal collapse is caused either by an obstruction to systemic blood flow (duct-dependent left-sided lesions) or cardiac failure due to cardiomyopathy, myocarditis, or arrhythmia. Lesions with a large left-to-right shunt such as ventricular septal defect (VSD), atrioventricular septal defect (AVSD), or an arteriovenous malformation (AVM) can cause cardiac failure, but these usually present beyond the neonatal period, when pulmonary pressures drop.

Duct-dependent left-sided lesions may have an obstruction to blood flow at any level; however, antenatal scans, which include a four-chamber view of the heart, should identify if there is a severe obstruction at the atrial or mitral level (e.g. mitral atresia) as the left ventricle is hypoplastic. Where antenatal screening has occurred, critical AS or coarctation of the aorta are more likely to present as neonatal collapse than HLHS as these may be harder to identify on antenatal imaging. As long as there is some forward flow through the aortic valve, the preductal saturations in these babies will be normal, although postductal saturations will be lower as blood is supplied to the body by shunting right to left through the duct. As the duct closes, systemic blood flow reduces and the patient presents with signs of shock. This is usually exacerbated by cardiac failure due to the heart having to pump against an obstruction e.g. AS. More blood is delivered to the pulmonary circulation while cardiac output from the left side is reduced, causing pulmonary oedema. These patients often present in extremis with signs of cardiac failure, including hepatomegaly, shock, and severe work of breathing due to pulmonary oedema and cardiac failure. Chest X-ray typically shows pulmonary congestion. Cardiomegaly is usually present but may be absent in HLHS.

Neonates with structurally normal hearts may present in this period with heart failure. Faced with a child in heart failure it can be difficult to determine the underlying cause: cardiomyopathy may be of genetic origin and can be associated with metabolic disease myocarditis may present with viral symptoms, a rash, or fever. The ECG classically demonstrates small QRS complexes, but these are not always present, and the trace may be fairly non-specific, often with sinus tachycardia.[7] ST segment depression or elevation is typically associated with myocarditis, but can also be present in other cardiac lesions due to myocardial ischaemia.

Arrhythmias in neonates may be primary or secondary to a congenital or acquired cardiac lesion. The commonest primary arrhythmia is neonatal supraventricular tachycardia (SVT). In this condition, there may have been concerns of 'a fast HR' in the antenatal period or at the time of presentation. Neonates with tachyarrythmias such as SVT are at risk of developing secondary cardiac failure due to arrythmogenic cardiomyopathy if not recognized early and treated promptly. Arrhythmias may be the primary cause of cardiac failure, but may also be symptomatic of cardiomyopathy or myocarditis

🎓 **Expert comment** Recording differential limb blood pressure

It is important to use the systolic pressure difference as it is this value that is most reduced by the resistance of the narrowed vessel.

Mean BP may sometimes be normal in children with cardiogenic shock, where this has developed over time: when there is reduced systemic blood flow over days, or even weeks, the body adapts via the sympathetic nervous and humoral systems so that urine output is reduced and the systemic vascular resistance (diastolic BP) is increased to compensate for reduced systemic cardiac output. On decompensation, patients often display signs of cardiogenic shock such as weak pulses or poor peripheral perfusion (pale, mottled skin, delayed capillary refill time) before their mean BP drops—which is typically a pre-terminal sign.

➕ **Clinical tip** Pre- and postductal pulses

Pulses on all limbs should be palpated and if femoral pulses are weaker than brachial pulses then this suggests coarctation with systolic BP in the legs typically being 20 mmHg less than in the right arm.

➕ **Clinical tip** Prostaglandin dosing

Prostaglandin is used to maintain the patency of the ductus arteriosus and reopen it if duct-dependent lesions are suspected. Dose-dependent side effects include vasodilation, apnoea, and pyrexia. If an infusion rate of ≥ 15 ng/kg/min is required then the patient should be intubated as the risk of apnoea is high.[8] Prostaglandin infusion errors can occur where there is unfamiliarity with the drug. Ensure that the dose is accurate (**ng**/kg/**min**) and that prostaglandin E2 (not D2) is prescribed and administered.

Dosing in suspected duct-dependent disease:

- Patient is hypoxic but stable, not shocked: **5ng/kg/min**, risk of apnoea low.
- Shocked, or hypoxic and shocked: start at **20ng/kg/min**. Intubate patient as high risk of apnoea with this dose.
- Peri-arrest: strong suspicion of duct-dependent lesion, e.g. coarctation and duct is closed: **50 ng/kg/min**, at this dose apnoea is expected and hypotension likely. Consult expert opinion— look to reduce dose to 20 ng/kg/min after 30 mins as by this point the drug is either ineffective or, if effective, the patency of the duct will be maintained on a lower dose.

⭐ **Learning point** Cyanotic cardiac lesions

Cyanotic lesions occur when there is reduced pulmonary flow or abnormal mixing.

Obstruction to pulmonary blood flow—before the lungs

Obstruction to blood flow can be identified on echocardiogram (echo) at any level, e.g. tricuspid atresia, severe tetralogy of Fallot, and pulmonary atresia. For these children to survive at delivery they all have an intracardiac communication, such as a VSD, that allows blood to shunt from right to left. The lungs are then supplied by a patent ductus arteriosus. Although cyanosis is present owing to right to left shunting, they are not shocked. These babies are well initially and could be identified on the postnatal ward by routine measurement of their oxygen saturations.[9] As this is not standard throughout the UK and elsewhere, these children may present as the duct closes with signs of increasing cyanosis and tachypnoea, which is driven by hypoxia. Pre- and postductal oxygen saturations will be low (<85%) and should be the same as blood shunts from right to left within the heart and mixes before it enters the aorta. There will be a minimal increment in response to high-flow oxygen. Work of breathing is less than would be expected for other causes of hypoxia such as lung disease or pulmonary oedema, and as there is obstruction to pulmonary blood flow, a chest X-ray will typically demonstrate oligaemic lung fields (see Figure 2.1).

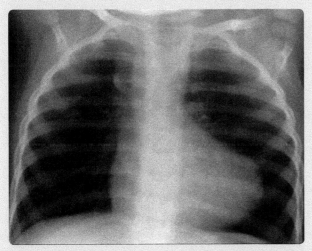

Figure 2.1 Chest X-ray of neonate with tetralogy of Fallot. Note the classic 'boot-shaped' heart due to the small pulmonary outflow tract, and the oligaemic lung fields due to reduced pulmonary blood flow.

Obstruction to pulmonary blood flow—in the lungs

Primary pulmonary hypertension is rare and usually presents to the neonatal unit in the first few hours of life, but pulmonary hypertension secondary to other pathologies, such as pneumonia or sepsis, is more common. Postductal oxygen saturations would be lower than preductal saturations in this situation as blood shunts away from the elevated pulmonary pressures. Chest X-ray may be congested if there is primary lung pathology, such as pneumonia, or oligaemic if pulmonary hypertension is primary.

It can be difficult to distinguish between pulmonary hypertension and structural cardiac disease, and prostaglandin should be started and continued until cardiac disease is excluded by echo. If the duct has closed and pulmonary hypertension develops, then the patient would present with signs of right heart failure: tachycardia, hepatomegaly, P pulmonale, and right ventricle hypertrophy on ECG.

Obstruction to pulmonary blood flow—leaving the lungs

Total anomalous pulmonary venous drainage (TAPVD) is a condition in which the pulmonary venous drainage returns to the right side of the heart rather than the left. The pulmonary veins may drain to the superior vena cava (supracardiac), inferior vena cava (infracardiac), heart (intracardiac), or rarely a mixture of these (mixed). All of these patients will be blue at birth as this condition is lethal unless there is a right to left shunt at birth. In *unobstructed* TAPVD, there is adequate right to left shunting through an atrial septal defect (ASD) and/or VSD, which both allows the right side of the heart to decompress and provides the left side of the heart with sufficient preload to deliver enough systemic blood flow to maintain organ function. *Obstructed* TAPVD occurs if any part of the pathway from pulmonary veins back to the left side of the heart is restrictive to flow. This may be present at birth or develop with time as pulmonary pressures drop and pulmonary blood flow increases. Obstruction to pulmonary venous blood flow leads to pulmonary congestion, further hypoxia, and hepatomegaly. Because the pulmonary veins drain to the right with no shunting, there is insufficient blood flow returning to the left side of the heart, which causes a reduced stroke volume and cardiac output leading to shock. These babies are both cyanosed and shocked and require urgent surgical intervention. Chest X-ray demonstrates congested lung fields and a cardiac silhouette suggesting a large right atrium but underfilled left side—classically described as 'a snowman in a snow storm' (see Figure 2.2). Obstructed TAPVD may present later as pulmonary pressures fall over the first month of life causing increasing pulmonary venous blood flow and volume overload to the right side of the heart.

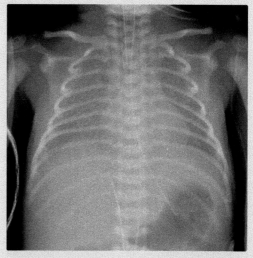

Figure 2.2 Chest X-ray of neonate with obstructed supracardiac total anomalous pulmonary venous drainage, demonstrating the classic features of 'a snowman in a snowstorm'.

> **✪ Learning point** Cyanosis due to inadequate mixing
>
> **Transposition of the great arteries**
>
> In transposition of the great arteries (TGA), the pulmonary artery arises from the left ventricle and the aorta from the right. This results in two circulations in parallel: the left ventricle receiving well-oxygenated blood from the lungs via the pulmonary veins and pumping it directly back to the lungs, via the pulmonary arteries, and the right side of the heart receiving deoxygenated blood from the body via the superior vena cava (SVC) and inferior vena cava (IVC) and pumping it directly back to the systemic circulation via the aorta without oxygenation. These parallel circulations would be fatal within a few minutes of birth without some mixing occurring. Although there is some mixing at a ductal level, shunting within the heart at the atrial or ventricular level allow for better mixing. If the patient has a large ASD or VSD in addition to TGA then these patients will be cyanosed but may appear otherwise well. If they have insufficient mixing within the heart then these patients will present when the duct closes or sometimes before this if mixing at ductal level is inadequate. Progressive systemic hypoxia leads to shock, and severe metabolic and lactic acidosis, which may be exacerbated by poor cardiac function due to coronary ischaemia.
>
> Diagnosis of TGA can often be made clinically without access to paediatric echo as it is the only cardiac lesion in which preductal saturations are lower than postductal saturations as the right arm blood supply stems from the deoxygenated right ventricle. Chest X-ray demonstrates the cardiac silhouette of 'an egg on a string' as the great arteries are parallel so there is no aortic knuckle.
>
> A neonate with collapse secondary to TGA should be resuscitated with inotropes, 100% oxygen, and ventilation but ultimately requires an urgent balloon atrial septostomy, which improves intracardiac mixing. Patients may require a time-critical transfer to a cardiac centre or a cardiologist may travel to the patient to perform the procedure if the diagnosis is certain.

Owing to concerns of cardiac failure as there was hepatomegaly and shock, fluid resuscitation was administered cautiously in 5 mL/kg aliquots. After 10 mL/kg his liver enlarged and he remained tachycardic and mottled so fluid resuscitation was stopped. Femoral pulses appeared weaker than the right brachial. ECG was examined and sinus rhythm was confirmed. Further intravenous access was difficult to obtain, so adrenaline was started via an IO needle at 0.2 µg/kg/min as signs of shock persisted. A blood culture was taken from the IO needle and broad-spectrum antibiotics were given along with aciclovir (in case of herpes infection).

> **✪ Learning point** Sepsis
>
> Sepsis in neonates commonly presents without fever and, even if another diagnosis is likely, cannot be excluded early on. Any collapsed neonate should therefore receive broad-spectrum antibiotics.[10]
>
> **Bacterial infection**
>
> The most common bacterial infections in neonates are group B streptococcus (GBS) and *Escherichia coli*, and are most often transmitted via the vaginal tract during birth (but can be acquired after birth). GBS is most likely to present as meningitis in the first week of life or as pneumonia later on. The site of infection may be occult in any bacteraemia. Time to antibiotics has been shown to correlate with survival,[11] so although culture of blood, urine, and cerebrospinal fluid (CSF) would ideally be taken prior to initiation of antibiotics, lumbar puncture (LP) is rarely possible when the child presents with collapse. Although LP is undoubtedly useful for confirming a diagnosis of meningitis and identifying the potential pathogen, there is a risk to the baby if there is raised intracranial pressure, coagulopathy, or thrombocytopenia. As these are all possible in the collapsed neonate and excluding these delays antibiotic administration, antimicrobials should be given prior to LP if septic shock is suspected. Blood and urine culture should be taken with the latter obtained by catheter (6 Fr nasogastric tube can be used if no catheter immediately available) or ultrasound-guided suprapubic aspiration. If only minimal blood is obtained intraosseously this should be prioritized and used for culture.
>
> Broad-spectrum antibiotics that penetrate the CSF are initiated: cefotaxime or benzylpenicillin/ gentamicin are commonly used in the UK. If listeria is suspected then intravenous amoxicillin is added (listeria is vertically transmitted and amniotic liquor is described as foul-smelling and green).

Viral infection

Many viruses can cause collapse, with herpes simplex virus (HSV) having the highest mortality of approximately 30% even if treated promptly with aciclovir.[12] Transmission can be vertical or acquired, and history should be sought for oral or genital lesions in caregivers, although in the majority of cases there is no relevant history.[13] Herpes can be localized, causing an encephalopathy, and characterized by reduced Glasgow Coma Scale score and/or seizures. Investigations classically show temporal lobe involvement on CT with this also reflected on EEG.

Enteroviruses can also cause collapse due to sepsis or myocarditis. Neonates infected by Parechovirus, a type of Enterovirus, can present with widespread erythema and rash and features of 'warm shock' with tachycardia, a wide pulse pressure that is not typical of other causes of neonatal sepsis. Parechovirus can be associated with a range of systemic features including seizures and gastrointestinal symptoms.[14]

⁶⁶ Expert comment Aciclovir

Disseminated herpes has a very poor prognosis and should be suspected where there is significant coagulopathy or liver failure in the presence of shock. Aciclovir should therefore be started if there is suspicion of sepsis with coagulopathy/liver involvement, or if there is encephalopathy.

Analysis of a blood gas sample demonstrated a lactate of 10 mmol/l and a glucose of 7 mmol/L. The rest of the blood gas did not demonstrate any electrolyte abnormalities and the haemoglobin was 140 g/L. Further examination showed no evidence of bleeding. A cranial ultrasound was performed and did not reveal any evidence of intraventricular haemorrhage.

✪ Learning point Bleeding and trauma

Historically, haemorrhagic disease of the newborn, caused by vitamin K deficiency, was the commonest cause of bleeding in neonates; however, the routine administration of vitamin K at birth has made this a rare disease. Haemorrhage is now more commonly caused by other bleeding disorders, perinatal trauma, or, sadly, secondary to physical abuse (see Case 16). Presentation may include a combination of anaemia, bleeding, and shock. Profound coagulopathy may also be secondary to other mechanisms such as HSV infection (see 'Learning Point: Sepsis').

The skin should be examined for signs of bruising (bearing in mind that Mongolian blue spots are common at birth and can be misdiagnosed as bruises). The umbilical cord may ooze on day 1 of life, but bleeding beyond this time is unusual and may indicate an underlying bleeding disorder. Bleeding sites are often occult and neonates can have significant blood loss due to intracranial, subgaleal, or intra-abdominal haemorrhage without obvious clinical signs.

✪ Learning point Cranial bleeding

The fontanelle must always be examined: a raised fontanelle suggests raised intracranial pressure. The sutures of the cranium may also be widened. Pupils may be dilated, asymmetrical, or poorly responsive. Absence of these signs does not exclude a significant bleed and if there is evidence of anaemia, concerns of trauma, or no cause identified for collapse then a head CT should be performed. If the child is too unstable to be moved to CT then a cranial ultrasound scan can be used to identify major bleeds.

Once an injury is identified then this should be immediately referred to the neurosurgical team who will decide if it is an emergency that requires immediate intervention. Survival in neurosurgical emergencies is improved by timely intervention, so, in these cases, urgent transfer to a paediatric neurosurgical centre is required (see Case 7).

Subgaleal/aponeurotic haemorrhage is defined as bleeding under the galea aponeurotica, the fibrous tissue layer covering the periosteum of the skull. Veins within this potential space can rupture and as this layer is not confined by the sutures of the skull, huge volumes of blood loss can occur before it is recognized. It is caused by birth trauma or bleeding disorders. Although these usually present before the baby is discharged, they can present later. The scalp should be examined for a fluctuant mass or fluid that crosses the sutures of the skull. Care should be taken to examine gravity-dependent areas such as the occiput and nape of the neck if the baby is supine.

✪ **Learning point** Non-accidental injury

Non-accidental injury is, unfortunately, a cause of neonatal collapse and death in infancy. Common injuries include intracranial haemorrhage, retinal haemorrhage, rib fractures, external bruising, and intra-abdominal pathology such as liver laceration. The mechanism of injury may be due to shaking of the baby or blunt trauma, e.g. a punch. If one injury is identified then others should be actively sought, with intra-abdominal and intracranial injuries most likely to cause death. In addition to resuscitating the patient with blood products as required (see 'Fluids, temperature, and bleeding'), surgical and safeguarding teams should be contacted immediately (see Chapter 16).

The team agrees that this patient has shock with signs of cardiac failure that is refractory to fluid and PEEP. It is agreed that the patient needs intubation and initiation of prostaglandin as a cardiac cause is likely.

The most experienced operator intubates the patient after the adrenaline is increased to 0.4 µg/kg/min to improve pulse volumes. Prostaglandin is started at a rate of 20 ng/kg/min and this is increased to 50 ng/kg/min after four-limb BP identifies unrecordable BP in both legs and a systolic BP of 80 mmHg in the right arm. Chest X-ray shows plethoric lung fields with cardiomegaly (see Figure 2.3). The baby is transferred to the Paediatric Intensive Care Unit (PICU).

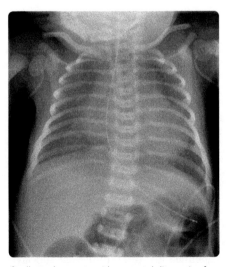

Figure 2.3 Chest X-ray of collapsed neonate with postnatal diagnosis of coarctation of the aorta, showing cardiomegaly and plethoric lung fields. Note deviation of trachea and oesophagus towards the right due to left atrial enlargement.

✦ Expert comment Algorithm for diagnosis of metabolic conditions

Figure 2.4 is a diagnostic algorithm for metabolic conditions in a collapsed neonate. As most of these conditions are genetic, family history of infantile deaths or miscarriages should be sought, although in the majority there is no family history. History should be sought of poor feeding, vomiting, diarrhoea, and lethargy/floppiness, and examination should include looking for dysmorphology and hepatomegaly (see Case 17).

★ Learning point Metabolic decompensation

Although there are several metabolic and endocrine diseases that present in infancy, the majority do not present in the neonatal period with collapse. However, those that do constitute a true emergency; thus, blood ammonia, lactate, glucose, and blood gas analyses should be part of all initial investigations in the shocked neonate unless an alternative diagnosis is certain, e.g. congenital cardiac lesion identified.

Metabolic diseases are caused by genetic defects in metabolic pathways that cause an accumulation of a product upstream of the defect and deficiency below it. The patient can be harmed therefore either by intoxication of a metabolite or by a deficiency or both. They can decompensate soon after birth as without maternal support, toxins rapidly build up, or they are unable to supply the body with the energy it needs (see Case 17)

★ Learning point Hypoglycaemia, hyponatraemia, and hyperkalaemia

Neonates often have poor glycogen reserves and are prone to hypoglycaemia if feeding poorly or systemically unwell so in the resuscitation phase it is appropriate to give 2 mL/kg dextrose 10% for hypoglycaemia and start maintenance fluid containing sodium chloride along with dextrose 10%. If the patient has further hypoglycaemia, then a hypoglycaemia screen should be sent (including lab glucose, ketones, lactate, cortisol, and acylcarnitine) and glucose delivery rapidly escalated until normoglycaemia is achieved. Metabolic conditions will often cause ongoing acidosis until sufficient glucose delivery is maintained at more than 6 mg/kg/min (see Clinical tip: calculating the glucose infusion rate in Case 17).

If hypoglycaemia is associated with high potassium and low sodium then adrenal insufficiency should be suspected with reduced levels of cortisol and aldosterone. This is most commonly caused by certain forms of congenital adrenal hyperplasia, which is an autosomal recessive condition. If both cortisol and aldosterone deficiency are present then presentation is with hypotension, hypoglycaemia, hyperkalaemia, and hyponatraemia. Significant volumes of fluid resuscitation and glucose are often required and the patient improves once hydrocortisone is given. Symptoms are non-specific and examination of genitalia may be helpful if androgen levels are abnormal as female genitalia may be virilized and male genitalia may be hyperpigmented.

★ Learning point Encephalopathy and seizures

Management of seizures should be as per local guidance, such as the APLS algorithm in the UK[1], and low glucose, calcium or sodium should be corrected in any seizing patients. Hyperammonaemia is another cause of seizure and blood ammonia should be checked in any infant with encephalopathy or seizure. The highest levels of ammonia intoxication are caused by urea cycle defects. Ammonia rapidly accumulates with initiation of feed and the baby becomes drowsy and then encephalopathic. While other metabolic conditions improve with supportive therapy and maintenance of normoglycaemia, hyperammonaemia does not and delay in treating this leads to devastating brain damage, cardiovascular failure, and death. Treatment is with specific metabolic drugs, which provide an alternative pathway for ammonia to be broken down and, most importantly, urgent dialysis or haemofiltration (see Case 17). Peritoneal dialysis, haemofiltration, and haemodialysis have increasing efficacy at clearing ammonia quickly, but, failure to send ammonia samples at presentation causes the biggest delay in treatment. Ammonia levels of >300 µmol/L have been shown to cause neurological injury; thus, levels above this should be treated aggressively. Advice should be sought from a metabolic consultant who will advise on the specific metabolic drugs, which should then be started as soon as possible (see Case 17).

✦ Expert comment Steroids

Hydrocortisone should be given if there is refractory shock with hypoglycaemia or the triad of hypoglycaemia, hyponatraemia, and hyperkalaemia. A cortisol level should be taken prior to giving hydrocortisone.

After admission to the PICU, the baby's lower limb perfusion and pulses improved with prostaglandin. An echo was performed by the paediatric cardiologist and a discrete coarctation was identified just distal to the left subclavian artery. The coarctation was repaired via thoracotomy the following day. However, the patient remained

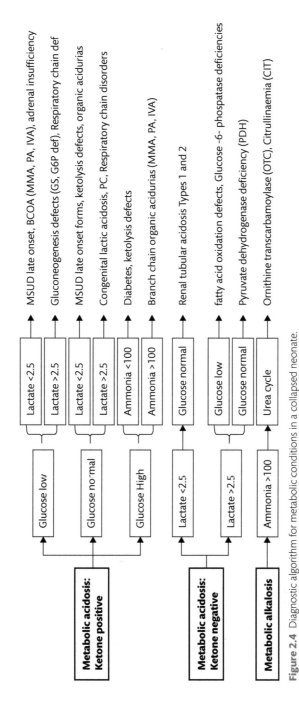

Figure 2.4 Diagnostic algorithm for metabolic conditions in a collapsed neonate.

MSUD, maple syrup urine disease; BCOA, branched chain organic aciduria; MMA, methylmalonic acidaemia; PA, propionic acidaemia; IVA, isovaleric acidaemia; GS, glycogen synthase; G6P, glucose-6-phosphatase; def., deficiency; PC, pyruvate carboxylase. Units for lactate are mmol/L and for ammonia are μmol/L

Figure reproduced with permission from: https://www.evelinalondon.nhs.uk/resources/our-services/hospital/south-thames-retrieval-service/metabolic-disorders-jan-2018.pdf

Figure 2.5 Main differential diagnoses of neonatal collapse, urgent assessment, and management steps.

TGA, transposition of the giant arteries; TAPVD, total anomalous pulmonary venous discharge; SVT, supraventricular tachycardia; PROM, prolonged rupture of membranes; GBS, group B streptococcus; GCS, Glasgow Coma Scale; ALT, alanine transaminase; WCC, white cell count; CXR, chest X-ray; HR, heart rate; IV, intravenous; FBC, full blood count; Tx, treatment; PCR, polymerase chain reaction; CT, computed tomography; NAI, non-accidental injury.

Figure reproduced with permission from: https://www.evelinalondon.nhs.uk/resources/our-services/hospital/south-thames-retrieval-service/neonatal-collapse-nov-2017.pdf

Category	Diagnosis	Clinical features	Management
Sepsis	Group B strep, E Coli	PROM, maternal GBS, fever in labour	Cefotaxime 50mg/kg IV and amoxicillin 100mg/kg IV
Sepsis	Herpes Simplex	↓GCS, coagulopathy, ↑ALT, herpes contact	Add Aciclovir 20 mg/kg IV. High index suspicion, history often absent
Sepsis	Pertussis	Apnoea, cough-pt. or contact, ↑WCC (lymph)	See pertussis guideline. Add macrolide. 6 hourly FBC - may need exchange Tx.
Cardiac	Coarctation aorta	Systolic arm/leg gradient > 20 mmHg	Urgent Prostin (may need high dose) and support (ventilation/inotropes)
Cardiac	Hypoplastic Left heart	Poor pulses - may be pink = pulm. overcirculation	Prostin. Avoid oxygen-can cause pulm. overcirculation. Target sats 75%
Cardiac	Transposition (TGA)	Preductal sats < post ductal sats	Urgent Prostin. If no response: urgent septostomy
Cardiac	TAPVD (obstructed)	Shocked & cyanosed/CXR plethoric	Prostin may make worse. Need echo confirmation and surgery
Cardiac	SVT	HR > 220 despite fluid, fixed HR, narrow QRS	See arrhythmia guideline. Adenosine, if shocked: ventilate + DC shock
Cardiac	Myocarditis	Cardiac failure, tachycardia, small QRS	Supportive (ventilation, inotropes). Consider immunoglobulin. Viral PCRs.
Metabolic	Urea cycle defect	↓GCS, Seizures, ↑ammonia, alkalosis	Ammonia >150mmol/L. Repeat to confirm. Metabolic opinion
Metabolic	Organic acidaemia	Profound metabolic acidosis, ketone positive	Supportive (inotropes, ventilation). May co-present with sepsis
Metabolic	Mitochondrial	↑Lactate, seizures, cardiomyopathy	Supportive (inotropes, ventilation). May co-present with sepsis
Trauma	Intracranial bleed	Focal neuro signs, fontanelle↑, retinal bleeds	Head CT to exclude neurosurgical problem/ ?NAI ?haemorrhagic disease
Trauma	Intra-abdominal bleed	Unexplained anaemia, abdominal bruising	Abdominal and head CT, ?non-accidental injury (NAI), ?haemorrhagic disease of newborn

ventilated for 5 days owing to concerns over poor cardiac function. Following this, the baby made a full recovery.

Discussion

Resources in neonatal resuscitation

It should be recognized that the management of neonatal collapse may stress any individual, team, or department to their maximum level. The on-call anaesthetist may not have recent experience of intubating a baby of that size; vascular access can be challenging at this age, especially if the child is shocked; it can be unnerving managing a resuscitation where the diagnosis is unknown; the situation can be extremely emotive, particularly if the family is distressed. Recognizing that neonatal collapse is often challenging, it is important to prepare for this by ensuring the team are knowledgeable, the correct equipment is available for neonatal resuscitation in the ED environment, and simulation is undertaken. The neonatal team usually do not respond to paediatric emergencies or arrest calls in the ED, but they are a resource with regard to intubation and vascular access that are often underutilized in this scenario.

A final word from the expert

Management of neonatal collapse must include generic resuscitation in tandem with early targeted investigations to facilitate diagnosis and guide subsequent urgent, specific therapeutic measures (e.g. balloon atrial septostomy for TGA with intact ventricular septum). The neonate with respiratory failure should be supported with PEEP and assessed for apnoea. It is crucial to examine for signs of cardiac failure along with signs of respiratory distress. For the child with seizures or encephalopathy, hypoglycaemia, hyponatraemia, and hypocalcaemia must be corrected, but ammonia should also be sent if the cause of neurological impairment is not entirely clear. If there are any neurological concerns then there should be a low threshold for imaging and excluding intracranial pathology. Figure 2.5 summarizes the main differential diagnoses of neonatal collapse and shows that by using clinical skills and targeted bedside tests an accurate diagnosis can be made.

References

1. Samuels M, Wieteska S. *Advanced Paediatric Life Support*. Hoboken, NJ: John Wiley & Sons; 2016.
2. Ventura AM, Shieh HH, Bousso A, et al. Double-blind prospective randomized controlled trial of dopamine versus epinephrine as firstline vasoactive drugs in pediatric septic shock. *Crit. Care Med*. 2015;43:2292–302.
3. Weiss SL, Peters MJ, Alhazzani W, et al. Surviving Sepsis Campaign international guidelines for the management of septic shock and sepsis-associated organ dysfunction in chilren. *Pediatr Crit Care Med*. 2020;21:e52-e106.
4. Maconochie I, Bingham R, Eich C, et al. European Resuscitation Council Guidelines for Resuscitation 2015 Section 6 Paediatric Life Support. *Resuscitation* 2015;95:222–47.

5. van der Linde D, Konings EEM, Slager MA, et al. Birth prevalence of congenital heart disease worldwide: a systematic review and meta-analysis. *J. Am. Coll. Cardiol.* 2011;58:2241–7.

6. Knowles RL, Ridout D, Crowe S, et al. Ethnic and socioeconomic variation in incidence of congenital heart defects. *Arch. Dis. Child.* 2017;102:496–502.

7. Durani Y, Egan M, Baffa J, Selbst SM, Nagar AL. Pediatric myocarditis: presenting clinical characteristics. *Am. J. Emerg. Med.* 2009;27:942–7.

8. Browning Carmo KA, Barr P, West M, Hopper NW, White JP, Badawi N. Transporting newborn infants with suspected duct dependent congenital heart disease on low-dose prostaglandin E1 without routine mechanical ventilation. *Arch. Dis. Child. Fetal Neonatal Ed.* 2007;92:F117–19.

9. Thangaratinam S, Brown K, Zamora J, Khan KS, Ewer AK. Pulse oximetry screening for critical congenital heart defects in asymptomatic newborn babies: a systematic review and meta-analysis. *Lancet* 2012;379:2459–64.

10. Lutsar I, Chazallon C, Carducci FI, et al. Current management of late onset neonatal bacterial sepsis in five European countries. *Eur. J. Pediatr.* 2014;173:997–1004.

11. Kumar A, Roberts D, Wood KE, et al. Duration of hypotension before initiation of effective antimicrobial therapy is the critical determinant of survival in human septic shock. *Crit. Care Med.* 2006;34:1589–96.

12. Kimberlin D, Lin C-Y, Jacobs RF, et al. The safety and efficacy of high-dose acyclovir in the management of neonatal herpes simplex virus infections. *Pediatrics* 2001;108:230–8.

13. Gardella C, Brown Z. Prevention of neonatal herpes. *BJOG* 2011;118:187–92.

14. Olijve L, Jennings L, Walls T. Human Parechovirus: an increasingly recognized cause of sepsis-like illness in young infants. *Clin Micr Rev.* 2017;31:e00047–17.

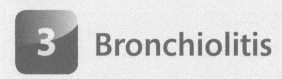

Bronchiolitis

Crawford Fulton

ⓘ **Expert commentary** by Kentigern Thorburn

Case history

A 6-month old infant was seen in the Emergency Department of a large district general hospital with a history of breathing difficulty. Clinical findings included a respiratory rate (RR) of 70 breaths per minute, crackles, and wheeze on auscultation. The paediatric team admitted him to the ward with a diagnosis of bronchiolitis.

On the paediatric ward, he was not feeding effectively and therefore was fed via a nasogastric tube (NGT). His work of breathing worsened on day 2 of admission and his oxygen saturations dropped to 84–88% in air, necessitating oxygen supplementation via nasal cannulae. The nasopharyngeal aspirate for respiratory pathogen polymerase chain reaction (PCR) tested positive for both respiratory syncytial virus (RSV) and human Metapneumovirus (hMPV).

> ✪ **Learning point** The burden of bronchiolitis and RSV on cells/children/hospital/Paediatric Intensive Care Unit
>
> Bronchiolitis in children results in a significant burden on primary and secondary care, in the winter months. It is the most common disease of the lower respiratory tract in children <1 year of age. RSV bronchiolitis is, in fact, the leading worldwide cause of admission to hospital in the same age group. Approximately one-third of all infants will develop bronchiolitis, but only 2–3% will require hospitalization. In 2015 in England, there were approximately 40,000 secondary care admissions for bronchiolitis and admissions are rising year on year.[1]
>
> RSV is responsible for up to 70% of bronchiolitis cases. The other less common pathogens include parainfluenza, adenovirus, influenza, hMPV, rhinovirus, and bocavirus. Figure 3.1 demonstrates the spectrum of respiratory viruses detected by multiplex PCR in children (of all ages) admitted to Alder Hey Children's Hospital from 2010 until 2019 and the seasonality of bronchiolitis.
>
> Bronchiolitis admissions to the Paediatric Intensive Care Unit (PICU) in autumn and winter account for a significant proportion of bed occupancy.
>
> In the UK between 2004 and 2012, infants aged <1 year accounted for 93% of all bronchiolitis admissions and 11.8% of admissions each year. The average length of PICU stay with bronchiolitis ranged from 5.4 to 6.7 days (mean 6.1 days). Over the 8 years there were 158 deaths, representing a PICU case fatality of 1.7% in infants aged <12 months and 4.4% in children aged ≥12 months.[1] Despite a substantial increase in hospital admissions for infants with bronchiolitis, the number requiring intensive care has changed little since 2004 (see Figure 3.2).

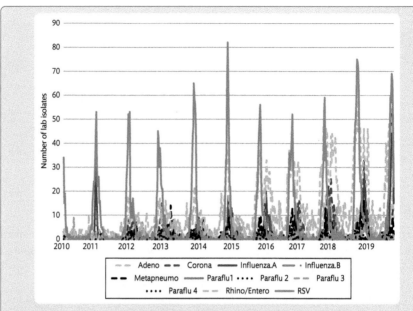

Figure 3.1 Respiratory viruses identified by multiplex polymerase chain reaction in Alder Hey Children's Hospital (2010–2019). The common respiratory viruses demonstrate predictable seasonality with peak numbers in December and January each year, impacting significantly on hospital capacity. Dual to multiple viral infection in bronchiolitis patients is not uncommon.

Adeno, adenovirus; corona, coronavirus; Metapneumo, metapneumovirus; Paraflu, parainfluenza; rhino, rhinovirus; Entero, enterovirus; RSV, respiratory syncytial virus.

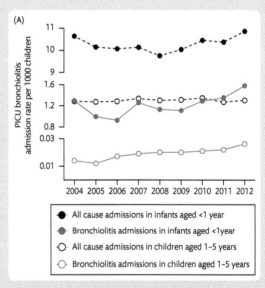

Figure 3.2 Paediatric intensive care unit (PICU) admissions with bronchiolitis and all causes from 2004 to 2012. (A) All-cause and bronchiolitis admission rates per 1000 children. (B) Mean age (months with 95% confidence interval (CI)) at admission for bronchiolitis. Between 2004 and 2006 the mean age rose significantly (**$p = 0.0004$, two-tailed Mann–Whitney). In more recent years the mean age has fallen significantly between 2008 and 2012 (*$p = 0.04$, two-tailed Mann–Whitney)

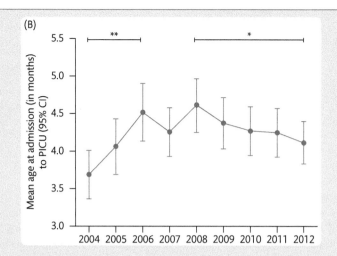

Figure 3.2 Continued

Infecting viruses cause the clinical features of bronchiolitis by having a cytopathic effect on respiratory endothelial cells, which results in loss of submucosal oedema, loss of cilial motility, infiltration by leukocytes, increased mucus secretion, necrosis, and sloughing of respiratory epithelial cells of the small airways. This results in loss of patency and reduction of gas flow through the small airways, and air trapping.[2] Air trapping itself can be exacerbated by ball-valve mechanism of airway obstruction due to mucus and cellular debris plugs. This gives rise to a clinical picture of pulmonary hyperinflation alongside atelectatic areas, combined with wheeze.

A detailed history during admission to the department revealed that he was an ex-premature infant born at 28 weeks' gestation and corrected gestational age of 3 months. His background included being ventilated with respiratory distress syndrome for his first 3 weeks of life. During this time he was also found to have oesophageal atresia with a tracheo-oesophageal fistula, which was repaired uneventfully. He had been discharged from the neonatal unit and was thriving at home, not requiring any supplemental oxygen.

⊕ **Learning point** Risk factors for severe disease

Of children admitted to hospital with bronchiolitis, only 3–10% will require admission to the PICU.[3] Those that are admitted to the PICU are thought to have more 'severe' disease and are likely to have predisposing risk factors. These risk factors that are associated with increased severity of disease can be placed into two groups: host and environmental risk factors

1. Host risk factors include age <6 months, chronic lung disease, prematurity, congenital heart disease, congenital and anatomical defects of the airways, neurological disease, and immunodeficiency.[3] Multiple viral pathogens and/or bacterial co-infection have also been shown to increase severity of disease as indicated by the need for PICU admission and mechanical ventilation.[4-6]
2. Environmental risk factors include poverty, overcrowding, malnutrition, older siblings, postnatal exposure to tobacco smoke, and nursery attendance.[3,4]

> **ℹ Expert comment** Risk factors
>
> Risk factors are not merely for severe disease, but also death. Although the mortality rate for those hospitalized with bronchiolitis is generally low, at 1–3%, it increases in children with severe bronchiolitis requiring PICU support.[7] Mortality is higher in those with comorbidity, especially underlying congenital heart disease, chronic lung disease, immunocompromise, neuromuscular disease, nosocomial infection,[7] and in developing/resource-limited regions.[8] RSV is the most common viral cause of death in children aged <5 years and especially in infants aged <1 year.[8] Bronchiolitis is not as innocuous as commonly assumed—certain subgroups deserve extra attentiveness.

Case history (continued)

Overnight, into day 3 of admission his oxygen requirement continued to rise. He was placed in a head box with oxygen delivering a fraction of inspired oxygen (FiO_2) of 0.6. His RR increased to 80 breaths per minute and his work of breathing increased. The general paediatric team stopped enteral feeding as it appeared to worsen his effort of breathing, and intravenous fluids were started. In view of his wheeze the doctors trialed nebulized bronchodilators (both salbutamol and ipratropium bromide). However, there was no improvement and therefore they were not continued.

Subsequently, in view of his worsening oxygen requirement and effort of breathing, he was commenced on humidified high-flow nasal cannula (HFNC) oxygen at a flow of 5 L/minute with a FiO_2 0.6. There did seem to be some response in that his effort of breathing appeared to improve temporarily. His oxygen saturations were around 92%, RR 75 breaths per minute, heart rate 140 beats per minute.

> **★ Learning point** Supportive care (pre-PICU) (oxygen, bronchodilators, and nebulized saline)
>
> The vast majority of babies with bronchiolitis who are admitted to hospital require very little support other than supplemental oxygen, if their oxygen saturations are <92%,[9] and supplementing feeds via a NGT, if they are not tolerating adequate oral feeds.
>
> **Oxygen**
>
> According to National Institute for Health and Care Excellence guidance,[9] oxygen supplementation should be given to maintain oxygen saturations at ≥92% but there is little reliable research data to support this cut off.

> **✓ Evidence base** Saturation targets
>
> One of the only randomized trials in infants with bronchiolitis (BIDS trial) comparing higher (94%) against lower targeted saturations (90%) showed it was safe and clinically effective to target lower saturations.[10]

> **★ Learning point** (continued)
>
> It is important to bear in mind that there are a number of factors that can influence saturation monitoring, including accuracy of oximeters themselves, poor peripheral perfusion, fever and acidosis.
>
> **Bronchodilators**
>
> Over the years the use of bronchodilators (generally beta agonists and ipratropium bromide) has been debated and researched without many, if any, positive clinical outcomes.

> ✔ **Evidence base** Bronchodilators
>
> Conclusions of a systematic review do not support the routine use of bronchodilators in infants with bronchiolitis. They do not improve oxygenation, overall outcome, hospital admission rate, or duration of hospitalization.[11]

> ✪ **Learning point** (continued)
>
> **Nebulized saline**
>
> In theory, nebulized hypertonic saline (3%) would appear to be useful in combatting the pathophysiological complications of bronchiolitis. Reducing mucus viscosity, enhancing mucus transport, and decreasing epithelial oedema are some of the mechanisms in which it may have a beneficial effect. There is an ambiguous collection of systematic reviews, meta-analyses, and reanalysis of meta-analyses suggesting that nebulized saline may have some beneficial outcomes, in particular reducing hospital admission and length of stay. But no clear conclusion can be pulled from these to support the use of hypertonic saline in every patient with bronchiolitis owing to the quality of evidence.[9,12]

His clinical condition continued to deteriorate further and he was now requiring FiO_2 0.8 on HFNC to maintain his saturations above 90%, despite increased flow on the HFNC to 8 L/minute. He had significant respiratory distress, bilateral crackles, and wheeze. A portable chest X-ray (CXR) showed bilateral patchy changes with areas of hyperinflation. There was no evidence of a pneumothorax. A capillary blood gas sample showed pH 7.2, partial pressure of carbon dioxide ($paCO_2$) 65 mmHg (8.7 kPa), base excess −3, and lactate 2.4. He was started on non-invasive ventilation (NIV) continuous positive airway pressure (CPAP) with a positive end expiratory pressure (PEEP) of 5 cmH_2O.

After a few hours on CPAP, the child remained unsettled and distressed by the CPAP mask. Therefore, he was given a small dose of chloral hydrate via the NGT. Subsequently, he was able to tolerate the CPAP mask well and his oxygen requirement fell to 65%. A repeat capillary blood gas on CPAP showed an improvement in his $paCO_2$ (down to 55 mmHg/7.3 kPa). Over the next 4 hours the baby appeared stable with CPAP.

By 8am the next morning (day 4), he had pauses in breathing and his oxygen requirement worsened again. The apnoeic pauses increased in frequency and duration requiring positive pressure support via a self-inflating bag and mask. The paediatric consultant reviewed the baby, who now appeared to be tiring. The consultant changed the NIV from continuous positive pressure to biphasic pressure mode and increased the pressure so the NIV was now providing a positive inspiratory pressure of 10 cmH_2O and an end expiratory pressure of 6 cmH_2O. In view of apnoeic episodes, they also opted to try a dose of caffeine.

> ✪ **Learning point** Humidified high-flow nasal cannuala and continuous positive airway pressure
>
> **HFNC**
>
> HFNC can be used to deliver high-flow humidified oxygen, which is thought to provide more comfortable and effective delivery of gases while maintaining airway humidity. In clinical practice it appears to be better tolerated by infants and children than NIV. It permits high gas flows (maximum flow rates depend on patient size) with or without increased oxygen concentration. Flow rates of

⊕ Clinical tip Biphasic NIV

In our institution we routinely use CPAP for infants with bronchiolitis. If a child has impending respiratory failure, despite CPAP, we may make a clinical judgement to use biphasic NIV (and providing a positive inspiratory pressure above the PEEP) as a next step to prevent intubation, but only in a setting where skilled practitioners and equipment are close to hand such as a paediatric high-dependency unit or PICU. There is much less evidence to support this step than CPAP alone.

>6 L/minute can generate positive expiratory pressures of up to 5 cmH$_2$O, although this pressure cannot routinely be measured in patients (unlike CPAP with NIV apparatus), which raises some concern among clinicians.

The use of this device is rapidly becoming widespread without demonstration of additional efficacy. Its role in the management of bronchiolitis is currently unclear—should it be used as a step before NIV, or be used instead of NIV?

⊘ **Evidence base** HFNC

A recent randomized controlled study trialled HFNC early in the bronchiolitis disease process, comparing the use of HFNC to nasal cannula oxygen.[13] They randomized 202 children with bronchiolitis and concluded that HFNC did not significantly reduce time on oxygen compared with standard therapy, suggesting that early use of HFNC did not modify the underlying disease process in moderately severe bronchiolitis. However, more recently there have been a number of larger randomized trials showing that HFNC may, in fact, reduce the need for escalation of respiratory support in babies with bronchiolitis.

✪ **Learning point** (continued)

In observational studies only, there is some indication that it may decrease rates of endotracheal intubation,[14] but there is a significant lack of robust evidence to support its current expanding use,[9] although further multicentre trials are in progress.

NIV–CPAP

There is supportive evidence that giving CPAP via mask or nasal prongs can be used in infants with bronchiolitis to decrease work of breathing, and prevent endotracheal intubation in infants with progressive hypoxaemia or hypercarbia.[15] By opening the airways, the positive pressure allows more expiratory flow, improves compliance, reduces work of breathing, and improves gas exchange.

✪ **Learning point** (continued)

In clinical practice CPAP tends to be trialled when either the infant appears to be in significant distress, is tiring, or has an increasing FiO$_2$ and/or increasing paCO$_2$. It is used as a modality to ultimately prevent intubation and mechanical ventilation. CPAP is used as standard practice in most units now. Despite its widespread use, systematic reviews have found the evidence regarding CPAP in bronchiolitis to be inconclusive owing to certain limitations in existing studies.[16,17]

❛❛ **Expert comment** Non-invasive respiratory support in bronchiolitis

What method of non-invasive respiratory support is best in bronchiolitis?

Is HFNC anything more than glorified nasal cannula oxygen therapy? Certainly the humidification element of this oxygen delivery device carries advantages over ordinary cold and dry nasal cannula oxygen in mucociliary transport, decreasing viscosity of airway secretions and energy expenditure. HFNC therapy washes CO$_2$-rich gas out of the respiratory anatomical dead space—replacing it with O$_2$-rich gas generates some (mild) positive airway pressure, and improves oxygenation by increasing end-expiratory lung volume (maybe even tidal volume), thereby increasing oxygen saturations and decreasing work of breathing. However, is HFNC superior to conventional CPAP generators that also humidify inhaled gases efficaciously? This question is more a tertiary-level quandary, in that often at secondary level it is more a case of what equipment is available. HFNC is becoming more widely available and utilized. Because of the cost of equipment, ease of setup and use, and an abundance of anecdotal benefits, I suspect that HFNC apparati will supplant CPAP flow drivers (both when replacing ageing machines and when 'business-casing' new equipment). Certainly in our children's hospital HFNC falls under ward management rather than critical care.

Case history (continued)

Despite these interventions, the baby continued to have significant apnoeas, requiring intermittent bag mask ventilation and, in view of this, the consultant paediatrician decided that he needed to be intubated. The team requested assistance from the anaesthetist. The on-call anaesthetic consultant felt uncomfortable having to anaesthetize and intubate the infant, as he was primarily an adult anaesthetist. The paediatrician also asked his registrar to refer the baby to the regional paediatric intensive care (PIC) transport team.

The transport team agreed that the infant should be intubated and ventilated as a matter of urgency. As neither the paediatrician nor the anaesthetist were confident in intubating infants, the transport team advised asking the neonatologist from the hospital's Neonatal Intensive Care Unit to assist. The neonatologist agreed to help. The PIC transfer team was mobilized but were 40 minutes away.

Meanwhile, the infant was fully monitored with electrocardiogram, pulse oximetry, and non-invasive blood pressure (NIBP) monitoring (set to record every 2 minutes). There was suction that was working close by, a range of endotracheal tube sizes, and an end-tidal CO_2 ($etCO_2$) monitor attached to the bagging circuit. The infant's stomach was emptied using the NGT.

After pre-oxygenation induction medications (fentanyl, ketamine, and rocuronium) were administered. The neonatologist intubated him with a size 4 endotracheal tube. Accurate tube position was confirmed by chest auscultation and the presence of $etCO_2$. Shortly after he was intubated, his NIBP dropped to 44/22; therefore, a 10 mL/kg bolus of saline was given, which improved his blood pressure. The neonatologist continued to hand ventilate the child while the paediatrician obtained a second intravenous access and sent off a blood culture. The infant was sedated using morphine and midazolam. Antibiotics were also given in view of the possibility of co-infection.

When the transport team arrived they confirmed position of the ET tube with a CXR, established the infant on their transport ventilator (settings of a peak inspiratory pressure (PIP) of 26, and PEEP of 7, rate of 35/minute in FiO_2 0.6.). After all checks were complete they transferred the infant uneventfully to the nearest PICU.

⊕ **Clinical tip** Intubating the infant with bronchiolitis—when and how?

Intubating infants in district general hospitals (DGHs) tends to cause significant angst and worry among the local team as, more often than not, the teams intubate these very unwell infants and children infrequently. Anaesthetists in the DGH tend to be more comfortable working with adults, which is why a team approach with the paediatrician, anaesthetist, and even neonatologist is ideal.

Regional PIC transport teams provide advice and training on managing critically unwell children, while stabilizing them and transferring them to PICUs.

While management of these infants with bronchiolitis is very much guided by the clinician at the bedside, regional PIC transport teams offer advice on decision making regarding escalation and about how to manage the intubation process. See the guidance illustrated in Figure 3.3.

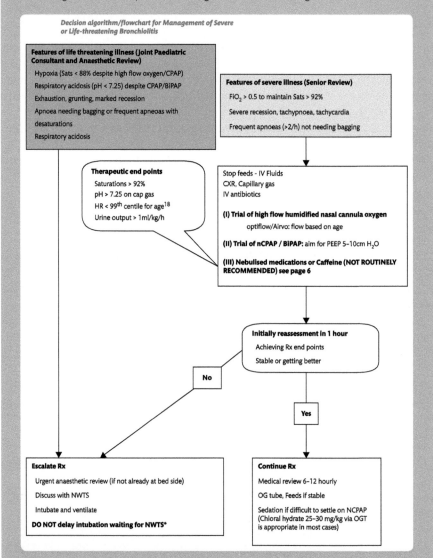

Figure 3.3 North West and North Wales Paediatric Transport Service (NWTS)—Guidelines—Managing Life Threatening Bronchiolitis 2016.

CPAP, continuous positive airway pressure; BiPAP, bilevel positive airway pressure; HR, heart rate; FiO₂, fraction of inspired oxygen; IV, intravenous; CXR, chest X-ray; nCPAP, nasal CPAP; PEEP, positive end expiratory pressure; NWTS, North West & North Wales Paediatric Transport Service; OG, orogastric; OGT, OG tube.

Reproduced from Shetty N, Phatak R, B—Managing Severe Life Threatening Bronchiolitis—16th June 2016, Copyright (2016), with permission from NWTS (North West & North Wales Paediatric Transport Service). Available at https://www.nwts.nhs.uk/_file/lUt7NWfWf6_272914.pdf

Expert comment Decision-making regarding escalation

There is a plethora of bronchiolitis scores (severity scores)—which usually signifies the weakness of the concept. Bronchiolitis scores are generally used in studies rather than ongoing everyday clinical practice. I would challenge whether they replace good old-fashioned basics like clinical assessment of effective oxygenation and ability to maintain effective oxygenation/work of breathing.

For me, it boils down to three key issues, each with two clinical considerations:

1. Hypoxia—saturations + FiO_2.
2. (Risk of) impending collapse/exhaustion—respiratory stamina (work of breathing) + substrate (patient type and/or comorbidities).
3. Apnoeas—'central' + lung parenchymal causes.

These clinical considerations combined with sound clinical acumen will answer any 'urgent' questions such as 'Should I escalate respiratory support?'; 'What type of support?'; 'Can I/they afford to sit tight?'; 'Can the patient?'; 'Should I intubate?'; 'Now?'

Regional guidelines, such as the included North West & North Wales Paediatric Transport Service Guidelines, need clarity of message and should be workable. They should be suitably designed to cover the more severe clinical spectrum of worsening bronchiolitis ('life-threatening bronchiolitis').

Clinical tip Is this really bronchiolitis?

In autumn and winter, when bronchiolitis admissions peak, there may be children admitted with a diagnosis of bronchiolitis that may have another pathology. Cardiac pathology and other infections such as pertussis may be confused with bronchiolitis. Moreover, there may be an underlying condition, which bronchiolitis may precipitate or exacerbate. It is important to identify when there is another pathology, especially if the child is deteriorating despite intervention.

Case history (continued)

After admission to PICU he required more oxygen and ventilation over the first 12 hours. His FiO_2 was 0.9 with a PIP of 28 cmH$_2$O and PEEP of 8 cmH$_2$O. His gases showed a worsening respiratory acidosis. A CXR revealed bilateral changes consistent with evolving acute respiratory distress syndrome (ARDS). Despite regular physiotherapy with hypertonic saline yielding thick secretions, he de-recruited recurrently, and took significant time to re-recruit back on the ventilator. Despite high ventilator pressures, the team was unable to achieve reasonable tidal volumes or good gas exchange, so they tried increased sedation and muscle relaxation, with no significant improvement.

Subsequently, it was decided that a trial of a high-frequency oscillatory ventilator (HFOV) would be attempted. The PICU team sited central venous and arterial lines, optimized cardiovascular status with a bolus of intravenous fluid, and drew up an adrenaline infusion in preparation for the changeover to HFOV. At the point of switching to HFOV, he required FiO_2 1.0, pressures 32/10. On HFOV he was started with an initial distending pressure of 24, which was increased gradually until there was a response in his oxygenation, guided by his saturations. He was cardiovascularly stable during this changeover. A CXR after initiation of HFOV revealed slightly improved aeration of the lung fields.

On day 2 in the PICU, he remained on HFOV, with a distending pressure of 28 in FiO_2 of 0.85. His oxygenation did improve, as did his CO_2 clearance. With these changes his oxygenation index (OI) was 36. The PICU team asked for an echocardiogram to ensure there was no structural abnormality of his heart, and to assess pulmonary pressures. The echocardiogram was difficult to perform owing to the HFOV and hyper-expanded lungs, but did reveal a structurally normal heart, with evidence of significantly raised pulmonary pressures. The team then decided to add in inhaled nitric oxide (iNO), which was started at 10 parts per million (ppm). This resulted in a transient improvement in oxygenation.

Clinical tip
Oxygenation index

Tracking the oxygenation index can be a useful tool in severe bronchiolitis to monitor escalating respiratory support and not overlook creeping hypoxaemia.

OI = mean airway pressure (in mmHg) × FiO_2 (in % oxygen)/ PaO_2 (in mmHg). An OI >25–30 is often used as trigger for discussions regarding extracorporeal membrane oxygenation (ECMO). A persistent OI >40 is used as a strong indication for ECMO support in an otherwise suitable candidate.

⚙ **Learning point** PICU management strategies

Much like the pre-PICU management options, there is a very poor evidence base to support much of the treatment used in PICU for children with severe bronchiolitis.

Mechanical ventilation

There is virtually no evidence to suggest which modes and methods of ventilation should by employed when ventilating babies with bronchiolitis, although there is some guidance (mostly extrapolated from adult evidence) on ventilating children with ARDS.[18] In particular, the use of increasing PEEP and the use of HFOV.

The use of HFOV remains controversial, especially after adult studies have suggested that treatment with HFOV may, in fact, be harmful.[19] However, it is still widely used in PICU, owing to a combination of anecdotal evidence, clinician experience, and the fact that HFOV on the whole is used differently. HFOV tends to be used in PICU as a rescue therapy, after the failure of conventional ventilation. There are no randomized controlled trials (RCTs) looking at the use of HFOV in children with bronchiolitis specifically, although an RCT from the 1990s comparing HFOV in respiratory failure with conventional ventilation suggests HFOV improves oxygenation and may be more 'lung protective', as evidenced by the reduced use of supplemental oxygen required at 30 days.[20]

iNO

iNO may offer some potential benefit as an add-on therapy in severe cases for a number of reasons. Not only can it be utilized for vasodilatory effects to improve blood flow within the lungs to improve oxygenation, there have also been theories that it may, indeed, have bronchodilatory properties, which would be useful in bronchiolitis. However, a single study using iNO compared with salbutamol in 12 ventilated infants with RSV bronchiolitis does not support that theory.[21]

Raised cardiac troponins have been described in infants with severe RSV infection. This is thought not to be as a direct myocarditis effect of the virus itself—instead, a reflection of right heart strain and insult, secondary to the lung parenchymal disease, and raised pulmonary vascular pressures.[22] In view of this aspect, iNO may have a role to play in managing the raised pulmonary vascular pressures suffered by infants with severe bronchiolitis. However, a Cochrane review found that other than a transient improvement in oxygenation, iNO did not demonstrate any statistically significant effect on mortality or ventilator-free days in patients with (non-specific) hypoxaemic respiratory failure.[23] Despite the lack of evidence, iNO is used relatively frequently in PICU when oxygenation is problematic. When a child remains hypoxic despite full ventilatory support and high FiO_2, then there are limited options for the clinician—ECMO being the ultimate intervention but this does not come without risk. Therefore, even with no significant evidence base, at the clinician's discretion, a trial of iNO may be appropriate when confronted with this difficult clinical hypoxaemic dilemma.

❝ **Expert comment** Bronchiolitis phenotypes

There are no RCTs on the level of PEEP or ventilatory strategies (e.g. volume-controlled vs pressure-controlled, or high-frequency vs conventional ventilation) for ventilated children with bronchiolitis-induced respiratory failure. This is not surprising seeing that bronchiolitis is not a homogenous clinical phenotype that can be uniformly addressed with a singular ventilation strategy.

Bronchiolitis is a heterogeneous lung disease with varying obstructive and restrictive elements—often within different parts of the same lung. Air trapping leads to increased end expiratory lung volume and decreased lung compliance compatible with an obstructive lung disease pattern. Lung consolidation and areas of atelectasis cause restrictive lung disease. In the severe end of the clinical spectrum solid ARDS-like lung disease may necessitate HFOV and even ECMO.

This clinical heterogeneity fuels my scepticism towards differentiating 'RSV bronchiolitis' from 'RSV pneumonia' by the presence of localized crackles and consolidation on chest radiograph.

Informed clinicians/intensivists, in the main, appreciate the pneumonic aspects of severe bronchiolitis, whether labelled 'RSV bronchiolitis', 'RSV pneumonia', or 'RSV pneumonitis'.

He deteriorated further on day 3 of PICU admission, despite the interventions by the intensive care team. His saturations were 88% on 90% oxygen and required a low-dose adrenaline infusion to maintain his blood pressure. The PICU team discussed him further, considering different treatment options, including recombinant human DNAse and use of endotracheal surfactant. They decided upon a trial of surfactant, which was given with a very limited response.

On day 4 his oxygenation worsened further, with an OI of 43. He continued on HFOV with 10 ppm iNO; therefore, he was turned prone to see if this could improve oxygenation.

> ### ✚ Clinical tip Prone positioning
>
> Placing intensive care patients with respiratory disease in the prone position has become fashionable and has a number of physiological benefits, including reducing atelectasis, optimizing V/Q matching, increasing functional residual capacity, and decreasing transpleural pressure. Within the research, it does appear to improve oxygenation significantly in adults with ARDS with a possible mortality benefit. The evidence to support this modality in children is, as usual, much less. However, most PICU clinicians would support its use, particularly when struggling with oxygenation in children with ARDS.

> ### ✚ Learning point Less common or less effective therapies
>
> #### Corticosteroids
>
> Using corticosteroids in bronchiolitis has been well debated and researched, owing to their acknowledged benefit in other airway diseases such as asthma, despite the fact that there has been a complete failure to demonstrate any significantly positive effect of systemic corticosteroids in children with bronchiolitis. A meta-analysis in 2013 showed no difference in hospital admission rate, length of stay, or readmission rate with systemic steroids;[24] therefore, their use in bronchiolitis is not recommended.
>
> Corticosteroid use in ARDS remains even more controversial. Most recently, in children, a prospective observational cohort study suggested that corticosteroid exposure (>24 hours) was associated with fewer ventilator-free days and longer duration of mechanical ventilation. The current guidance discourages the routine use of steroids in paediatric ARDS.[18]
>
> There is currently a large RCT being undertaken in Australia and New Zealand comparing systemic steroids and nebulized adrenaline with standard treatment in infants admitted to the PICU with bronchiolitis.
>
> #### Surfactant
>
> The quantity and quality of endogenous surfactant in children with severe bronchiolitis may be abnormal. A Cochrane review found very few studies and patients to include in the review and therefore was insufficient to establish the effectiveness of surfactant. They did, however, find that surfactant seemed to reduce days of both mechanical ventilation and PICU admission, and improve oxygenation and $paCO_2$ elimination.[25] The forthcoming 'BESS' trial (Bronchiolitis Endotracheal Surfactant Study), studying efficacy and mechanism of surfactant therapy for critically ill infants with bronchiolitis, will hopefully provide more answers.
>
> #### Ribavarin
>
> Ribavarin is believed to interfere with viral nucleic acid function and therefore inhibit RSV replication. It is expensive and difficult to deliver as nebulized droplets stick to the ventilator circuits. A systematic review in ventilated children has shown no convincing evidence for its use[26] and therefore its routine use is not recommended.

Case history (continued)

He remained in FiO_2 1.0, HFOV with mean airway pressure of 28 cmH_2O, and iNO 10ppm. His saturations remained around 86% with PaO_2 63 mmHg/8.4 kPa (OI 44). In view of the critical condition and maximum mechanical ventilatory support, he was discussed with the local ECMO coordinator to decide whether he would be a candidate for ECMO were he to deteriorate further. It was decided that he would be a candidate for ECMO, and pre-emptive preparation was made by sending bloods for cross-match and a cranial ultrasound scan to exclude any haemorrhage.

ⓘ Expert comment New therapies

Antivirals

Novel small-molecule antivirals (e.g. fusion inhibitory RNAs) that inhibit viral fusion by interacting with the F protein that mediates the fusion of viral envelope with host cell membrane (RSV and hMPV) are currently under investigation.

Immunoprophylaxis (passive immunity)

Palivizumab was the original humanized monoclonal antibody (IgG11K) produced using recombinant DNA techniques in mouse myeloma host cells—directed against an epitope in the A antigenic site of the F protein of RSV. Second-generation (motavizumab) and third-generation (numax-YTE) monoclonal antibody variants, derived from palivizumab, are being evaluated in clinical trials.

Vaccine

There is currently no licensed RSV vaccine, but reportedly >50 vaccine candidates in development. The World Health Organization (WHO) instigated a process as an extension of the Global Vaccine Action Plan (endorsed by the 194 member states of the World Health Assembly in May 2012) to provide guidance aiming to accelerate timelines to development and licensure of high quality, safe, and effective RSV vaccines. The WHO's focus is on geographical areas where global disease burden is focused (i.e. low- and middle-income countries).

Over the following day his oxygenation improved as did his ventilation without ECMO. His mean airway pressure was able to be reduced over the next 3 days along with his oxygen requirement until he was changed back to conventional ventilation. He was eventually extubated to NIV after further 4 days of conventional ventilation, at which stage he was discharged from PICU to the ward under the respiratory physicians.

Discussion

Bronchiolitis is common, and is responsible for a mammoth secondary care and PICU workload over the 'bronchiolitis season' annually. The children that require intensive care support not only are thought to have more severe disease, but also are likely to be more vulnerable with comorbidities, and so on.

Paediatricians and intensivists are experienced in caring for children with bronchiolitis. However, the evidence base for pre-PICU and PICU management strategies is universally poor. Therefore, as with so many conditions in the PICU, clinical management is derived from experience and anecdotal evidence. Ultimately, good supportive care and appropriate respiratory support are the essential elements to managing these children, be it from feeding support and supplementary oxygen, through to ECMO.

ECMO is being utilized with increasing frequency for a range of conditions in PICU, and this also applies to bronchiolitis. There is very little, if any, recent published data reporting ECMO use and outcomes for children with bronchiolitis. New data from the Extracorporeal Life Support Organization (ELSO) regarding the use of ECMO for bronchiolitis are presented in Figure 3.4. Worldwide, ECMO, for patients aged < 1 year, with a primary diagnosis of bronchiolitis, only makes up a very small proportion when compared to the total ECMO runs for all conditions. These data, however, do not include those with a primary diagnosis of ARDS secondary to viral aetiology.

Despite the diminutive numbers, it is clear that, since 2000, ECMO is being utilized increasingly for bronchiolitis. According to ELSO, with the previous 15 years of data, the overall average time on ECMO for survivors is 233 hours. With increased use comes what appears to be a more consistent survival, around 70% over the past 10 years.

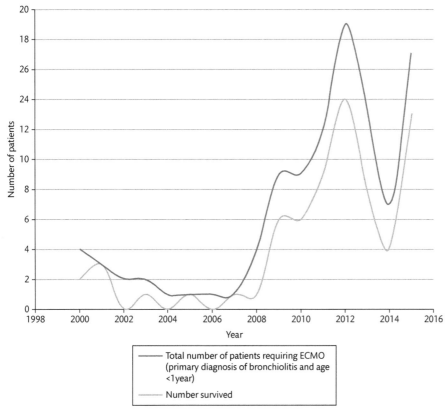

Figure 3.4 Total number of patients (<1 year old) who required extracorporeal membrane oxygenation (ECMO) with a primary diagnosis of bronchiolitis, plotted with number of survivors per year (2000–2015)
Source: data from Extracorporeal Life Support Organization (ELSO).

A final word from the expert

Not all children are equal when it comes to bronchiolitis—those with underlying chronic conditions/comorbidity carry an additional risk of severe disease and death. This vulnerable subgroup merits added vigilance.

The old adage: 'All that wheezes ain't asthma'—should be extended to: 'All that wheezes ain't necessarily asthma or bronchiolitis'. Do not forget to remain a discerning clinician and intensivist. Once you have won the day and exercised the ABCDs, as with all illness, always ask the '3 Wise Whys': Why this child? Why now? Why so severely? With bronchioles size does matter—as does Poiseuille, Laplace, Bernoulli, and friends. However, it is not uncommon for the severity of disease (i.e. requiring PICU admission) to expose a previously unappreciated underlying comorbidity, especially cardiac. I am not suggesting that every PICU admission for bronchiolitis deserves an echocardiogram, but the threshold should be lower.

Keep an eye out for (1) hypoxia; (2) (risk of) impending collapse/exhaustion; and (3) apnoea. A basic supportive management approach for evolving bronchiolitis remains the cornerstone of our treatment. It is therefore reliant on clinical acumen and attentiveness.

References

1. Green CA, Yeates D, Goldacre A, et al. Admission to hospital for bronchiolitis in England: trends over five decades, geographical variation and association with perinatal characteristics and subsequent asthma. *Arch. Dis. Child* 2016;101:140–6.
2. Welliver TP, Garofalo RP, Hosakote Y, et al. Severe human lower respiratory tract illness caused by respiratory syncytial virus and influenza virus is characterized by the absence of pulmonary cytotoxic lymphocyte responses. *J. Infect. Dis.* 2007;195:1126–36.
3. Smyth RL, Openshaw PJ. Bronchiolitis. *Lancet* 2006;368:312–22.
4. Hall CB, Weinberg GA, Iwane MK, et al. The burden of respiratory syncytial virus infection in young children. *N. Engl. J. Med.* 2009;360:588–98.
5. Thorburn K, Harigopal S, Reddy V, Taylor N, van Saene HK. High incidence of pulmonary bacterial co-infection in children with severe respiratory syncytial virus (RSV) bronchiolitis. *Thorax* 2006;61:611–15.
6. Richard N, Komurian-Pradel F, Javouhey E, et al. The impact of dual viral infection in infants admitted to a pediatric intensive care unit associated with severe bronchiolitis. *Pediatr. Infect. Dis. J.* 2008;27:213–17.
7. Thorburn K. Pre-existing disease is associated with a significantly higher risk of death in severe respiratory syncytial virus infection. *Arch. Dis. Child.* 2009;94:99–103.
8. Nair H, Nokes DJ, Gessner BD, et al. Global burden of acute lower respiratory infections due to respiratory syncytial virus in young children: a systematic review and meta-analysis. *Lancet* 2010;375:1545–55.
9. National Institute for Health and Care Excellence. Bronchiolitis in children: diagnosis and management. Available from: https://www.nice.org.uk/guidance/ng9/resources/bronchiolitis-in-children-diagnosis-and-management-pdf-51048523717 (last accessed 3 April 2020).
10. Cunningham S, Rodriguez A, Adams T, et al. Oxygen saturation targets in infants with bronchiolitis (BIDS): a double-blind, randomised, equivalence trial. *Lancet* 2015;386:1041–8.
11. Gadomski AM, Scribani MB. Bronchodilators for bronchiolitis. *Cochrane Database Syst. Rev.* 2014;(6):CD001266.
12. Zhang L. Hypertonic saline for bronchiolitis—a meta-analysis reanalysis. *J. Pediatr.* 2016;176:221–4.
13. Kepreotes E, Whitehead B, Attia J, et al. High-flow warm humidified oxygen versus standard low-flow nasal cannula oxygen for moderate bronchiolitis (HFWHO RCT): an open, phase 4, randomised controlled trial. *Lancet* 2017;389:930–9.
14. Schibler A, Pham TM, Dunster KR, et al. Reduced intubation rates for infants after introduction of high-flow nasal prong oxygen delivery. *Intensive Care Med.* 2011;37:847–52.
15. Thia LP, McKenzie SA, Blyth TP, Minasian CC, Kozlowska WJ, Carr SB. Randomised controlled trial of nasal continuous positive airways pressure (CPAP) in bronchiolitis. *Arch. Dis. Child.* 2008;93:45–7.
16. Donlan M, Fontela PS, Puligandla PS. Use of continuous positive airway pressure (CPAP) in acute viral bronchiolitis: a systematic review. *Pediatr. Pulmonol.* 2011;46:736–46.
17. Jat KR, Mathew JL. Continuous positive airway pressure (CPAP) for acute bronchiolitis in children. *Cochrane Database Syst. Rev.* 2015;(1):CD010473.
18. Pediatriac Acute Lung Injury Consensus Conference Group. Pediatric acute respiratory distress syndrome: consensus recommendations from the Pediatric Acute Lung Injury Consensus Conference. *Pediatr. Crit. Care Med.* 2015;16:428–39.
19. Ferguson ND, Cook DJ, Guyatt GH, et al. High-frequency oscillation in early acute respiratory distress syndrome. *N. Engl. J. Med.* 2013;368:795–805.
20. Arnold JH, Hanson JH, Toro-Figuero LO, Gutiérrez J, Berens RJ, Anglin DL. Prospective, randomized comparison of high-frequency oscillatory ventilation and conventional mechanical ventilation in pediatric respiratory failure. *Crit. Care Med.* 1994;22:1530–9.

21. Patel NR, Hammer J, Nichani S, Numa A, Newth CJ. Effect of inhaled nitric oxide on respiratory mechanics in ventilated infants with RSV bronchiolitis. *Intensive Care Med.* 1999;25:81–7.

22. Thorburn K, Eisenhut M, Shauq A, Narayanswamy S, Burgess M. Right ventricular function in children with severe respiratory syncytial virus (RSV) bronchiolitis. *Minerva Anestesiol.* 2011;77:46–53.

23. Sokol J, Jacobs SE, Bohn D. Inhaled nitric oxide for acute hypoxemic respiratory failure in children and adults. *Cochrane Database Syst. Rev.* 2003;(1):CD002787.

24. Fernandes RM, Bialy LM, Vandermeer B, et al. Glucocorticoids for acute viral bronchiolitis in infants and young children. *Cochrane Database Syst. Rev.* 2013;(6):CD004878.

25. Jat KR, Chawla D. Surfactant therapy for bronchiolitis in critically ill infants. *Cochrane Database Syst. Rev.* 2015;(8):CD009194.

26. Davison C, Ventre KM, Luchetti M, Randolph AG. Efficacy of interventions for bronchiolitis in critically ill infants: a systematic review and meta-analysis. *Pediatr. Crit. Care Med.* 2004;5:482–9.

4 Cardiac arrest

Andrew J. Lautz and Ryan W. Morgan

🕐 **Expert commentary** by Vinay M. Nadkarni

Case history

A 3-year-old previously healthy boy was pulled unconscious from a backyard swimming pool after an unknown submersion time. His mother, who was the only adult at home, called emergency medical services after pulling him from the pool. The dispatcher asked if an automated external defibrillator was available, but the nearest one was located 1 km away at the child's school. The boy's mother was directed to assess his responsiveness and check for breathing. He was unresponsive and apnoeic, so the dispatcher guided his mother to deliver 30 chest compressions followed by two rescue breaths. After his mother delivered both rescue breaths, the boy started coughing and gasping, vomited and initiated spontaneous breaths at regular intervals. His mother appropriately stopped cardiopulmonary resuscitation (CPR) and placed him on his side in the recovery position. When paramedics arrived to the scene shortly thereafter, he had strong carotid pulses and was breathing spontaneously, although he remained somnolent. Paramedics connected him to an automated external defibrillator and a monitor. His heart rate (HR) was 132 beats per minute (bpm), blood pressure was 90/52 mmHg, and oxygen saturation was 91%. He was started on 15 L/minute oxygen via a non-rebreather facemask and was transported to the nearest Emergency Department (ED).

> ✅ **Evidence base** Compression-only CPR
>
> Compression-only CPR has gained traction as an effective modality in bystander-initiated CPR in adult out-of-hospital cardiac arrest (OHCA). However, the preponderance of asphyxiation as the aetiology of cardiac arrest in children makes extrapolation of adult data to paediatric cardiac arrest problematic. A paediatric OHCA registry study in Japan examining dispatcher-assisted bystander CPR between 2008 and 2010 found an association between conventional CPR and 1-month survival with favourable neurological outcome on multivariate analysis, but no such association with compression-only CPR.[1] A second Japanese paediatric OHCA registry study from 2011 to 2012 attempted to more directly address the efficacy of compression-only CPR in this population. In the unadjusted analysis, conventional CPR was associated with a higher likelihood of neurologically favourable survival, as compared to compression-only CPR, but differences between compression-only and conventional CPR disappeared in children >1 year of age with multivariate adjustment and propensity matching. Importantly, both groups outperformed those who received no bystander CPR.[2] A US registry study of paediatric OHCA from 2013 to 2015 examined compression-only versus conventional bystander CPR. Only conventional CPR was associated with improved survival with favourable neurological outcome on multivariate analysis; among infants, in particular, compression-only CPR had outcomes similar to no bystander CPR.[3]

⊕ Clinical tip Compression to ventilation ratio

The recommended ratio of compressions to ventilations differs based upon the number of rescuers and with the placement of an advanced airway. For patients with a natural airway, single rescuers should utilise a ratio of 30 compressions followed by two ventilations, while a ratio of 15 compressions per two ventilations is preferred with multiple rescuers. For intubated patients continuous ventilation at a rate of 8–10 breaths per minute is recommended.[5] Compression of at least one-third of the anterior–posterior chest diameter is recommended in infants and prepubertal children, equating to about 4 cm in infants and 5 cm in children, while a compression depth of 5–6 cm is advised in adolescents and adults.[6]

On arrival to the paediatric ED, the patient's temperature was 35.9°C. He remained tachycardic with a HR of 135 bpm, and he was tachypnoeic with a respiratory rate of 38 breaths per minute. He was in respiratory distress, characterized by nasal flaring and subcostal retractions. His oxygen saturation was 95% on 15 L/minute oxygen via non-rebreather facemask. Blood pressure was 88/48 mmHg, and his extremities were warm with capillary refill of 1–2 seconds. He opened his eyes to trapezius pinch and localized to the painful stimulus by reaching his ipsilateral hand above his clavicle. He occasionally uttered single words. His pupils were 4 mm and briskly reactive bilaterally. An arterial blood gas was notable for a pH of 7.17, partial pressure of carbon dioxide ($paCO_2$) of 45 mmHg (6 kPa), partial pressure of oxygen (paO_2) of 72 mmHg (9.6 kPa), bicarbonate of 11 mmol/L, and lactate of 3.0 mmol/L. Serum glucose was 242 mg/dL (13.4 mmol/L). Electrolytes were unremarkable. Blood urea nitrogen was 16 mg/dL, and serum creatinine was 0.3 mg/dL. A chest radiograph demonstrated bilateral interstitial oedema but no focal opacification. He was admitted to the Paediatric Intensive Care Unit (PICU) for further management.

Shortly after arrival to the PICU, he developed worsening tachypnoea with increased accessory muscle use, accompanied by progressive hypoxaemia with an oxygen saturation of 77%. The patient received manual ventilation with bag and mask with 100% fraction of inspired oxygen (FiO_2) with improvement in oxygen saturation to 91%, and the decision was made to proceed with tracheal intubation. A nasal cannula was placed to administer 10 L/minute of 100% FiO_2 for apnoeic oxygenation, and bag–mask ventilation was continued preceding intubation. Owing to the risk for cardiac arrest with tracheal intubation and transition to invasive positive pressure ventilation, defibrillator pads were pre-emptively placed on the patient and connected to a defibrillator. After assuring adequate vascular access with two peripheral intravenous (IV) catheters, IV fentanyl and midazolam were administered for induction, followed by neuromuscular blockade with rocuronium. Direct laryngoscopy yielded easy visualization of the glottis, although copious frothy secretions were present. Successful tracheal tube placement was confirmed with auscultation and capnography, with an initial end-tidal CO_2 ($etCO_2$) measurement of 50 mmHg, and the patient was hand-ventilated with a bag–mask system. His oxygen saturation nadir during laryngoscopy was 82%, which improved to 93% within the first minute after intubation. The first blood pressure measured after tracheal intubation revealed hypotension with blood pressure of 72/38 mmHg. Progressive bradycardia developed over the next 30 seconds with a HR of 54 bpm and loss of detectable pulses. Chest compressions were rapidly initiated.

> **✦ Learning point** Bradycardia with poor perfusion
>
> Adult victims of IHCA are much more likely to have myocardial ischaemia or a cardiac dysrhythmia as the proximate cause of the arrest, while children more often present with hypoxaemia or shock prior to arrest.[7] As infants and children with circulatory shock or progressive respiratory failure generally develop bradycardia with poor perfusion prior to the onset of pulselessness, paediatric guidelines recommend initiation of CPR for bradycardia with poor perfusion.[8] In fact, children with IHCA who receive CPR for bradycardia with poor perfusion have better survival to hospital discharge relative to those whose rhythm is pulseless electrical activity (PEA) or asystole.[8]

> **✚ Clinical tip** DOPE
>
> **Di**splacement of the tracheal tube— $etCO_2$ during chest compressions and stable securement to the patient.
>
> **O**bstruction—suction catheter passed easily through the tracheal tube.
>
> **P**neumothorax—bilateral chest movement with ventilation.
>
> **E**quipment, including the bag and mask, the fresh oxygen source, and ventilator.

The code leader rapidly identified herself and assigned roles to all team members utilizing closed-loop communication. She assigned a specific CPR coach to focus on the five tenets of high-quality CPR: (1) chest compression depth of at least one-third of the anterior–posterior chest diameter (approximately 5 cm); (2) chest compression rate between 100 and 120 compressions per minute; (3) limitation of interruptions in chest compressions; (4) full chest recoil between compressions; and (5) avoidance of overventilation with a target rate of 10 breaths per minute.[6] With an advanced airway confirmed in place, the team provided continuous chest compressions and ventilation with an end-tidal capnograph at a rate of 10 breaths per minute. To avoid fatigue, compressors were rotated every 2 minutes, or earlier when a decrement in chest compression quality was detected. These changes were timed to occur during pulse checks to minimize interruptions to CPR. Invasive haemodynamic monitoring was not in place, but quantitative end-tidal capnography was utilized to monitor CPR quality, targeting a goal $etCO_2$ of at least 20 mmHg (2.7 kPa). The initial electrocardiogram (ECG) rhythm was a narrow-complex bradycardia without associated pulses, identified as PEA, and the team considered reversible causes. The DOPE mnemonic was utilized to assess the airway and exclude problems.

At the first pulse check, the patient was still in PEA cardiac arrest with absent pulses. $etCO_2$ dropped from 20 mmHg during chest compressions to zero when compressions were paused. Compressions were rapidly resumed, limiting the interruption in chest compressions to < 10 seconds for pulse checks and < 2 seconds for change of compressors. With resumption of high-quality CPR, $etCO_2$ rose to 24 mmHg. IV epinephrine (0.01 mg/kg) (adrenaline) was administered, and the time-keeper assisted the code leader in directing the team to repeat doses of epinephrine every 3–5 minutes during the resuscitation. Doses of IV lidocaine (1 mg/kg) were prepared in the event that shock-refractory ventricular fibrillation (VF) or ventricular tachycardia (VT) developed. Repeat arterial blood gas revealed a metabolic acidosis with a pH of 7.23, $paCO_2$ of 50 mmHg, pO_2 of 68 mmHg, bicarbonate of 15 mmol/L, and lactate of 4.2 mmol/L. Serum glucose was 212 mg/dL, while serum sodium and potassium were 144 and 4.9 mEq/L, respectively. Serum magnesium was 2.0 mg/dL, and the ionized calcium was 1.32 mmol/L. In the absence of hypocalcaemia or hyperkalaemia, no calcium or bicarbonate were administered. CPR was continued with ECG and pulse checks every 2 minutes.

> **✚ Clinical tip** Reversible causes (6 H's and 5 T's)
>
> - Hypoxia.
> - Hypovolaemia.
> - Hypothermia.
> - Hydrogen ion (acidosis).
> - Hypo-/hyperkalaemia.
> - Hypoglycaemia.
> - Tension pneumothorax.
> - Tamponade (cardiac).
> - Thrombosis (pulmonary).
> - Thrombosis (coronary).
> - Toxins.

> **✦ Learning point** $ETCO_2$ and invasive blood pressure monitoring
>
> $EtCO_2$ and invasive haemodynamic monitoring during paediatric IHCA (p-IHCA) have the potential to provide real-time feedback on the quality of CPR. $etCO_2$ is the partial pressure of carbon dioxide at the end of exhalation. As changes in pulmonary blood flow affect the clearance of carbon dioxide, $etCO_2$ reflects both pulmonary blood flow and cardiac output. In fact, a rapid increase in the $etCO_2$ to above 40 mmHg is often suggestive of the return of spontaneous circulation (ROSC) during resuscitation. However, persistently low $etCO_2$ (<10 mmHg) has been associated with inability to attain

ROSC in some adult studies.[9] Data for specific etCO$_2$ targets to guide CPR are lacking in paediatrics, however. Expert panels have suggested targeting a goal etCO$_2$ of >20 mmHg, but guidelines have been more circumspect and have only suggested consideration of etCO$_2$ to monitor the quality of CPR.[10] As a large proportion (>95%) of p-IHCAs occur in the PICU where arterial line blood pressure monitoring is often either present or readily attainable (in >60%), invasive haemodynamic monitoring is a second potential avenue for intra-arrest CPR feedback.

⊕ **Clinical tip** Avoidance of empiric calcium and bicarbonate

Routine administration of calcium or sodium bicarbonate during paediatric cardiac arrest is not recommended. Calcium administration (as calcium chloride or calcium gluconate) is only recommended in the setting of known calcium channel blocker overdose or documented hypocalcaemia, hypermagnesaemia, or hyperkalaemia. In general, administration of calcium has no proven benefit and may be associated with worse outcomes.[11] Similarly, sodium bicarbonate may be beneficial in special resuscitation conditions, such as hyperkalaemia or known sodium channel blocker overdose. Excessive sodium bicarbonate utilization may cause hypokalaemia, hypocalcaemia, hypernatraemia, and hyperosmolality.[11]

At the fourth pulse check 8 minutes into the resuscitation, the rhythm was noted to be VF. Compressions were resumed while the defibrillator was charged to minimize interruption in chest compressions. When the defibrillator was charged, the code leader called for everyone to clear the patient. The ventilation bag and oxygen source were disconnected from the tracheal tube, and the compressor paused compressions and stepped back from the patient. Defibrillation was attempted at 2 J/kg, followed by immediate resumption of chest compressions and manual ventilation via the tracheal tube. Quantitative capnography continued to display an etCO$_2$ between 20 and 25 mmHg with high-quality CPR

At the next pulse check 10 minutes into the resuscitation, the rhythm continued to be VF. Chest compressions were resumed while the defibrillator was again charged. After clearing the patient, defibrillation was attempted at 4 J/kg followed by resumption of CPR and administration of IV epinephrine with a plan to administer IV lidocaine after the next defibrillation attempt. At this point the team activated the extracorporeal membrane oxygenation (ECMO) team for initiation of extracorporeal CPR (E-CPR).

✪ **Learning point** E-CPR

E-CPR is the initiation of ECMO to restore circulation when prolonged conventional CPR fails to achieve ROSC and the underlying cause of arrest is believed to be reversible. With CPR ongoing, venous and arterial cannulas are placed for veno-arterial ECMO. While femoral cannulation is feasible in adolescents and adults, cannulation via the neck or chest may be required in infants and young children owing to size constraints in the femoral vessels. After successful cannulation and connection to a primed ECMO circuit, chest compressions are stopped as circuit flow takes over circulatory support. A 2016 multicentre registry study of IHCA in children with both cardiac and non-cardiac diagnoses who received CPR for at least 10 minutes found improved survival to hospital discharge and survival with favourable neurological outcome in those who received E-CPR versus conventional CPR only.[12] As with all ECMO utilization, E-CPR is meant as a bridge to recovery in patients with reversible underlying conditions. Put another way, ECMO is a support modality and not a curative treatment.

Given the complexity of ECMO support, guidelines continue to emphasize that ECMO be utilized 'in settings that allow expertise, resources, and systems to optimize the use of ECMO during and after resuscitation'.[4]

ⓘ Expert comment   Duration of resuscitation

Longer durations of CPR have been linked to worse outcomes in paediatric cardiac arrest, and CPR was historically considered futile after 20 minutes of chest compressions or after the administration of more than two doses of epinephrine. More recently published data suggest that when high-quality CPR is provided, survival with favourable neurological outcome is possible with much longer resuscitations. A 2013 Get With The Guidelines–Resuscitation (GWTG-R) registry study of p-IHCA found a negative linear association with survival during the first 15 minutes of CPR, with an overall survival to hospital discharge of 44% in children who received 15 minutes or less of CPR versus 16% in children who received more than 35 minutes of resuscitation. However, 60% of survivors of p-IHCA who received prolonged CPR (>35 minutes) had favourable neurological outcomes.[13] In a GWTG-R registry study of E-CPR between 2000 and 2011, 25% of children with in-hospital paediatric cardiac arrest who survived to hospital discharge with a favourable neurological outcome had received more than 37 minutes of CPR.[12] Although many children with prolonged duration of resuscitation do not have favourable outcomes, these data clearly demonstrate that long periods of CPR are not universally futile. As such, the duration of CPR should not be the only factor in decisions to terminate resuscitation.

At the next pulse check, the patient remained in VF. Defibrillation was again attempted at 4 J/kg, and IV lidocaine (1 mg/kg) was administered in the setting of refractory VF. The resuscitation continued with pulse checks every 2 minutes with attempted defibrillation at 4 J/kg in the setting of ongoing VF and with alternating doses of IV epinephrine and lidocaine over the next 8 minutes. etCO$_2$ remained 20–25 mmHg during chest compressions. Twenty minutes into the resuscitation, the ECMO team arrived, and preparations for E-CPR were ongoing. With the next pulse check, the patient remained in VF. Defibrillation was again attempted at 4 J/kg after clearing the patient, and chest compressions were immediately resumed. The etCO$_2$ rapidly increased to 45 mmHg shortly after restarting compressions, suggesting ROSC, so compressions were held. The ECG revealed a narrow-complex tachycardia with a HR of 135 bpm, and femoral pulses were readily palpated. The blood pressure was 84/46 mmHg, and the oxygen saturation was 86%. The patient was transitioned from manual ventilation to a ventilator set to target a tidal volume of 6–8 mL/kg with a positive end expiratory pressure (PEEP) of 6 cm H$_2$O on an FiO$_2$ of 100%. Quantitative capnography revealed an etCO$_2$ of 48 mmHg. The ECMO team remained on standby in the immediate post-arrest period for possible cannulation in the event of a second cardiac arrest.

The patient remained unconscious, intubated, and mechanically ventilated, and the team transitioned to goal-directed post-cardiac arrest management. He was unresponsive to verbal or painful stimulation, and pupils remained bilaterally reactive to light. Repeat chest radiograph demonstrated a well-positioned tracheal tube with unchanged bilateral interstitial oedema and with new patchy subsegmental atelectasis. An arterial blood gas was drawn to assess oxygenation and ventilation. The pH was 7.25 with a paCO$_2$ of 52 mmHg and a pO$_2$ of 50 mmHg. The serum bicarbonate was 16 mmol/L with a lactate of 5.8 mmol/L. Repeat serum glucose was 145 mg/dL, with serum sodium

145 mEq/L, potassium 3.7 mEq/L, and ionized calcium 1.21 mmol/L. The oxygen saturation remained at 86%, despite 100% FiO_2, so the PEEP was increased to 10 cm H_2O. Additionally, in the setting of hypercarbia, the minute ventilation was augmented by increasing the ventilator rate. Over the next 30 minutes, his oxygen saturation improved to 96%, and the FiO_2 was weaned serially targeting the minimum FiO_2 to achieve normoxia with oxygen saturation 94–98%. The $etCO_2$ decreased during this time period to 38 mmHg, and repeat arterial blood gas demonstrated improvement in the pH and $paCO_2$ to 7.32 and 42 mmHg, respectively. Trends in $etCO_2$ were monitored, targeting normocapnia with a goal $paCO_2$ of 35–45 mmHg. The patient was started on dextrose-containing isotonic IV fluids, and serial blood glucose measurements were ordered with stated plan to target normoglycaemia with serum glucose levels between 80 and 180 mg/dL.

A peripheral arterial line was placed in the right radial artery after ROSC for continuous invasive blood pressure monitoring, and central venous access was obtained in the right internal jugular vein under ultrasound guidance. Hypotension developed within the first hour of ROSC with a systolic blood pressure of 70 mmHg and a mean arterial pressure (MAP) of 45 mmHg. The patient's extremities remained cool, and capillary refill was 3–4 seconds. Continuous central venous pressure (CVP) monitoring revealed a CVP of 4 mmHg. He received a rapid bolus of IV isotonic sodium chloride 20 mL/kg; and he was started on an epinephrine infusion, which was titrated to 0.2 μg/kg/min. With these interventions, blood pressure measured on the arterial line improved to 92/52 with a MAP of 65 mmHg, and his capillary refill improved to 2–3 seconds. The epinephrine infusion was titrated to maintain a systolic blood pressure greater than the fifth percentile for age.

As the patient remained comatose and intubated, he was started on continuous electroencephalogram (EEG) monitoring for subclinical seizures. A seizure action plan was developed with a plan for first-line IV levetiracetam 50 mg/kg and second-line IV lorazepam 0.1 mg/kg. The team discussed targeted temperature management and planned to initiate controlled normothermia. After achievement of haemodynamic stability, he was transported to the computed tomography (CT) scanner to obtain non-contrast CT imaging of his brain to assess for occult traumatic brain injury in the setting of drowning. He was manually ventilated assuring adequate chest rise and maintenance of PEEP, while monitoring oxygen saturation and $etCO_2$ during transport and for the duration of the CT scan. He remained on the epinephrine infusion and invasive blood pressure monitoring for the duration of the transport. The CT scan showed no haemorrhage or mass, and there was no evidence of cerebral oedema, mass effect, or herniation in this immediate post-arrest imaging. Bilateral cerebral near-infrared spectroscopy was connected to monitor trends in cerebral perfusion.

> **✪ Learning point** Post-cardiac arrest syndrome
>
> The post-cardiac arrest syndrome is characterized by four key processes: (1) post-arrest brain injury; (2) post-arrest myocardial dysfunction; (3) systemic ischaemia–reperfusion injury; and (4) persistence of the precipitating pathology.[14] Post-arrest brain injury manifests as a spectrum from altered consciousness or coma to persistent vegetative state or brain death. Ischaemic strokes can occur, and myoclonus and seizures are common. Survivors may have persistent neurocognitive deficits. Pathophysiological mechanisms of brain injury include initiation of apoptotic and necrotic neuronal cell death, cerebral microvascular thrombosis preventing reflow after ROSC, impairment in cerebral blood flow autoregulation post-arrest, and cerebral oedema. Post-arrest myocardial dysfunction is marked by transient global ventricular hypokinesis, often

termed myocardial stunning, reaching a nadir of ventricular function around 8 hours post-arrest and typically normalizing within 24–72 hours. In this time period, children often require inotropic support to support cardiac output. The systemic ischaemia–reperfusion injury of cardiac arrest with ROSC manifests clinically with impaired vasoregulation, hypercoagulability with microvascular thromboses, and intravascular volume depletion. Accumulated tissue oxygen debt may lead to endothelial activation and systemic inflammation with multiorgan dysfunction. Adrenal insufficiency and immune dysregulation can also occur. Finally, the inciting pathology that resulted in cardiac arrest, whether it be hypoxemic respiratory failure, trauma with resulting haemorrhage, septic shock, or a toxic ingestion, will frequently persist in the post-arrest period and contribute to ongoing organ dysfunction.

⑪ Expert comment   Post-cardiac arrest management

Post-cardiac arrest management strategies are focused on treating the post-cardiac arrest syndrome and mitigating further injury after ROSC. The emphasis on strict normoxia avoids tissue hypoxia or hyperoxia post-cardiac arrest. Importantly, hyperoxia may exacerbate neurological injury by promoting generation of additional free radicals and oxidative damage. In fact, animal studies and observational data in adults suggest worse neurological outcomes in the presence of post-arrest hyperoxia, although this association has not been found in several small paediatric studies.[4,15] Despite impairment in cerebral blood flow autoregulation to blood pressure, cerebrovascular sensitivity to carbon dioxide tension is thought to be intact post-cardiac arrest; thus, avoidance of hypercarbia and hypocarbia may be particularly important. Hypercarbia may increase cerebral blood flow and exacerbate cerebral oedema and intracranial hypertension. Conversely, hypocarbia may cause cerebral vasoconstriction and further ischaemic damage. Hyper- or hypoglycaemia may aggravate post-arrest brain injury, so serum blood glucose monitoring and management is key. Close attention to haemodynamics during the expected period of myocardial dysfunction, generally with continuous invasive arterial blood pressure monitoring, is imperative. Post-arrest hypotension often necessitates inotropic support; and vasoactive infusions should be expectantly available at the bedside, even in the presence of haemodynamic stability. To date, there are no paediatric studies evaluating the efficacy of specific vasoactive agents post-arrest, and vasoactive infusions should instead be selected based on underlying pathophysiology, physical examination, and echocardiographic findings.[10] Lastly, prompt identification and treatment of seizures may ameliorate post-arrest brain injury, so prospective surveillance with EEG monitoring may be beneficial where feasible.

After CT imaging, the patient returned to the PICU, cooling blankets were placed underneath and on top of the patient, and continuous temperature monitoring was accomplished via bladder catheter. The team targeted controlled normothermia, with a set temperature of 36°C and a goal temperature of 35–37°C over the next 5 days. He was not started on any continuous sedative infusions owing to his apparent lack of awareness or interactivity. However, intermittent boluses of sedatives were made available in the event he developed awareness or agitation, and sedatives plus neuro-muscular blockade were prepared in case of shivering.

✔ Evidence base   Therapeutic normothermia and hypothermia

Hyperthermia after cardiac arrest has been associated with poor neurological outcome. Active targeted temperature management has been recommended following both adult and paediatric cardiac arrest, but specific temperature thresholds have not been defined in children. Two paediatric randomized controlled trials attempted to address this knowledge gap: the out-of-hospital Therapeutic Hypothermia after Pediatric Cardiac Arrest (THAPCA) trial and the in-hospital THAPCA trial. The out-of-hospital THAPCA trial randomized 295 children who remained unconscious after OHCA to 5 days of controlled normothermia (36.8°C) or 2 days of therapeutic hypothermia to 33°C followed by slow rewarming and controlled normothermia at 36.8°C over the subsequent 3 days. There was no statistically significant difference in the primary outcome of survival with good neurological outcome at 12 months between groups.[16] However, the study was underpowered for survival, and there was a strong trend towards improved survival with therapeutic hypothermia. The in-hospital THAPCA trial was terminated early due to futility after 329 patients were randomized to similar groups as in the out-of-hospital trial. Again, there was no significant difference in survival with favourable neurological outcome at 12 months between patients who received therapeutic hypothermia as compared with those treated with controlled normothermia.[17]

The patient's hypotension improved over the course of the first 24 hours after ROSC, and he was weaned off the epinephrine infusion by the second hospital day with blood pressures remaining within the expected range for age. With ongoing invasive mechanical ventilation with higher mean airway pressures, oxygenation improved, and the FiO_2 was weaned to <40%. His pupils remained symmetrically reactive to light, and he developed no seizure activity by EEG. He developed purposeful movements approximately 36 hours after ROSC and required sedation to treat agitation and maintain safety as he made repeated attempts to grasp the tracheal tube. He received bolus doses and was started on continuous infusions of IV fentanyl and midazolam to achieve light sedation and to prevent unintentional extubation, while monitoring for delirium. Magnetic resonance imaging (MRI) of the brain with and without IV contrast was performed on the fourth hospital day, which showed no abnormalities. The cooling blanket was discontinued after 5 days, and he maintained a normal temperature in the range of 36–37°C without developing fevers. The temperature-sensing bladder catheter was removed at this time, and he was able to void spontaneously. Physical and occupational therapy were consulted for evaluation for early mobility. Hypoxemic, hypercarbic respiratory failure manifesting as acute respiratory distress syndrome after drowning necessitated ongoing invasive mechanical ventilation until the seventh hospital day. As his lung compliance improved, the PEEP, pressure support, and ventilator rate were all weaned to minimal settings over the course of several days. He tolerated a trial of continuous spontaneous ventilation with PEEP and pressure support, both set at 5 cm H_2O. The sedative infusions were discontinued, and he opened his eyes and followed simple commands prior to extubation. He was extubated to nasal cannula with his parents at the bedside on the seventh hospital day. The arterial line and central venous catheter were removed. He was able to speak and sit at the edge of the bed with assistance, and he was monitored in the PICU for an additional 24 hours prior to transfer to the general ward. He required an additional week of hospitalization while being weaned off supplemental oxygen and while working on enteral feeding and rehabilitation. As part of his rehabilitation, he received ongoing support with physical and occupational therapy and was able to transition back to full feeding by mouth with the aid of speech therapists.

Discussion

Outcomes after p-IHCA have improved dramatically over the past two decades. Survival to hospital discharge in survivors of p-IHCA increased from 24% in 2001 to 39% in

2009 and 45% in 2016, although children with OHCA fare worse.[18–20] Widespread implementation of early, high-quality CPR coupled with targeted post-arrest care has the potential to further improve patient outcomes.

Prognostication after paediatric cardiac arrest has been studied with some success. EEG tracings in the first week post-arrest have been used to estimate neurological prognosis, with continuous and reactive tracings associated with a higher likelihood of survival with a favourable neurological outcome, while discontinuous or isoelectric tracings have been associated with worse neurological outcomes. Pupillary reactivity 12–24 hours after cardiac arrest has been associated with survival to hospital discharge and favourable neurological outcome, although non-reactive pupils early in the post-arrest course are not necessarily predictive of poor outcome.[21] Early loss of grey–white matter differentiation or effacement of the sulci or basilar cisterns on CT imaging have been associated with poor outcomes, although normal imaging within the first 24 hours does not necessarily translate to favourable neurological outcomes. Finally, changes in somatosensory-evoked potentials or diffusion restriction in the cortex or basal ganglia on MRI have been associated with worse neurological outcomes after hypoxic–ischaemic injury.[22]

A final word from the expert

High-quality CPR and targeted post-cardiac arrest management save lives and preserve brain function. Intra-arrest efforts should focus on adequate depth and rate of chest compressions, minimization of interruptions in compressions, allowance of full chest recoil, and avoidance of overventilation. Utilization of quantitative capnography to target an etCO$_2$ of at least 20 mmHg during compressions and invasive arterial blood pressure monitoring to target a DBP of at least 25 mmHg in infants and 30 mmHg in children during the relaxation phase of chest compressions offer promise as markers of effective, high-quality CPR. Meticulous post-cardiac arrest monitoring and management are paramount in reducing secondary injury after resuscitation from cardiac arrest. Particular attention should be paid to target normoxia, normocarbia, normotension for age, and normoglycaemia. Active cooling with targeted temperature management should be instituted to prevent and treat hyperthermia, and seizures should be aggressively identified and treated. In centres with expertise in paediatric ECMO, E-CPR should be considered in refractory cardiac arrest as a bridge to recovery in children whose cardiac arrest resulted from potentially reversible conditions.

We have seen vast improvement in the rates of survival with favourable neurological outcome after p-IHCA over the past two decades. However, neurological morbidity and mortality remain substantial, particularly after OHCA. Further research is urgently needed to better understand mechanisms of injury and identify potential cellular or molecular targets for resuscitation from paediatric cardiac arrest. Further clinical research may help delineate optimal resuscitative targets in children, including haemodynamic targets during CPR and post-arrest, etCO$_2$ thresholds for high-quality CPR, and temperature targets in the post-arrest period.

References

1. Goto Y, Maeda T, Goto Y. Impact of dispatcher-assisted bystander cardiopulmonary resuscitation on neurological outcomes in children with out-of-hospital cardiac arrests: a prospective, nationwide, population-based cohort study. *J. Am. Heart Assoc.* 2014;3:e000499.
2. Fukuda T, Ohashi-Fukuda N, Kobayashi H, et al. Conventional versus compression-only versus no-bystander cardiopulmonary resuscitation for pediatric out-of-hospital cardiac arrest. *Circulation* 2016;134:2060–70.
3. Naim MY, Sutton RM, Friess SH, et al. Blood pressure- and coronary perfusion pressure-targeted cardiopulmonary resuscitation improves 24-hour survival from ventricular fibrillation cardiac arrest. *Crit. Care Med.* 2016;44:e1111–17.
4. de Caen AR, Maconochie IK, Aickin R, et al. Part 6: Pediatric basic life support and pediatric advanced life support: 2015 international consensus on cardiopulmonary resuscitation and emergency cardiovascular care science with treatment recommendations. *Circulation.* 2015;132(16 Suppl. 1):S177–203.
5. Berg MD, Schexnayder SM, Chameides L, et al. Part 13: Pediatric basic life support: 2010 American Heart Association Guidelines for Cardiopulmonary Resuscitation and Emergency Cardiovascular Care. *Circulation* 2010;122(18 Suppl. 3):S862–75.
6. Atkins DL, Berger S, Duff JP, et al. Part 11: Pediatric basic life support and cardiopulmonary resuscitation quality: 2015 American Heart Association Guidelines Update for Cardiopulmonary Resuscitation and Emergency Cardiovascular Care. *Circulation* 2015;132(18 Suppl. 2):S519–25.
7. Nadkarni VM, Larkin GL, Peberdy MA, et al. First documented rhythm and clinical outcome from in-hospital cardiac arrest among children and adults. *JAMA* 2006;295:50–7.
8. Donoghue A, Berg RA, Hazinski MF, et al. Cardiopulmonary resuscitation for bradycardia with poor perfusion versus pulseless cardiac arrest. *Pediatrics* 2009;124:1541–8.
9. Meaney PA, Bobrow BJ, Mancini ME, et al. Cardiopulmonary resuscitation quality: [corrected] improving cardiac resuscitation outcomes both inside and outside the hospital: a consensus statement from the American Heart Association. *Circulation* 2013;128:417–35.
10. de Caen AR, Berg MD, Chameides L, et al. Part 12: Pediatric advanced life support: 2015 American Heart Association Guidelines Update for Cardiopulmonary Resuscitation and Emergency Cardiovascular Care. *Circulation* 2015;132(18 Suppl. 2):S526–42.
11. Kleinman ME, Chameides L, Schexnayder SM, et al. Part 14: Pediatric advanced life support: 2010 American Heart Association Guidelines for Cardiopulmonary Resuscitation and Emergency Cardiovascular Care. *Circulation* 2010;122(18 Suppl. 3):S876–908.
12. Lasa JJ, Rogers RS, Localio R, et al. Extracorporeal cardiopulmonary resuscitation (E-CPR) during pediatric in-hospital cardiopulmonary arrest is associated with improved survival to discharge: a report from the American Heart Association's Get With The Guidelines-Resuscitation (GWTG-R) Registry. *Circulation* 2016;133:165–76.
13. Matos RI, Watson RS, Nadkarni VM, et al. Duration of cardiopulmonary resuscitation and illness category impact survival and neurologic outcomes for in-hospital pediatric cardiac arrests. *Circulation* 2013;127:442–51.
14. Neumar RW, Nolan JP, Adrie C, et al. Post-cardiac arrest syndrome: epidemiology, pathophysiology, treatment, and prognostication. A consensus statement from the International Liaison Committee on Resuscitation (American Heart Association, Australian and New Zealand Council on Resuscitation, European Resuscitation Council, Heart and Stroke Foundation of Canada, InterAmerican Heart Foundation, Resuscitation Council of Asia, and the Resuscitation Council of Southern Africa); the American Heart Association Emergency Cardiovascular Care Committee; the Council on Cardiovascular Surgery and Anesthesia; the Council on Cardiopulmonary, Perioperative, and Critical Care; the Council on Clinical Cardiology; and the Stroke Council. *Circulation* 2008;118:2452–83.
15. Topjian AA, Berg RA, Taccone FS. Haemodynamic and ventilator management in patients following cardiac arrest. *Curr. Opin. Crit. Care* 2015;21:195–201.

16. Moler FW, Silverstein FS, Holubkov R, et al. Therapeutic hypothermia after out-of-hospital cardiac arrest in children. *N Engl J Med* 2015;372:1898–908.

17. Moler FW, Silverstein FS, Holubkov R, et al. Therapeutic hypothermia after in-hospital cardiac arrest in children. *N Engl J Med* 2017;376:318–29.

18. Girotra S, Spertus JA, Li Y, et al. Survival trends in pediatric in-hospital cardiac arrests: an analysis from Get With the Guidelines-Resuscitation. *Circ. Cardiovasc. Qual. Outcomes* 2013;6:42–9.

19. Berg RA, Nadkarni VM, Clark AE, et al. Incidence and outcomes of cardiopulmonary resuscitation in PICUs. *Crit. Care Med.* 2016;44:798–808.

20. Sutton RM, Case E, Brown SP, et al. A quantitative analysis of out-of-hospital pediatric and adolescent resuscitation quality—a report from the ROC epistry-cardiac arrest. *Resuscitation* 2015;93:150–7.

21. Abend NS, Topjian AA, Kessler SK, et al. Outcome prediction by motor and pupillary responses in children treated with therapeutic hypothermia after cardiac arrest. *Pediatr. Crit. Care Med.* 2012;13:32–8.

22. Abend NS, Licht DJ. Predicting outcome in children with hypoxic ischemic encephalopathy. *Pediatr. Crit. Care Med.* 2008;9:32–9.

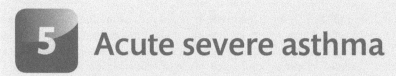

5 Acute severe asthma

Andrew Nyman

🕐 **Expert commentary** by Andrew Durward

Case history

A 10-year-old girl with a background history of mild exercise-induced asthma controlled with an intermittent 'reliever' (salbutamol metered-dose inhaler) presented to the Emergency Department (ED) of a tertiary hospital following a 3-day illness with coryza, fever, coughing, and wheeze. She had been referred by her general practitioner (GP) as two salbutamol nebulizers 30 minutes apart and an ipratropium nebulizer failed to improve her respiratory distress. The GP had also given her a 2 mg/kg dose of prednisone. Her mother gave a history of worsening cough over the last few days with lack of response of the metered-dose salbutamol inhalers at home. She had several hospital admissions for acute asthma in the previous year, requiring escalation of bronchodilators and short course oral steroids on each occasion. However, she had never required admission to a paediatric intensive care unit (PICU) for asthma exacerbation. She had no written rescue plan for an acute asthma attack.

> ❖ **Learning point** What is asthma?
>
> Asthma is the most commonly diagnosed long-term medical condition in the UK, affecting over 5 million people, of whom over 1 million are children.[1] It is a long-term inflammatory disease of the bronchi and bronchioles thought to be caused by a combination of genetic and environmental factors. Asthma is characterized by recurring symptoms resulting in reversible airflow obstruction due to bronchospasm and mucous plugging. The symptoms may include episodes of wheezing, coughing, chest tightness, and shortness of breath, as well as acute life-threatening airway obstruction. The severity of asthma varies, with a worsening quality of life and higher mortality risk if poorly controlled. 'Brittle' asthma is a type of asthma distinguishable from other forms by recurrent, severe attacks.[2]
>
> The underlying pathology varies, but, in general, there is a complex chronic inflammatory process that leads to the release of inflammatory mediators, which trigger the smooth muscle of the airway to contract and narrow the air passages, with subsequent increased production of intraluminal mucous. An important feature of asthma is that the airway obstruction is potentially reversible with medical treatment in the form of bronchodilators. Most people with asthma have an episodic illness with periods of reasonable health interspersed with periods of increased symptoms, which occasionally progresses to an acute exacerbation—an 'asthma attack'.
>
> The acute exacerbation is usually caused by exposure to a trigger to which the person is sensitive. Common triggers are viral infections, environmental tobacco smoke, aeroallergens, or exercise. The cause of asthma is unclear, but a combination of genetic and environmental factors is thought to make a person more susceptible to triggers that lead to airway narrowing. National guidelines stress the importance of prevention strategies as two-thirds of asthma deaths in the UK were found to have been precipitated by factors that are preventable.[3]

On admission to the ED, the patient was hypoxic with saturations of 80% in air. This improved to 90% following the application of high-flow oxygen via a face mask. Work of breathing was increased with respiratory accessory muscle use. Clinical examination revealed markedly prolonged bilateral wheezing but no evidence of pneumothorax. Blood pressure was normal, and she had a heart rate of 180 beats per minute during a salbutamol and ipratropium nebulizer. A diagnosis of acute severe asthma, exacerbated by a viral illness, was made. C-reactive protein was 40 mg/L and intravenous co-amoxiclav was started for community-acquired pneumonia. Owing to the high work of breathing and lack of response to back-to-back nebulizers, an intravenous (IV) bolus of salbutamol (5 µg/kg), followed by a continuous infusion at 1 µg/kg/min and 40 mg/kg IV magnesium sulfate were given with marginal improvement in work of breathing. She received an additional dose of steroid (IV hydrocortisone) in the ED. Within 20 minutes, no clinical response was noted and salbutamol infusion rate was escalated to a maximum of 2 µg/kg/min. She started to show signs of exhaustion and respiratory fatigue, and was unable to speak. Attempts at obtaining an arterial blood gas failed but a venous blood sample showed a partial pressure of carbon dioxide ($paCO_2$) of 8 kPa. Oxygen saturations were 88% in 10 L/min of oxygen via a face mask re-breath bag. The high-dose salbutamol was also associated with marked tachycardia (190/min). A chest X-ray (CXR) was performed and demonstrated severe hyperinflation and some patchy areas of consolidation. The anaesthesia team was called to assess the patient for intubation and ventilation. Physical examination confirmed the patient had severe asthma with respiratory fatigue, difficulty maintaining oxygen saturations above 94%, and lack of response to inhaled or IV bronchodilators and magnesium.

> ⭘ **Learning point** Asthma and Paediatric Intensive Care Unit admission
>
> As progressive fatigue develops patients may not demonstrate signs of agitation or tachypnoea so the severity of asthma maybe underappreciated, The British Thoracic Society (BTS)/Scottish Intercollegiate Guidelines Network (SIGN) guidelines for severe asthma provide guidance on criteria for admission to hospital, for secondary care management and definitions of 'acute severe' and 'life-threatening' asthma based on clinical assistance, but, do not provide guidance for management of life-threatening asthma *once invasive ventilation is required*. In addition, there is markedly wide variation across the world with respect to the management and monitoring of acute severe asthma that requires Paediatric Intensive Care Unit (PICU) admission.[4]

> ⊕ **Clinical tip** Salbutamol toxicity
>
> It is important to be mindful of limiting salbutamol dose in older children, as weight-based calculations can lead to inappropriately high infusion rates. We recommend a **maximum** of infusion rate of 20 µg/min. Significant side effects include tachycardia, metabolic acidosis, myocardial injury, tremor, agitation, and nausea, which may respond favourably to reducing or pausing the salbutamol if side effects occur.[9]

> ❝ **Expert comment** The role of bronchodilators in acute severe asthma
>
> The first-line treatment of acute severe asthma according to BTS guidelines is bronchodilation with inhaled salbutamol. Therapeutic salbutamol levels between 5 and 20 ng/mL can be easily achieved using back-to-back nebulizers or a low-dose intravenous salbutamol infusion (<1 µg/kg/min). Higher infusion rates (>1 µg/kg/min) may result in signs of toxicity (tachycardia and lactic acidosis) without further benefit.[7] Prevention of salbutamol toxicity is important as robust evidence is still lacking to support IV salbutamol in addition to inhaled salbutamol in acute severe asthma.[8]
>
> Failure to respond to salbutamol often raises the question about other bronchodilators. BTS/SIGN guidelines [https://www.brit-thoracic.org.uk/quality-improvement/guidelines/asthma/] recommend aminophylline for children with severe or life-threatening asthma which remains unresponsive at this stage. The British National Formulary for Children (BNFc: https://bnfc.nice.org.uk/) suggests a dose of

5 mg/kg followed by an infusion. Aminophylline should, however, be administered with caution, as it has a narrow therapeutic range and can precipitate tachycardia and arrhythmias. Close monitoring of both clinical parameters and drug levels is required.

However, in patients who are already receiving oral theophylline as part of asthma management, prior to commencing aminophylline, we would recommend a blood theophylline level is taken to ensure safe dosing. Although a single randomized controlled trial in Australia suggested improved saturations within 6 hours following the addition of aminophylline to inhaled salbutamol, it is worth noting the increased side effects. In addition, the dose used in that study was twice the currently recommended dose in the UK and there appears to be no apparent reduction in symptoms, number of nebulized treatments, and length of hospital stay.[10] Currently, there is insufficient evidence to recommend aminophylline to reduce PICU admission and or mechanical ventilation.[11]

If higher-dose bronchodilation (salbutamol or aminophylline) fails to produce a clinical response, it suggests the mechanism of airflow obstruction is small or large airway mucus plugs rather than bronchospasm. It is worth remembering that up to a third of patients with acute severe asthma requiring intubation and ventilation fail to respond to IV salbutamol bronchodilation.

Mucus plugging with widespread airway occlusion is a common mechanism of death in acute fatal asthma.[12] Typically, mucus plugs develop over days and the patients report increasing use of bronchodilators or nebulizers at home with less and less effect. This is characterized by widespread patchy areas of air trapping and atelectasis, which results in ventilation perfusion mismatch and hypoxia.[13] In contrast, sudden asphyxial asthma has a very rapid onset, which in minutes to hours produces severe bronchospasm and life-threatening silent chest on auscultation.[14] This is usually rapidly reversible and has a good outcome if pre-hospital cardiopulmonary resuscitation (CPR) is not required.

On clinical review by anaesthesia, intubation and mechanical ventilation was deemed necessary for both patient fatigue (hypercarbia) and hypoxia (saturations remained below 92% despite facemask oxygen). Ketamine (1 mg/kg) and fentanyl (2 µg/kg) were used for induction of anaesthesia after a 10 ml/kg saline IV fluid bolus was administered. Neuromuscular blockade was achieved with rocuronium (1 mg/kg). Manual hand-bagging at high pressure was required to move the chest with difficulty at a low rate. End tidal CO_2 (etCO$_2$) was 8 kPa with a prolonged expiratory slope. The patient was rapidly transferred to PICU for mechanical ventilation. Pressure-control ventilation was used and muscle relaxation maintained. A peak pressure of 57 cmH$_2$O was required to move the chest (6–8 mL/kg tidal volume). Positive end expiratory pressure (PEEP) was set to 5 cmH$_2$O and a rate of 25 breaths per minute set in pressure-control mode, with an inspiratory time of 0.8 seconds and expiratory time of 1.6 seconds. In 50% oxygen, saturations were 98%. An arterial blood gas showed pH 6.87; paCO$_2$ 20.1; partial pressure of oxygen (paO$_2$) 36; base excess (BE) –3.1; HCO$_3$ 27 mmol/l; and lactate 4.5 mmol/l. The etCO$_2$ was 10 kPa. A CXR (Figure 5.1) showed severe hyperinflation and some patchy consolidation but no air leaks. The cuffed endotracheal tube was in a good position.

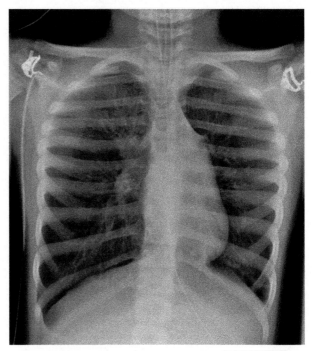

Figure 5.1 Chest X-ray postintubation demonstrating severe hyperinflated lung fields. Haemodynamic instability would be expected based on the radiological evidence of cardiac compression.

🔆 **Expert comment** Managing acute severe asthma without invasive ventilation

Many adjunctive therapies have been tried in order to avoid intubation in acute severe asthma, such as the use of inhaled helium–oxygen mixtures ('heliox'), as well as non-invasive ventilatory support.[5,6] Non-invasive face mask ventilation may improve dyspnoea by offloading the respiratory muscles, but its effects are not predictable and are strongly influenced by many factors, including the mask's fit and the patient's acceptance and cooperation. There is insufficient or conflicting evidence to advocate the use of these therapies routinely in children.

✚ **Clinical tip** Induction of anaesthesia for acute severe asthma

During induction of anaesthesia, it is important to ensure that cardiac preload is adequate by considering the need for an IV fluid bolus. Hypotension is a frequent complication of mechanical ventilation in asthmatic patients, often responding to fluid and/or inotropic support.[15] Ketamine and fentanyl are ideal induction of anaesthesia agents in this scenario as they have a good haemodynamic profile. Propofol, for example, may depress cardiac output and cause significant hypotension when preload is limited by high intrathoracic pressures.

⭐ **Learning point** Indications for ventilation in asthma

There are three main indications for ventilation in asthma. First, is *arterial hypoxaemia*. Ventilation perfusion (V/Q) mismatch is universal in acute asthma but is usually not severe owing to an effective hypoxic pulmonary vasoconstriction response.[13] Normalization of V/Q mismatch has considerable lag, even as the patient's ventilatory status improves and airflow obstruction resolves. The second indication is *fatigue with hypercarbia*. Work of breathing in asthma is high when airflow obstruction is severe and is inefficient with lung hyperinflation due to poor diaphragmatic efficiency at near maximal flattening. There is no threshold value for pH or $paCO_2$, as the requirement for intubation and ventilation is usually multifactorial. If transfer to a regional PICU is required, intubation is often undertaken at a lower threshold to facilitate safe transport, especially over long distances. The third indication is *confusion and obtundation*. This may occur with both hypoxia and hypercarbia. In this subgroup of patients, work of breathing and respiratory distress may not appear severe as respiratory drive is blunted. This is one of the pitfalls of clinical asthma severity scores where high respiratory rate (RR) and accessory muscle use are scored as high risk.

🔆 **Expert comment** Pitfalls in intubation of patients for acute severe asthma

Multiple studies demonstrate that a frequent complication in children following intubation for life-threatening asthma is haemodynamic instability (requiring significant fluid resuscitation and inotropic support). Positive-pressure ventilation and the consequent decrease in systemic venous return due to increased intrathoracic pressure (hyperinflation) is known to negatively affect cardiac output.[15] A good representation of this can be seen in a screenshot of the patient's bedside monitor (Figure 5.2). The dramatic decrease in pulse pressure (arterial waveform), as indicated by the stars, corresponds to the mandatory breaths delivered by the ventilator. Fluid depletion due to dehydration, combined with intrinsic PEEP, loss of endogenous catecholamines, and the vasodilating properties of anaesthetic induction agents may cause severe hypotension. If this persists after the administration of a fluid bolus, temporarily disconnecting the patient from the ventilator (up to 60 seconds with close monitoring of oxygen saturations) with a resulting increase in blood pressure confirms the need to adjust the ventilator. Usually decreasing the ventilator rate allowing adequate time for expiration improves this.

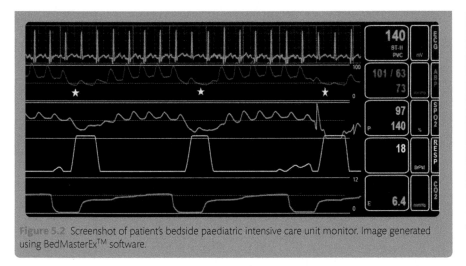

Figure 5.2 Screenshot of patient's bedside paediatric intensive care unit monitor. Image generated using BedMasterEx™ software.

⊕ Clinical tip End-tidal CO_2 in asthma

Use of $etCO_2$ monitoring is essential to confirm endotracheal placement especially if chest movement is difficult. In severe asthma, dead space can be around 50% and the $etCO_2$ can underestimate true arterial CO_2 by up to 50%. The point is illustrated in this case where arterial $paCO_2$ was 20 kPa and $etCO_2$ was only 10 kPa. Inspection of the end-tidal wave trace shows the end-expiratory plateau is not reached. For this reason, it is advisable to obtain an arterial blood gas to assess not only $paCO_2$, but also quantify alveolar dead space.

Following intubation, the major problem was persisting hypercarbia rather than hypoxia, and there was concern about the need for high ventilatory pressures (> 35 cmH$_2$O). There was still marked wheezing, despite muscular relaxation and sedation. The relatively high RR (25/min) used initially caused progressive air trapping as visual inspection of the flow time curve on the ventilator showed expiratory flow had not completed with each new breath. Ventilation was optimized, reducing the RR to 17/min, resulting in a longer expiratory time of 3.5 seconds and ensuring expiratory flow had returned to zero before each breath (Figure 5.3). A blood gas on the lower rate of 17/min showed pH 6.98; paCO$_2$ 16.5 kPa; paO$_2$ 32.7 kPa; BE –4.1; HCO$_3$ 29 mmol/l; lactate 1.2 mmol/l; haemoglobin 95 g/l; saturation 98%. Tidal volumes were between 6 and 8 mL/kg and paCO$_2$ remained static (i.e. was not increasing). Lactate had improved to 1.2 mmol/L since reducing salbutamol to 0.5 µg/kg/min as there was no benefit to the higher dose. At a RR of 17/min, expiratory flow terminated before each new breath (see arrow in Figure 5.3).

⊕ Clinical tip Flow-time curve

Inspection of the flow time curve is important to prevent air stacking and hyperinflation.[16]

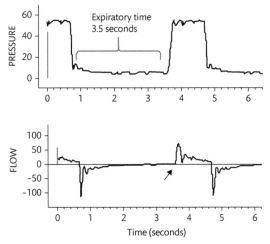

Figure 5.3 Ventilator waveforms showing pressure and flow over time (seconds). Reproduced courtesy of AD/AN.

The most important goal in ventilating severe asthma is to ensure progressive air trapping is avoided as this will rapidly lead to a spiral of escalating airway pressures, dynamic hyperinflation, and barotrauma. In many historical paediatric series, normal or near-normal gases were targeted and/or bicarbonate was added to keep pH >7.2.[17]

Historically, mortality was 25% in children ventilated for asthma.[18] Darrioli and Perret were the first to show zero mortality in asthma with a controlled hyperventilation strategy that avoided progressive air trapping.[19] The strategy involves using lower RRs that allow sufficient time for expiration to occur and using high enough airway pressures to move the chest to achieve an adequate minute ventilation that prevents CO_2 from *rising*. The aim is not to normalize CO_2 (as hypercarbia is well tolerated in acute severe asthma), but to ensure it does not rise further while other therapies (e.g. mucolytic agents or physiotherapy) are used to treat the cause of mechanical airway obstruction. The safety of this strategy lies in the measurement of the plateau pressure via an inspiratory hold manoeuvre to ensure alveoli are not exposed to excessive pressure (<30 cmH_2O) and auto-PEEP is not generated (expiratory hold). High peak pressures <50 cmH_2O may be required to achieve gas exchange.

Leatherman demonstrated that the most effective rate was allowing 3–4 seconds for expiration.[16] If the RR was too low (<12), the benefit of longer expiratory time was too marginal to compensate for a lowered minute ventilation. In a hypothetical patient with 8 mL/kg tidal volume and an inspiratory time of 0.8 seconds, a rate of 10 as a baseline (5.2 seconds expiratory time) will have 40% less minute ventilation than a rate of 15 where expiration is shorted (3.2 seconds) but adequate to avoid dynamic hyperinflation. Hence, the *fastest* rate that avoids dynamic hyperinflation is ideal. If this setting is correct, CO_2 should not keep increasing.

An inspiratory and expiratory pause were measured to estimate plateau pressure and auto-PEEP, respectively. On an inspiratory hold, pressure fell from 57 cmH_2O to a plateau pressure of 27 cmH_2O (Figure 5.4).

A flexible bronchoscope was performed at the bedside and demonstrated extensive thick tenacious adherent mucous plugs in the large and first- and second-degree bronchi (similar in appearance to plastic bronchitis). Endotracheal DNAse (2.5 mg in a 20 mL saline solution) was instilled directly into each lung under bronchoscopic vision. Chest physiotherapy was performed cautiously to disperse DNAse into the smaller airways. Within an hour, large mucus plugs and cellular debris were suctioned from the airway, with a progressive increase in tidal volume to 8 mL/kg and then 10 mL/kg. CO_2 clearance also improved (paCO$_2$ 8 kPa, etCO$_2$ 5 kPa; Figure 5.6). Ventilatory pressures were progressively reduced from 57 to 30 cmH_2O over the next few hours (Figure 5.7) ensuring the RR was not changed to allow sufficient time for expiration (3.5 seconds expiration). After stopping sedation and neuromuscular blockade, the ventilation was converted from pressure-controlled to pressure-supported, to better facilitate spontaneous respiration.

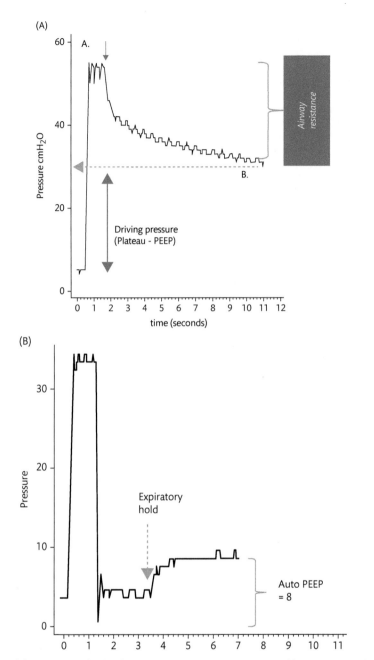

Figure 5.4 (A) An *inspiratory hold*. Peak pressure to pause pressure is measured by an inspiratory hold (in which the patient is muscle relaxed with no leak around the endotracheal tube by inflating the cuff). Although the peak pressure is 57 cmH$_2$O, only 27 cmH$_2$O is transmitted to the distal airways (driving pressure = 27–5 = 22 cmH$_2$O) as approximately 30 cmH$_2$O of pressure is lost overcoming major resistance (mucus plugs) in large and small airways. (B) An expiratory hold showing an auto-positive end expiratory pressure (PEEP) of 8 cmH$_2$O.
Reproduced courtesy of AD/AN.

> **✪ Learning point** Inspiratory flow limitation in asthma
>
> Figure 5.5. Shows a peak airway pressure of 57 mmH$_2$O (point A) at the endotracheal tube tip. As
> the pressure is driven through the central trachea and bronchi, mucus plugs create a resistance to
> airflow. Some of the pressure is dissipated overcoming this resistance. Alveoli at point C experience
> a pressure of 40. At point D, the airways are completely plugged and closed and receive no pressure.
> Alveoli in point E are exposed to a pressure of 35 cmH$_2$O (the pressure left over from what dissipated
> on reaching this point. Alveoli at point G experience an even lower pressure of 32 as there is partial
> mucus obstruction at the sub-segmental level. Asthma is therefore a *patchy non-homogenous disease
> of the airways with many different areas of different ventilation and perfusion.* The inspiratory hold
> with determination of plateau pressure determines how much of the airway pressure (on average) is
> transmitted to the alveoli. In this case, although the peak pressure is 57 cmH$_2$O, the majority of alveoli
> are only receiving pressure of 27 cmH$_2$O. This is not sustainable, however, as exposing the airways to
> persistent high pressures over time risks air leaks, so urgent strategies are required to overcome this
> airway obstruction.

> **✪ Learning point** Auto-PEEP
>
> During an expiratory hold, alveolar units empty at different rates depending on the degree of small
> airway obstruction (mucous plugs). In totally obstructed segments (Figure 5.6 point B) there is no
> expiratory flow. In others (points A, D, and C) there are various degrees of obstruction such that
> alveolar emptying may be markedly prolonged (point A has an expiratory pressure of 15 cmH$_2$O).
>
> The sum pressure of all ventilated alveoli measured at the endotracheal tube is the auto-PEEP (point
> A). In this case it is 10 cmH$_2$O.

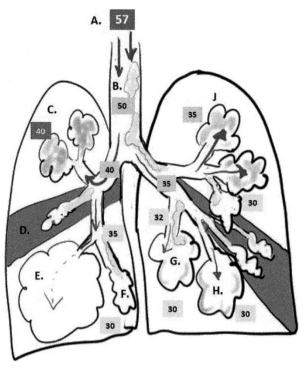

Figure 5.5 Diagram showing non-homogeneous lung regions during inspiration.

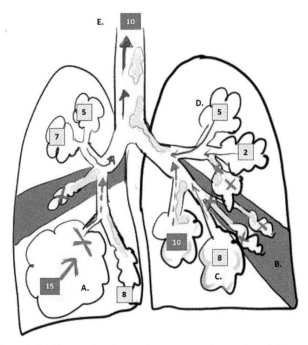

Figure 5.6 Expiratory hold. Diagram showing non-homogeneous lung regions during expiration.

> **⊕ Clinical tip Managing auto-PEEP**
>
> Various degrees of auto-PEEP can be present in acute severe asthma. However, attempts to 'match' PEEP with auto-PEEP are not consistent. On some occasions, increasing PEEP to equal auto-PEEP measured by an expiratory hold can reduce dynamic hyperinflation. The response can also be paradoxical with a worsening of airflow.[20] As there are always some partially obstructed airways in severe asthma, setting PEEP to 5 cmH$_2$O is a reasonable starting point. It can be adjusted in steps of 2 cmH$_2$O with visual inspection of flow curves to titrate for benefit. Manual decompression of the chest to forcibly reduce hyperinflation may have significant adverse cardiorespiratory consequences and is not recommended.[3] As the mucous plugs remain *in situ*, dynamic hyperinflation will recur within a few breaths.

The patient was successfully extubated within 24 hours and re-commenced regular salbutamol inhalation via a spacer. She was referred to the specialist asthma clinic to ensure she received appropriate follow-up and a written rescue asthma plan.

> **⊕ Clinical tip Ventilation modes, strategies, and extracorporeal support in acute severe asthma**
>
> There are many different ventilatory modes and ventilators currently available. In general, pressure control modes are more suitable for the paediatric population as tidal volume estimates are variable and may be unreliable in paediatrics, especially in smaller children and neonates. Pressure control has numerous well described advantages in asthma.[23] Recently a number of auto-regulating modes that aim to target lower volumes such as adaptive support ventilation or pressure regulated volume control have gained popularity. As they rely on algorithms to constantly adjust to the lowest pressure delivery settings, these have not been tested at the extreme end of the dynamic spectrum in asthma where airway resistance may be highly variable and may change from breath to breath in a heterogeneously diseased airway/lung. When alveolar ventilation is extremely borderline and critical (CO$_2$ >15 kpa), not knowing exactly what the ventilator is doing as mucus plugs shift or obstruct maybe be a disadvantage. The case discussed shows a simple approach of targeting pressure and measuring the

> **❝ Expert comment**
> Intratracheal DNAse in acute severe asthma
>
> Bronchoscopic evidence of dense mucous plugging in asthma is well reported,[12] and intratracheal DNAse has been used in plastic bronchitis, cystic fibrosis, and asthma as a safe, non-irritant, and effective mucolytic agent.[21,22] Employing this therapy safely and effectively, however, requires acquisition of skills and experience by both medical and physiotherapy staff.

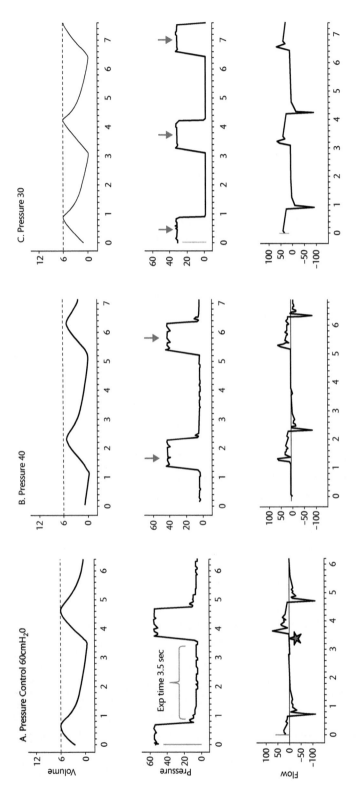

Figure 5.7 Reduction in ventilation with reduction in peak pressure from (A) 57 cmH$_2$O to (B) 40 cmH$_2$O to (C) 25 cmH$_2$O as airway resistance and expiratory flow limitation resolved. Note tidal volume remained 6 mL/kg (pressure control mode with progressive reduction in peak pressures following DNAse therapy). Images generated using Stata® software.

resultant tidal volume. As the airflow limitation improves, the pressure is lowered into a safer zone while preserving an adequate tidal volume and RR to deliver an effective minute ventilation ('pressure regulated doctor in control mode'). High-frequency oscillation has been used in acute severe asthma. This mode in experienced hands may be effective, but its potential to hyperinflate and over-distend the lung in an unpredictable manner remains a concern, especially in a heterogeneously diseased lung where ventilation is not uniform. Refractory hypoxia or hypercarbia may be an indication for extracorporeal membrane oxygenation (ECMO) support (especially veno-venous) and survival in this group of patients is in excess of 80%.[24] It is important to recognize that refractory airflow obstruction in severe cases is more likely due to extensive small and large airway mucus plugging than bronchospasm.[12] Ventilatory assistance provides time to institute the appropriate therapy and DNase can be a lifesaving, non-irritant mucolytic that is potentially ECMO sparing.[21,22]

A final word from the expert

Acute severe asthma continues to impose a significant global burden on the healthcare services despite advances in diagnosis and treatment.[1] Almost 6% of the UK population suffers from asthma, making it one of the most common childhood diseases. It is estimated that up to 10% of asthmatic children require hospital admission with a mortality estimated at 0.27 per 100,000.[1] Shortcomings in all levels of care (primary, secondary, and tertiary) were identified in the 2014 UK national review of asthma deaths. In this study 75% of children died before receiving hospital care.[3] Mortality risk has been associated with several factors, including poor disease control, overuse of bronchodilators, underuse of systemic steroids, differential access to care, exposure to pollutants, and cigarette smoke.[25]

The outcome is typically poor in patients with acute severe asthma who suffer a cardiorespiratory arrest prior to hospitalization, with death or neurological disability secondary to hypoxic-ischaemic brain injury. In contrast, international studies suggest very low mortality rates (<1%) in acute severe asthma where there is no CPR prior to admission to the ICU.[26] If asthmatic patients require invasive mechanical ventilation, survival from ICU should be expected. The aim of ventilation is to allow time for resolution of the acute asthma and airway inflammatory process. Ventilation strategies that facilitate controlled hypoventilation, avoiding progressive and excessive hyperinflation, should be employed. Aggressive treatment of mucous plugging should be encouraged, in addition to considering reducing or stopping IV bronchodilators where the physiology is related to mucus plugging rather than bronchospasm, such as in this case. In rare instances where these measures prove inadequate, ECMO should be employed (See Case 14 for more on ECMO). In order to reduce the wide variation in management and outcomes for children admitted to PICU for life-threatening asthma, especially for those who require invasive ventilation, further research is warranted urgently.

References

1. Anderson HR, Gupta R, Strachan DP, Limb ES. 50 years of asthma: UK trends from 1955 to 2004. *Thorax* 2007;62:85–90.
2. Doeing DC, Solway J. Airway smooth muscle in the pathophysiology and treatment of asthma. *J. Appl. Physiol.* 2013;114:834–43.
3. Levy M, Andrews R, Buckingham R, Evans H. Why asthma still kills: the National Review of Asthma Deaths (NRAD) Confidential Enquiry Report. Available at: https://www.rcplondon.ac.uk/projects/outputs/why-asthma-still-kills (last accessed 9 April 2020).

4. Bratton SL, Newth CJL, Zuppa AF, et al. Critical care for pediatric asthma: wide care variability and challenges for study. *Pediatr. Crit. Care Med.* 2012;13:407–14.

5. Fernández MM, Villagrá A, Blanch L, Fernández R. Non-invasive mechanical ventilation in status asthmaticus. *Intensive Care Med.* 2001;27:486–92.

6. Schaeffer EM, Pohlman A, Morgan S, Hall JB. Oxygenation in status asthmaticus improves during ventilation with helium-oxygen. *Crit. Care Med.* 1999;27:2666–70.

7. Starkey ES, Mulla H, Sammons HM, Pandya HC. Intravenous salbutamol for childhood asthma: evidence-based medicine? *Arch. Dis. Child.* 2014;99:873–7.

8. Travers AH, Milan SJ, Jones AP, Camargo CA, Rowe BH. Addition of intravenous beta(2)-agonists to inhaled beta(2)-agonists for acute asthma. *Cochrane Database Syst. Rev.* 2012;(12):CD010179.

9. Sarnaik SM, Saladino RA, Manole M, et al. Diastolic hypotension is an unrecognized risk factor for β-agonist-associated myocardial injury in children with asthma. *Pediatr. Crit. Care Med.* 2013;14:e273–9.

10. Yung M, South M. Randomised controlled trial of aminophylline for severe acute asthma. *Arch. Dis. Child.* 1998;79:405–10.

11. Mitra A, Bassler D, Goodman K, et al. Intravenous aminophylline for acute severe asthma in children over two years receiving inhaled bronchodilators. *Cochrane Database Syst. Rev.* 2005;(2):CD001276.

12. Kuyper LM, Paré PD, Hogg JC, et al. Characterization of airway plugging in fatal asthma. *Am. J. Med.* 2003;115:6–11.

13. Rodriguez-Roisin R. Acute severe asthma: pathophysiology and pathobiology of gas exchange abnormalities. *Eur. Respir. J.* 1997;10:1359–71.

14. Wasserfallen JB, Schaller MD, Feihl F, Perret CH. Sudden asphyxic asthma: a distinct entity? *Am. Rev. Respir. Dis.* 1990;142:108–11.

15. Dehò A, Lutman D, Montgomery M, et al. Emergency management of children with acute severe asthma requiring transfer to intensive care. *Emerg. Med. J.* 2010;27:834–7.

16. Leatherman J. Mechanical ventilation for severe asthma. *Chest* 2015;147:1671–80.

17. Cox RG, Barker GA, Bohn DJ. Efficacy, results, and complications of mechanical ventilation in children with status asthmaticus. *Pediatr. Pulmonol.* 1991;11:120–6.

18. Seddon PC, Heaf DP. Long term outcome of ventilated asthmatics. *Arch. Dis. Child.* 1990;65:1324–7.

19. Darioli R, Perret C. Mechanical controlled hypoventilation in status asthmaticus. *Am. Rev. Respir. Dis.* 1984;129:385–7.

20. Blanch L, Bernabé F, Lucangelo U. Measurement of air trapping, intrinsic positive end-expiratory pressure, and dynamic hyperinflation in mechanically ventilated patients. *Respir. Care.* 2005;50:110–23.

21. Nyman A, Puppala K, Colthurst S, et al. Safety and efficacy of intratracheal DNase with physiotherapy in severe status asthmaticus. *Crit. Care* 2011;15(Suppl. 1):P185.

22. Durward A, Forte V, Shemie SD. Resolution of mucus plugging and atelectasis after intratracheal rhDNase therapy in a mechanically ventilated child with refractory status asthmaticus. *Crit. Care Med.* 2000;28:560–2.

23. Sarnaik AP, Daphtary KM, Meert KL, et al. Pressure-controlled ventilation in children with severe status asthmaticus. *Pediatr. Crit. Care Med.* 2004;5:133–8.

24. Zabrocki LA, Brogan TV, Statler KD, et al. Extracorporeal membrane oxygenation for pediatric respiratory failure: survival and predictors of mortality. *Crit. Care Med.* 2010;39:364–70.

25. Watson L, Turk F, James P, Holgate ST. Factors associated with mortality after an asthma admission: a national United Kingdom database analysis. *Respir Med* 2007;101:1659–64.

26. Triasih R, Duke T, Robertson CF. Outcomes following admission to intensive care for asthma. *Arch. Dis. Child.* 2011;96:729–34.

6 Paediatric acute respiratory distress syndrome

Christiane S. Eberhardt

🎔 **Expert commentary** by Peter C. Rimensberger

Case history

A 13-year-old girl, weighing 28 kg, with a background of cerebral palsy and scoliosis, was fed via percutaneous endoscopic gastrostomy (PEG), and had a history of gastro-oesophageal reflux without specific treatment. She presented to the Emergency Department with 7 days of cough, coryza, and fever. In the 24 hours prior to presentation, she developed mild signs of respiratory distress and several episodes of vomiting. She had been treated by her general practitioner since day 4 after onset of symptoms with co-amoxicillin and clarithromycin for suspicion of a community-acquired pneumonia.

Nasopharyngeal swabs and peripheral blood cultures were taken. The septic work-up showed an inflammatory syndrome (white blood cells 24.5 10^9/L; neutrophils 12.6 10^9/L; C-reactive protein 110 mg/L; remaining investigations were normal). Antibiotics were switched to the intravenous (IV) route (ampicillin and clarithromycin) and IV fluids started at 100% maintenance. Because of hypoxaemia (SpO$_2$ at 88% at room air), supplemental oxygen via a facial mask was initiated at 4 L/min. However, during the night, this had to be increased to up to 8 L/min to maintain saturations over 88%.

> ✪ **Learning point** Definition of paediatric acute respiratory distress syndrome
>
> **Definition and severity assessment**
>
> The American–European Consensus Conference issued the first definition of acute respiratory distress syndrome (ARDS) in 1994, which was updated in 2012 with the Berlin definition.[1] For children, the validity of these criteria was then confirmed by a multicentre evaluation.[2]
>
> In 2015, the Paediatric Acute Lung Injury consensus conference (PALICC) adapted the adult criteria to the paediatric population to improve reliability and feasibility of the definition, to predict outcome, and allow for comparison between centres. PALICC based the definition on retrospective outcome data analysis of paediatric ARDS, and the severity grading to predict outcome was subsequently confirmed by a large prospective data set.[3]
>
> As detailed in Table 6.1, the main modification is the assessment of oxygen failure in intubated patients when the oxygenation index (OI) or the oxygen saturation index (in the absence of an arterial line) is used instead of the P/F ratio criterion. Also, the definition of paediatric ARDS (PARDS) now includes non-invasive respiratory support without stratification of severity.

Table 6.1 Paediatric Acute Lung Injury Consensus Conference criteria for paediatric acute respiratory distress syndrome (PARDS)

Age	Exclude patients with perinatal-related lung disease			
Timing	Within 7 days of known clinical insult			
Origin of oedema	Respiratory failure not fully explained by cardiac failure or fluid overload			
Chest imaging	Chest imaging findings of new infiltrate(s) consistent with acute pulmonary parenchymal disease			
Oxygenation	Non-invasive mechanical ventilation	Invasive mechanical ventilation		
	PARDS (no severity stratification)	Mild PARDS	Moderate PARDS	Severe PARDS
	Full face-mask bi-level ventilation or CPAP ≥5 cmH$_2$O PF ratio ≤300 SF ratio ≤264	4≤OI<8 5≤OSI<7.5	8≤OI<16 7.5≤OSI<12.3	OI >16 OSI >12.3
Special populations				
Cyanotic heart disease	Standard criteria above for age, timing, origin oedema, and chest imaging with an acute deterioration in oxygenation not explained by underlying cardiac disease			
Chronic lung disease	Standard criteria above for age, timing, and origin oedema with chest imaging consistent with new infiltrate and acute deterioration in oxygenation from baseline, which meet oxygenation criteria above			
Left ventricular dysfunction	Standard criteria for age, timing, and origin oedema with chest imaging changes consistent with new infiltrate and acute deterioration in oxygenation, which meet criteria above not explained by left ventricular dysfunction			

CPAP, continuous positive airway pressure; PF, PaO$_2$ (mmHg)/FiO$_2$; SF, SpO$_2$/FiO$_2$; OI, oxygenation index (FiO$_2$ × mean airway pressure × 100)/PaO2 (mmHg);
OSI, oxygen saturation index (FiO$_2$ × mean airway pressure × 100)/SpO$_2$; PaO$_2$, arterial oxygen pressure; SpO$_2$, transcutaneous oxygen saturation; FiO$_2$, fraction of inspired oxygen.

Source: Data from *Pediatr Crit Care Med.*, 16(5), Pediatric Acute Lung Injury Consensus Conference Group. Pediatric acute respiratory distress syndrome: consensus recommendations from the Pediatric Acute Lung Injury Consensus Conference, pp. 428–39, Copyright (2015), The Society of Critical Care Medicine and the World Federation of Pediatric Intensive and Critical Care Societies.

⊕ Clinical tip Risk factors of PARDS

When taking care of a patient within 7 days of a known clinical insult or a worsening of respiratory symptoms (not solely due to fluid overload or cardiac failure), the following criteria help to identify patients at risk of PARDS (Table 6.2).

Table 6.2 Risk factors for development of paediatric acute respiratory distress syndrome (PARDS)

	Lung affecting conditions	General conditions
Risk factors for ARDS in infancy and early childhood* **Score of relevance (indicated by number; 5 = maximum)**	Near-drowning (3.9) Thoracic trauma (3.7) Flu (3.4) Pneumonia—LRTI (3.3) Bronchiolitis (3.3) Pertussis (2.9) BPD (2.6) Milk aspiration (2.4)	Sepsis (4.4) Congenital immunodeficiency (3.8) Paediatric cancer (2.6) Major surgery (1.7) GOR (1.7)

(continued)

Table 6.2 Continued

	Lung affecting conditions	General conditions
Chest X-ray (4)	New infiltrates consistent with acute pulmonary parenchymal disease	
Oxygenation support requirements to maintain SpO$_2$ ≥88% (4):	Non-invasive mechanical ventilation	Invasive mechanical ventilation
	Mask, nasal cannula or high-flow nasal cannula	Nasal mask CPAP or BiPAP	
	Minimum flow[†]: <1 year: 2 L/min 1–5 years: 4 L/min 5–10 years: 6 L/min >10 years: 8 L/min	FiO$_2$ ≥ 40%	OI <4 or OSI <5

ARDS, acute respiratory distress syndrome; LTRI, lower respiratory tract infection; BPD, bronchopulmonary dysplasia; GOR, gastro-oesophageal reflux; FiO$_2$, fraction of inspired oxygen; OI, oxygenation index (FiO$_2$ × mean airway pressure × 100)/PaO2; OSI, oxygen saturation index (FiO$_2$ × mean airway pressure × 100)/SpO$_2$; CPAP, continuous positive airway pressure; BiPAP, bilevel positive airway pressure.

*Score (mean) represents the relevance of each comorbidity in terms of pathogenesis and frequency in PARDS (0 = minimum and 5 = maximum), evaluated by members of the Respiratory Section of the European Society of Paediatric and Neonatal Intensive Care.[2]

[†]Calculation of flow-at-risk rate if use of oxygen blender: minimum flow = FiO2 × flow rate (L/min)
Source: Adapted from *Intensive Care Med*, 39(12), De Luca D, Piastra M, et al., The use of the Berlin definition for acute respiratory distress syndrome during infancy and early childhood: multicenter evaluation and expert consensus, pp. 2083–2091, Copyright (2013), with permission from Springer Nature.

In the early morning (day 8 from onset of symptoms), she deteriorated with increased work of breathing, oxygen saturation of 60%, and drowsiness. She was transferred to the Paediatric Intensive Care Unit (PICU), where facial mask continuous positive airway pressure (CPAP) of 6 cm H$_2$O and fraction of inspired oxygen (FiO$_2$) 0.6 was started. Because of persisting high oxygen requirements, she was switched rapidly to non-invasive positive pressure ventilation (NIPPV), with a positive end expiratory pressure (PEEP) of 6 cmH$_2$O and a pressure support above a PEEP of 8 cmH$_2$O. On NIPPV, saturations were hardly maintained over 88%. The blood gas from arterial puncture was as follows: pH 7.27; partial pressure of carbon dioxide 6.8 kPa (51 mmHg); partial pressure of oxygen (PaO$_2$) 6.1 kPa (45 mmHg); base excess –3.6 mmol/L; HCO$_3^-$ 23.4 mmol/L (P/F ratio (PaO$_2$ (mmHg)/FiO$_2$): 45/0.6 = 76).

✪ Learning point Pathophysiology of PARDS

The pathophysiology of ARDS can be divided into three phases: the acute exudative phase during the first week, which is followed by the recovery stage that itself is divided into the proliferative and fibrotic phases.

During the exudative phase, mostly innate immune cells (neutrophils, macrophages) damage alveolar epithelial and endothelial cells. Alveolar fluid transport is compromised. Plasma proteins and cells accumulate in the interstitium and alveolar spaces. The inflammatory exudate leads to inactivation of surfactant, and damage of type II alveolar cells, and supports the formation of hyaline membranes. The loss of type I alveolar cells and their ion channels impedes the osmotic gradient necessary to reabsorb the oedema fluid from the alveolar spaces into the interstitium. Altogether, this contributes to compromised gas exchange. The impairment of alveolar vascularization (vasomotor tone and microthrombi) results in pulmonary hypertension. All this leads to a ventilation/perfusion (V/Q) mismatch and failure to vasoconstrict hypoxic areas of the lung with subsequent refractory hypoxia.

The proliferative phase is characterized by a regeneration of the alveolar cells with consecutive clearance of exudative fluid and production of surfactant. Normalization of vasomotor tone and absorption of microthrombi contribute to diminish pulmonary hypertension. A reduction in shunts improves oxygenation and pulmonary compliance slowly recovers.

Finally, the fibrotic phase can evolve if alveolar collagen is not removed and cystic changes limit functional recovery.

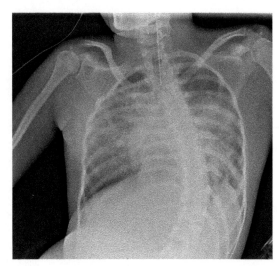

Figure 6.1 Chest X-ray after intubation.

In the absence of an oxygenation response to NIPPV within the next hour, she was orally intubated with a cuffed endotracheal tube (ETT), size 6.5. Chest X-ray showed bilateral infiltrates (see Figure 6.1). Conventional invasive ventilation was commenced (initial settings: pressure control, PEEP 6 cmH_2O; peak inspiratory pressure (PIP) 24 cmH_2O, resulting in tidal volumes (Vt) of 5 mL/kg body weight, respiratory rate (RR) 20 breaths per minute, FiO_2 0.7) and a SpO_2 of 89% could be achieved. In order to improve oxygenation PEEP was titrated up to 8 and then to 10 cmH_2O, resulting in PIPs of 26 and 28 cmH_2O, respectively. With this, SpO_2 improved to 92%, while the FiO_2 could be lowered to 0.5.

> ⭐ **Learning point** Lung-protective ventilation
>
> Treatment for PARDS is merely supportive rather than curative. Therefore, measures should be taken to avoid iatrogenic complications and provide the best lung protective ventilation strategies.
>
> Ventilator-induced lung injury can be induced by alveolar distension (barotrauma, volutrauma) and ventilation at low lung volumes (atelectrauma). The cyclic stretching (shear stress) of alveolar cells releases inflammatory mediators and leads to an additional biotrauma. High FiO_2, having a toxic effect, may further contribute to this inflammatory response.
>
> Thus, lung-protective ventilation strategies consist of the use of adequate PEEP settings (by slow titration), pressure limitation, and/or delivery of low tidal volumes clearly below physiological values. This might necessitate some degree of permissive hypercapnia. In a lung condition where active alveoli can be recruited, a FiO_2 below 0.6 (values above are considered to be toxic) can be maintained, even without the need for permissive hypoxaemia. In that case, an appropriate PEEP level should prevent collapsing and re-opening of alveoli and thus reduce subsequent biotrauma. An increase in PEEP will then also reduce the oxygen requirements by reduction of the intrapulmonary shunt. This was the rationale for developing a PEEP/FiO_2 table in the Acute Respiratory Distress Syndrome Clinical Network (ARDSNet) trial, which has also been beneficial in the paediatric population.[4,5] Although PALICC recommended recruitment manoeuvres (weak agreement), PEEP titration has to be used with caution; few data are available; potential for lung recruitment is not always predictable, and varies from patient to patient, depending on the aetiology and severity of PARDS.

In children, the role of tidal volumes and their association with mortality remains unclear. There is not a single study showing a direct relationship between the Vt applied (in the range of 6 to 12 mL/kg) and mortality. However, an initial target range of 5–8 mL/kg ideal body weight (IBW) can be recommended. In situations of poor lung compliance (smaller residual inflatable lung volumes = 'baby lung') when high inspiratory pressures are required, Vt should be further reduced to 3–6 mL/kg IBW, according to disease severity and its further evolution.

In any case, inspiratory pressure limitation to 28 cmH$_2$O, independent of the PEEP level, is strongly recommended by the PALICC.[6]

⊕ Expert comment Role of non-invasive ventilation in PARDS

Although CPAP and bi-level non-invasive ventilation (NIV) can be considered to be the first approach when respiratory support is required, they should be used only with careful monitoring of the response to the intervention.[1] There are no data available on the use of CPAP for PARDS with the exception of patients with viral bronchiolitis for whom CPAP reduces work of breathing (low-quality evidence) but does not reduce intubation rates (reviewed in Sinha et al.[7]). Clear failure criteria for CPAP have not been defined yet.

Non-invasive ventilation (NIV) is increasingly being used in paediatric patients with acute hypoxaemic respiratory failure. Published data come from uncontrolled prospective or retrospective studies in acute respiratory failure. To date, there are only two paediatric randomized controlled trials (RCTs) comparing the effects of NIV versus standard therapy (i.e. oxygen supplementation),[8,9] with one of them showing a reduced intubation rate in the NIV group in 50 patients mainly with viral lower respiratory tract disease.[9] Therefore, there are insufficient data to recommend the use of NIV, although it might have its role in mild-to-moderate PARDS. In severe PARDS it might increase adverse outcome following delayed intubation, as has been observed in adults, and therefore cannot be recommended. In any case, the success of NIV should be assessed 1 hour after initiation by observing measures such as HR and RR, the SpO$_2$/FiO$_2$ ratio, acidosis, level of consciousness, and presence of more than one organ failure.[9,10] In general, persisting unchanged, or even increased FiO2 requirements over more than 1 hour are considered as NIV-failure criterion.

A radial arterial line was placed and a blood pressure (BP) of 85/47 mmHg (mean arterial pressure (MAP) 59 mmHg) was recorded. She was febrile (39°C), tachycardic (heart rate (HR) 130 beats per minute), had a capillary refill time of 4–5 seconds, no urine output for the last 4 hours, and peripheral oedema. A saline fluid bolus of 10 mL/kg did not have any effect on HR or BP. She was started on an adrenaline infusion at a rate of 0.05 μg/kg/min, which was increased up to 0.1 μg/kg/min to maintain MAP above 60 mmHg.

During the first night in the PICU, she gradually required more respiratory support and PEEP had to be titrated up to maintain saturations above 88% (FiO$_2$ 0.8, PEEP 12 cmH$_2$O, PIP 28 cmH$_2$O, RR 40 breaths per minute, I/E ratio 1:1, OI 23.5). Slight CO$_2$ retention was observed. The decision was made to convert to high-frequency oscillatory ventilation (HFOV). Initial settings were mean airway pressure (mPaw) 22 cmH$_2$O (set 2 cmH$_2$O above the observed mPaw during conventional ventilation), frequency 10 Hz, ΔP 46 cmH$_2$O, and FiO$_2$ 0.8, which was slowly reduced to a FiO$_2$ of 0.6.

In addition, on day 9 (day 2 after admission), the results of the NPA were positive for influenza A and the blood culture revealed a *Streptococcus pyogenes* bacteraemia.

⊕ Clinical tip Recommended goals of ventilation in PARDS

Permissive hypoxaemia and hypercapnia for moderate-to-severe PARDS

- After optimizing PEEP, target SpO$_2$ 88–92% if PEEP ≥ 10 cmH$_2$O.
- When SpO$_2$ <92%, monitor central venous saturation.
- No routine bicarbonate supplementation.
- Maintain pH 7.15–7.3.
- Contraindications: intracranial hypertension, severe pulmonary hypertension, selected congenital heart disease lesions, haemodynamic instability, and significant ventricular dysfunction.

➕ **Clinical tip** Conventional mechanical ventilation

The following are the recommended ventilation targets and settings for conventional ventilation (modified from the PALICC recommendations)[4]:

- target tidal volumes 5–8 mL/kg, lower if poor compliance;
- PIP ≤28 cmH_2O, higher (29–32 cmH_2O) if reduced chest wall compliance;
- elevated levels of PEEP (10–15 cmH_2O) if tolerated to decrease FiO_2;
- PEEP >15 cmH_2O may be needed for severe PARDS;
- cuffed ETT is preferred.

➕ **Clinical tip** High-frequency oscillatory ventilation (HFOV)

- Consider if plateau pressures >28 cmH_2O.
- Optimal lung volume: recruitment by stepwise increase and decrease of mPaw (monitor oxygenation, CO_2 response, and haemodynamics).
- Allow ETT air leak around the ETT/cuff to augment CO_2 wash-out if needed.

✓ **Evidence base** Mode of ventilation

Conventional ventilation

There are no data on outcome depending on mode of ventilation (control or assisted). Most studies have evaluated the advantage of an open lung strategy that consisted of additional aspects of ventilation and thus confounding interventions. However, lung-protective ventilation with low tidal volumes and lower peak pressures improves outcome in adults.

HFOV

A recent Cochrane review based on 10 identified RCTs (1850 adults), showed that patients on HFOV had better oxygenation during the first 24–72 hours, but this was not associated with any differences in length of ventilation or mortality. Data on the use of HFOV in PARDS come mainly from retrospective studies, which showed either no benefit or even an increased mortality in the HFOV group.[11,12] These data must be interpreted with caution as, in most patients, HFOV was used as a rescue mode when continuous mandatory ventilation was considered to have failed. This limits the validity of declaring HFOV as not potentially lung protective. However, when patients were switched from continuous mandatory ventilation to HFOV by the attending physicians early after the onset of PARDS, lower mortality could be observed, with the odds ratio for death increasing exponentially with any additional day longer on continuous mandatory ventilation. Nevertheless, these observations are insufficient to recommend the early use of HFOV in PARDS.[4]

NIV

A large observational study (LUNG SAFE (Large observational study to Understand the Global impact of Severe Acute respiratory FailurE)) analysed outcomes in 2813 adults with ARDS, of whom 436 were only treated with NIV. NIV patients showed a higher mortality during their stay in the Intensive Care Unit than continuous mandatory ventilation patients with the same disease severity. This was not significant when assessing the overall mortality during the hospital stay. In children with acute respiratory failure, NIV could improve hypoxaemia;[9] however, more robust and paediatric data are needed.

Other modes of ventilation

To date, there are no data to support the routine use of high-frequency jet ventilation, high-frequency percussive ventilation, or liquid ventilation in PARDS.[4]

Respiratory extracorporeal membrane oxygenation

The evidence for the use of veno-venous extracorporeal membrane oxygenation (ECMO) in PARDS is weak. Results in favour are from one of the only RCTs in adults (CESAR (Conventional ventilatory support vs extracorporeal membrane oxygenation for severe adult respiratory failure)), comparing the outcome after conventional management with ECMO referral. However, there was no protocol for the conventional management, mostly performed in small hospitals and standard of care was not certain. Secondly, only 75% of the referred patients underwent ECMO and missing data from three patients could reverse significance.[13] During the H1N1 pandemic, the use of ECMO in ARDS was described in observational studies and increased the interest in performing trials in non-refractory ARDS to assess the value of early ECMO. However, data in children are sparse.

In the absence of clear evidence, PALICC recommends initiating ECMO in experienced centres, if the underlying cause for PARDS is reversible when lung protective ventilation strategies do not obtain a sufficient gas exchange, or as a bridge to transplant.[4]

> **ⓘ Expert comment** Tidal volume or peak pressure?
>
> Lung protective ventilation with low Vt and/or low PIP has been associated with better outcome in adults. In a systematic Cochrane review that included five randomized trials assessing ventilation strategies with different target tidal volumes and plateau pressures, the following was found: lower Vt or low airway driving pressure (plateau pressure 30 cmH$_2$O or less), resulting in Vt ≤7 mL/kg IBW was compared to ventilation that used Vt in the range of 10–15 mL/kg. There was no beneficial effect of low Vt if a plateau pressure ≤31 cmH$_2$O was used. These findings suggest strongly that plateau pressure elimination seems to be the more important determinant for improving outcome. More recent data from retrospective individual patient data analysis of the same trials indicates that the main determinant of lung protection directly correlated to mortality seems to be distending pressure (PIP-PEEP) with a cut-off level of 15 cmH$_2$O independent of the PEEP setting chosen.[14] This goes along with the 'baby lung' concept as described by Gattinoni and Pesenti[15] several years ago, suggesting that the less compliant a lung is, the smaller the residual lung volume that can be aerated. In other words, a functionally small poorly compliant lung supports only lower Vt than a functionally larger, better compliant lung.
>
> For children, robust data is not available on any of these lung-protective concepts. In fact, a relationship between tidal volumes and outcome has never been shown. However, in a small study, Panico et al. identified an independent association between distending pressure and mortality in 84 children with acute lung injury/ARDS after adjusting for disease severity and number of organ dysfunction at admission.[16]

After adrenaline infusion, her haemodynamics stabilized and the urine output was around 0.5–1 mL/kg/h. Intermittent desaturations and difficulties with ventilation resolved with an increase in sedation with morphine (20 µg/kg/h), midazolam (0.2 mg/kg/h), and neuromuscular blockade (vecuronium bolus doses). Over the next 24 hours she was weaned from adrenaline. Fluids were decreased to 60% maintenance to achieve a negative balance. The antibiogram reported a multisensitive *S. pyogenes* bacteraemia, and the subsequent blood cultures remained sterile. Antibiotics were continued. During the following night, her oxygen requirements increased (FiO2 = 1.0). An air leak was ruled out on X-ray. She was proned, which improved her oxygenation. She also required twice-daily chest physiotherapy due to thick and copious secretions.

> **⊘ Evidence base** Adjuvant therapies
>
> There is little evidence for the benefit of adjuvant strategies to improve PARDS.
>
> **Fluid restriction**
>
> In the adult population, a restrictive fluid management decreased duration of ventilation and ICU stay.[17] In children, a recent systematic review showed that a lower cumulative fluid balance led to reduced mortality and length of ventilation.[18] However, study populations were small and further trials are warranted.
>
> **Neuromuscular relaxants**
>
> The short-term use (48 hours) of neuromuscular relaxants reduced hospital mortality and barotrauma in adult ARDS, as evidenced by a meta-analysis of three French RCTs.[19] In an explorative paediatric study measuring their immediate effect (15 minutes after beginning of infusion), it improved oxygenation and allowed reduction in the mean airway pressure.[20]
>
> **Prone position**
>
> The rationale of prone positioning is to improve lung mechanics and gas exchange in the dependent lung regions by improving the ventilation-perfusion coupling. According to a Cochrane review, prone

positioning can lead to a slightly (non-significant) improved mortality rate in patients with severe ARDS, especially if prone positioning was started during the first 48 hours and lasted for at least 16 hours per day. However, tube obstruction and pressure sores rates were increased. To date—and in children—the evidence is weak to support prone positioning but it should be considered in severe PARDS,[21] as recommended by PALICC.[4]

Corticosteroids

The use of steroids to counteract the inflammatory response in PARDS is not recommended in the face of insufficient paediatric data.[21] In adults, results are ambiguous, but starting steroids early and in the patient subgroups with steroid-responsive lung pathologies (e.g. chronic lung disease of prematurity, asthma) could improve their outcome. However, more studies on neuromuscular outcomes, steroid-related complications, different dosages, and delivery methods are needed.

Inhaled nitric oxide

The aim of inhaled nitric oxide (iNO) is to induce vasodilatation in the aerated lung areas and to decrease the ventilation/perfusion mismatch typical in PARDS. An RCT in children did show a benefit in the oxygenation index and pulmonary vascular resistance index, but not a reduction in mortality.[21] This was in line with a Cochrane review and the routine use is thus not recommended.[21] However, in some cases with severe hypoxaemia, iNO may lead to improvement of oxygenation allowing reduction of FiO_2 to less toxic levels. iNO might help to avoid right ventricular failure due to pulmonary hypertension.

Exogenous surfactant

Outcomes after the use of surfactant in ARDS are inconsistent depending on the type of surfactant used and its posology. Short-term improvement in oxygenation may occur. Effect on a decreased mortality in the paediatric population with direct lung injury could not be reproduced in a consecutive trial.[22,23] To date, there is not enough evidence for the use of surfactant to decrease mortality or lengths of ventilation.[21]

❝ Expert comment Adjuvant therapies

Many adjuvant treatment approaches have been thought and trialled over the years. Besides a general concept of fluid restriction in any inflammatory disease process outside life-saving resuscitation, however, there are only three interventions that have been shown to be effective in some selected patients with ARDS: corticoids; prone position; and neuromuscular blockade.

Out of all tested pharmacological interventions and after many conflicting results, only corticoids have shown, in a recent individual meta-analysis, some benefits, i.e. shorter ventilation times and lower mortality when patients were treated early (before 14 days of ARDS onset) at high doses and for a prolonged time. Whether these encouraging observations can be transposed to children remains questionable, given the big variety of aetiologies of ARDS in children that are sometimes distinctly different from those in adults.

Prone positioning and neuromuscular blockade within the first 48 hours showed a positive effect on outcome in adult patients with severe ARDS, as defined by a P/F ratio of ≤100. In such, these two treatments should rather be considered as rescue treatment strategies. There are no sufficient paediatric data to confirm these observations and clinical trials are currently underway.

✪ Learning point NAVA

The principal of NAVA is to detect the electrical activity of the diaphragm (Edi, measured in microV) and to deliver pressure in synchrony with the diaphragm and in proportion depending on the magnitude of the patient's electrical signal. A special Edi catheter, similar to a nasogastric tube, is inserted with its detection electrodes close to the diaphragm. The detected Edi is then amplified by the NAVA level to provide respiratory support.

On day 12 and after 3 days of HFO ventilation her ventilation parameters were stable (mPaw 14 cmH_2O, frequency 10 Hz, ΔP 38 cmH_2O, FiO_2 0.4) and chest X-ray was improving. She was changed to conventional ventilation (pressure control, PEEP 8 cmH_2O, PIP 24 cmH_2O, RR 20 breaths per minute, FiO_2 0.5, Vt 6 mL/kg). PEG feeding was resumed at 60% of maintenance. On day 13 she had a negative fluid balance from admission, and her ventilation and sedation were weaned towards extubation. She had a good gag and cough reflex, and a respiratory drive but synchronization with the ventilator became challenging. She was therefore switched to invasive neurally adjusted ventilatory assist (NAVA) (PEEP 8 cmH_2O, NAVA level 1.5 cmH_2O/microV, FiO_2 0.4) and stabilised with little work of breathing and an Edi max around 15-20 microV.

❻ Expert comment Role of NAVA

NAVA as an assist mode has gained a lot of interest over the last years as this mode can reduce patient–ventilator asynchrony (inspiratory and expiratory) importantly and therefore improve patient comfort. Furthermore, the proportional assistance to the patient's effort, as measured by the electromyography signal of the diaphragm (Edi), allows to titrate an adequate pressure support level through a closed loop feedback by the patients respiratory drive: matching the support offered to the breath-to-breath demand made by the diaphragm. This closed-loop concept allows the patient to dictate his/her optimal Vt, i.e. the lower the respiratory system compliance, the lower the Vt but faster the breathing rate, and the better the compliance the larger the Vt and the lower the rate. These clinical observations from adults, children and neonates with and without a lung pathology renders the mode interesting for lung protective ventilation, as well as for gradually weaning the patient from the ventilator, especially in patients with acquired respiratory muscle fatigue. However, robust clinical data showing the superiority of this mode compared to other ventilation modes are still lacking.

➕ Clinical tip NAVA

If the patient's Edi is 16 microV and the chosen NAVA level 0.5 cmH$_2$O/microV, the delivered pressure over PEEP will be 8 cm H$_2$O (16 microV × 0.5 cmH$_2$O/microV). In order to adapt the NAVA level (range usually between 0.5 and 2 cmH$_2$O/microV), the Edi max should not exceed 20–25 microV, the achieved peak pressures sufficient, and the patient clinically comfortable with only little or no work of breathing.

On day 14, 7 days from admission, her ventilation support was low (PEEP 7 cmH$_2$O, NAVA level 0.6 cmH$_2$O/microV, FiO$_2$ 0.4, achieved PIPs 20 cmH$_2$O) and she was extubated to NIV NAVA (facial mask, PEEP 6 cmH$_2$O, NAVA level 1 cmH$_2$O/microV, FiO$_2$ 0.5, Edi max 20 microV, PIP achieved 14 cmH$_2$O) and woke up to her premorbid state. On day 16, she was weaned to a facial mask (2 L/min), which was stopped at day 19. She was finally discharged home at day 21, 14 days after admission and completed her course of antibiotic treatment for 14 days after the first negative blood culture.

❻ Expert comment Challenges

Since 1967, when David Ashbaugh first described ARDS, enormous technical advances in mechanical ventilation have been made and many experimental and clinical studies have addressed various ventilation strategies aiming to protect the lungs from further injury. However, we still struggle to know how to define and best treat this syndrome. This happened for several reasons:

1. It took a long time to understand mechanical characteristics of an ARDS lung, which was thought for many years to be stiff (poorly compliant), calling for the use of high airway pressure in an attempt to normalize gas exchange. We had to learn that the lung is not only stiff, but certainly functionally small (small aerable lung area). This warrants the use of smaller tidal volumes and airway pressure limitation, and therefore sometimes the need to allow for permissive hypercapnia.
2. Ashbaugh had observed in a 12-year-old boy for the first time that moderately adjusting the PEEP level might help to improve blood gases. Nonetheless, the use of higher PEEP levels remained uncommon in association with large tidal volumes and/or high inspiratory pressures, because of the associated risk of major barotrauma. It is only with the implementation of lower tidal volume targets that this risk has been drastically reduced and that PEEP and PEEP titration are being used more.
3. Repeated calls for unified simple guidelines on ventilator management (one number for all, e.g. one target tidal volume/kg body weight for all patients) have led to recommendations that still miss good evidence.[24,25] Additionally, these guidelines give misleading confidence and thus make it more difficult to question many claims regarding so-called lung protective ventilation strategies.
4. Various new and advanced ventilation modes (e.g. HFOV and various assist modes, including NAVA) have appeared over time and have been rapidly introduced in clinical practice without having any relevant outcome studies. This led to the use of multiple modes in various units, the individual unit's preference being based mainly on local routines and best beliefs of care providers. Designing good, meaningful, and well-powered multicentre trials is therefore extremely difficult.
5. In the absence of an appropriate severity scoring it has been difficult to stratify study populations optimally to render intervention studies more meaningful and to predict outcome. Recent revisions of ARDS definitions distinct for adults, children, and neonates may help to overcome this problem for future trials.
6. Studies investing into adjuvant strategies for PARDS have been weakened by various uncontrolled confounding factors (e.g. missing strictly applied ventilation protocols) and the absence of appropriate patient and disease severity stratification.

Discussion

Outcome of PARDS and recommended follow-up

PARDS mortality varies between 8% and 35%, but is, in general lower than in adults and PARDS is often not the (main) cause of death.[26] Adult long-term survivors have increased rates of post-traumatic stress disorder, depression, poor neurocognitive, and also poor pulmonary functions.[26] However, no substantial studies have been conducted to assess pulmonary and neurocognitive outcomes in children.

Therefore, PALICC recommends the following follow-ups in survivors of PARDS:[4]

Assessment of pulmonary outcome
- 1-year follow up (questionnaire, pulse oximetry; spirometry if possible).

Assessment of neurocognitive outcome:
- Evaluation of socio/physical/neurocognitive outcome after 3 months (or prior to school start).

Others outcome measures to be evaluated are suggested:[26]
- long-term mortality (e.g. 90 days); however, no substantial change compared to short-term survival is expected;
- new/progressive organ dysfunction;
- long-term emotional health, neurocognitive function, and quality of life;
- biometric outcomes.

A final word from the expert

Although the ARDSNet volume- and pressure-limited approach seems to be useful and might give, at least at this moment, the best information on how to guide mechanical ventilation in PARDS, more data are still needed to customize mechanical ventilation strategies in relation to the patient's individual condition. The most recently proposed concept of primarily limiting distending pressure (P_{dist} = PIP-PEEP),[16] ending up with relative wide, but patient- or disease-specific Vt ranges, and to dial in PEEP according to the oxygenation response following the PEEP/FiO_2 table from the ARDSNet, seems to be promising for PARDS.[4] However, it remains to be proven whether this might reduce mortality and improve functional outcome. Unfortunately, this will most likely be undertaken only on retrospective analyses from large registries, given the difficulties to do proper, well-powered RCTs in this field in children.

References

Suggested further reading **

** 1. Force ADT, Ranieri VM, Rubenfeld GD, et al. Acute respiratory distress syndrome: the Berlin Definition. *JAMA* 2012;307:2526–33.
  2. De Luca D, Piastra M, Chidini G, et al. The use of the Berlin definition for acute respiratory distress syndrome during infancy and early childhood: multicenter evaluation and expert consensus. *Intensive Care Med.* 2013;39:2083–91.
  3. Khemani RG, Thomas NJ, Venkatachalam V, et al. Comparison of SpO2 to PaO2 based markers of lung disease severity for children with acute lung injury. *Crit. Care Med.* 2012;40:1309–16.

4. Khemani RG, Parvathaneni K, Yehya N, Bhalla AK, Thomas NJ, Newth CJL. PEEP lower than the ARDS Network protocol is associated with higher pediatric ARDS mortality. *Am. J. Respir. Crit. Care Med.* 2018;198:77–89.

5. ARDSnet. ARDS Clinical Network Mechanical Ventilation Protocol Summary 2008. Available from: http://www.ardsnet.org/files/ventilator_protocol_2008-07.pdf (accessed 16 February 2017).

6. Pediatric Acute Lung Injury Consensus Conference Group. Pediatric acute respiratory distress syndrome: consensus recommendations from the Pediatric Acute Lung Injury Consensus Conference. *Pediatr. Crit. Care Med.* 2015;16:428–39.

7. Sinha IP, McBride AK, Smith R, Fernandes RM. CPAP and high-flow nasal cannula oxygen in bronchiolitis. *Chest* 2015;148:810–23.

8. Fioretto JR, Ribeiro CF, Carpi MF, et al. Comparison between noninvasive mechanical ventilation and standard oxygen therapy in children up to 3 years old with respiratory failure after extubation: a pilot prospective randomized clinical study. *Pediatr. Crit. Care Med.* 2015;16:124–30.

9. Yanez LJ, Yunge M, Emilfork M, et al. A prospective, randomized, controlled trial of noninvasive ventilation in pediatric acute respiratory failure. *Pediatr. Crit. Care Med.* 2008;9:484–9.

10. Piastra M, De Luca D, Marzano L, et al. The number of failing organs predicts non-invasive ventilation failure in children with ALI/ARDS. *Intensive Care Med.* 2011;37:1510–16.

11. Gupta P, Green JW, Tang X, et al. Comparison of high-frequency oscillatory ventilation and conventional mechanical ventilation in pediatric respiratory failure. *JAMA Pediatr.* 2014;168:243–9.

12. Bateman ST, Borasino S, Asaro LA, et al. Early high-frequency oscillatory ventilation in pediatric acute respiratory failure. a propensity score analysis. *Am. J. Respir. Crit. Care Med.* 2016;193:495–503.

13. Wallace DJ, Milbrandt EB, Boujoukos A. Ave, CESAR, morituri te salutant! (Hail, CESAR, those who are about to die salute you!). *Crit. Care* 2010;14:308.

14. Amato MB, Meade MO, Slutsky AS, et al. Driving pressure and survival in the acute respiratory distress syndrome. *N. Engl. J. Med.* 2015;372:747–55.

15. Gattinoni L, Pesenti A. The concept of "baby lung". *Intensive Care Med.* 2005;31:776–84.

16. Panico FF, Troster EJ, Oliveira CS, et al. Risk factors for mortality and outcomes in pediatric acute lung injury/acute respiratory distress syndrome. *Pediatr. Crit. Care Med.* 2015;16:e194–200.

17. Wiedemann HP, Wheeler AP, Bernard GR, et al. Comparison of two fluid-management strategies in acute lung injury. *N. Engl. J. Med.* 2006;354:2564–75.

18. Ingelse SA, Wosten-van Asperen RM, Lemson J, Daams JG, Bem RA, van Woensel JB. Pediatric acute respiratory distress syndrome: fluid management in the PICU. *Front Pediatr.* 2016;4:21.

19. Alhazzani W, Alshahrani M, Jaeschke R, et al. Neuromuscular blocking agents in acute respiratory distress syndrome: a systematic review and meta-analysis of randomized controlled trials. *Crit. Care* 2013;17:R43.

20. Wilsterman ME, de Jager P, Blokpoel R, et al. Short-term effects of neuromuscular blockade on global and regional lung mechanics, oxygenation and ventilation in pediatric acute hypoxemic respiratory failure. *Ann. Intensive Care* 2016;6:103.

21. Tamburro RF, Kneyber MC. Pulmonary specific ancillary treatment for pediatric acute respiratory distress syndrome: proceedings from the Pediatric Acute Lung Injury Consensus Conference. *Pediatr. Crit. Care Med.* 2015;16(5 Suppl. 1):S61–72.

22. Willson DF, Thomas NJ, Markovitz BP, et al. Effect of exogenous surfactant (calfactant) in pediatric acute lung injury: a randomized controlled trial. *JAMA* 2005;293:470–6.

23. Willson DF, Thomas NJ, Tamburro R, et al. Pediatric calfactant in acute respiratory distress syndrome trial. *Pediatr. Crit. Care Med.* 2013;14:657–65.

24. Rimensberger PC, Cheifetz IM, Kneyber MCJ. The top ten unknowns in paediatric mechanical ventilation. *Intensive Care Med.* 2018;44:366–70.

25. Kneyber MCJ, de Luca D, Calderini E, et al. Recommendations for mechanical ventilation of critically ill children from the Paediatric Mechanical Ventilation Consensus Conference (PEMVECC). *Intensive Care Med.* 2017;43:1764–80.
26. Yehya N, Thomas NJ. Relevant outcomes in pediatric acute respiratory distress syndrome studies. *Front Pediatr.* 2016;4:51.

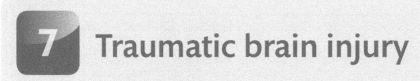

7 Traumatic brain injury

Lisa A. DelSignore

⏱ **Expert commentary** by Robert C. Tasker

Case history

A 10-year-old boy is brought into the Emergency Department (ED) by paramedics after a motor vehicle collision. He was a restrained backseat passenger in the car that was hit by another vehicle at an estimated speed of 40 miles per hour. He was unconscious at the scene, breathing shallowly, and was noted to have multiple facial lacerations and a frontal scalp contusion. Paramedics initiated assisted bag-mask ventilation en route to the hospital. A pulse was present. Upon arrival to the ED, his vital signs were temperature 37.7°C, heart rate (HR) 62 beats per minute (bpm), blood pressure (BP) 130/90 mmHg, respiratory rate (RR) 12 breaths per minute (assisted), pulse oximetry oxygen–haemoglobin saturation (SpO_2) 96% in room air. Neurological assessment revealed a Glasgow Coma Scale (GCS) score of 6 (motor response 4, verbal response 1, eye opening response 1) and symmetric, but sluggishly reactive pupils, sized 6 mm bilaterally.

⊗ **Learning point** Definition and epidemiology of traumatic brain injury

Traumatic brain injury (TBI) remains a major cause of morbidity and mortality in children, specifically in infants and older adolescents.[1] It is estimated that between 600 and 700 per 100,000 of the child population suffer from TBI annually, as estimated by ED populations from Western countries.[1] Based on the GCS at time of initial injury, TBI can be classified as mild (GCS ≥13), moderate (GCS 9–12), or severe (GCS ≤8).[2]

The primary injury in TBI is a direct result of trauma. This can involve a range of effects, including concussive symptoms (i.e. brain contusion), intracranial bleeding, or traumatic axonal injury. Secondary injuries after TBI include clinical problems, such as vasospasm, seizures, and refractory intracranial hypertension from cerebral oedema. Cerebral oedema is common in children with severe TBI, and therapy is targeted at reducing it by supporting optimal cerebral perfusion pressure (CPP). The type of cerebral oedema observed in TBI is multifactorial, reflecting a combination of vasogenic oedema and cellular oedema. Cerebral swelling peaks 24–72 hours after injury, but it can continue or worsen despite treatment depending on the severity and extent of brain injury.[3]

He was successfully intubated using rapid-sequence induction for airway protection, after which the head of his bed was placed upward at 30 degrees. He was ventilated to an end-tidal CO_2 ($etCO_2$) value of 35–40 mmHg, which correlated with the partial pressure of carbon dioxide ($paCO_2$) on his initial blood gas of 35–40 mmHg. His oxygen saturation by pulse oximetry post-intubation was 100% on a fraction of inspired oxygen (FiO_2) of 0.30 via mechanical ventilation. His initial laboratory work revealed a sodium level of 133 mEq/L (mmol/L), with otherwise normal electrolytes.

✪ Learning point Intracranial compliance, intracranial hypertension, and cerebral perfusion pressure

The skull can be imagined as having a fixed volume, one in which three components exist: brain tissue; blood vessels; and cerebrospinal fluid (CSF). If one of these components increases in volume, there may be some accommodation while maintaining a normal intracranial pressure (ICP). This concept is known as the Monro–Kellie hypothesis and involves intracranial compliance.[3] This adaptation results in transitioning cerebral venous blood volume (CBV) into the extracranial spinal plexus. However, once this accommodation is lost, a small increase in the volume of the contents within the skull will result in dramatic increases in ICP. In the brain, CPP is determined by inflow arterial pressure (mean arterial pressure (MAP)) and outflow pressure. The downstream pressure is taken as the ICP or jugular venous pressure (JVP), whichever is higher (CPP = MAP – ICP or JVP). Hence, increased ICP will lead to decreased CPP, and puts the brain at risk of hypoperfusion, ischaemia, and tissue infarction.

✪ Learning point Cerebral perfusion pressure and autoregulation

What becomes important to the brain during the stress of intracranial hypertension is its ability to maintain the cerebral metabolic rate for oxygen ($CMRO_2$).[4] Intracranial hypertension (or elevated ICP) necessitating treatment in acute settings is defined in both children and adults as an ICP >20 mmHg.[5,6] In contrast, we use age-specific CPP targets, as CPP is dependent on age-appropriate MAP. Optimal targets for CPP in children remain controversial. The most recent paediatric guidelines for severe TBI[5] suggest that a minimum CPP of 40 mmHg should be considered. In general, an overall goal range of 40–65 mmHg is accepted with the lower end target for infants and the upper end target for adolescents.[5]

Another important concept is cerebral autoregulation and the relationship between CPP and cerebral blood flow (CBF). Cerebral autoregulation is the brain's ability to maintain a constant CBF in order to ensure adequate oxygenation and nutrient delivery to tissues over a wide range of MAPs.[4] When the limits of lower and higher CPPs are exceeded, the brain loses its ability to maintain a constant CBF. When the lower limit of autoregulation is not maintained or achieved, CBF becomes directly related to CPP. As such, significant decreases in CBF can lead to brain tissue ischaemia and infarction. In contrast, large increases in CBF, which result from exceeding the upper limit of autoregulation, can lead to increased CBV, which negatively affects intracranial compliance and worsens intracranial hypertension.[4]

❖ Expert comment Cerebral blood flow and brain penumbra

Normal CBF ranges between 45 and 60 mL/100 g tissue/minute.[4,7] There are well-known neuronal time-dependent events that occur in response to significant decreases in CBF. For example, a CBF of less than 20 mL/100 g tissue/minute is associated with decreased consciousness but without impairment of electroencephalographic (EEG) activity. Once CBF drops below a critical threshold of 18 mL/100 g tissue/minute, neurons begin to convert from aerobic to anaerobic metabolism, EEG activity is altered, and tissue ischaemia is evident.[4,7] This degree of hypoperfusion may be reversible for up to 4 hours. Further decline in CBF to <10 mL/100 g tissue/minute results in disruption of neuronal cell membranes, loss of EEG activity, and time-dependent cell death. Extremely low values of CBF (e.g. 5 mL/100 g tissue/minute) result in neuronal death and tissue infarction if sustained.[7] Thus, timing of injury and quick management are crucial to preserving and providing adequate CBF and CPP.

Back to case

Given the patient's vital signs were consistent with increased ICP and impending brain herniation, in addition to a low serum sodium, a dose of 3% hypertonic saline was administered and cranial computed tomography (CT) imaging was obtained. The CT scan revealed a large right-sided subdural haematoma with associated midline shift, decreased ventricular size, and diffuse effacement of brain architecture (i.e. sulci and gyri). He was taken emergently to the operating suite by the neurosurgical team for subdural haematoma evacuation.

> **⊘ Learning point** Initial management strategies
>
> The key principles guiding initial management of children with severe TBI are optimization of CPP and an overall reduction of $CMRO_2$ to prevent further secondary brain injuries. Management of ongoing intracranial hypertension is essential and may mitigate brain herniation syndromes and death.
>
> There are both initial medical and surgical approaches to severe TBI management that should be enacted simultaneously. Immediate neurosurgical consultation is essential to determine if there is a need for emergency life-saving surgery, such as intracranial haematoma evacuation, or external ventricular drain (EVD) placement. An EVD will help augment CSF removal, in addition to functioning as an ICP monitor. The neurosurgical approaches mentioned will be discussed in further detail subsequently.
>
> With regard to managing intracranial hypertension, the paediatric guidelines for severe TBI[7] support targeting treatment of sustained (>5 minutes) ICP >20 mmHg. Evidence supporting this is relatively weak.[8] Given that there is no readily available and direct way of measuring a patient's CPP, ICP monitoring remains a surrogate target for the mainstay of treatment. However, it should be recognized that lower ICP, per se, is not necessarily a guarantee of better outcomes.
>
> **Medical approaches**
>
> A stepwise approach to normalization of physiological parameters that affect CBF, CBV, and $CMRO_2$ is imperative. Targeting a normal SpO_2 of 95–100% and normal ventilation, as defined by an arterial $paCO_2$ of 35–40 mmHg (4.7–5.3 kPa) with a pH of 7.35–7.4, are important to maintain appropriate CBF. Hypoxia can lead to cerebral vasodilation and thereby increase both CBF and CBV, which may exacerbate ongoing intracranial hypertension.[4,7]
>
> Hypercarbia and respiratory acidosis have a similar effect to hypoxia on cerebral blood vessels. Hypocarbia and respiratory alkalosis have the opposite effect and result in vasoconstriction. As such, both extremes of CO_2 balance and pH balance can be detrimental to CPP. Vasodilation will increase CBF and CBV, which can exacerbate elevated ICP. Vasoconstriction will decrease CBF and CBV, which can predispose the brain tissue to ischaemia and infarction.[9]
>
> Factors that primarily affect CBV include the position of the head of the bed, hyperosmolar therapy, and serum sodium levels. The patient's head of bed should be at 30 degrees up, to promote optimal venous drainage to help reduce oedema.[5,6] Hyperosmolar therapy using either hypertonic saline or mannitol helps to remove extra fluid from brain tissue. Overall, serum sodium balance is important to reduce cerebral oedema. Avoidance of hyponatraemia and targeting a serum sodium level of 140–155 mEq/L (mmol/L) are the current recommendations.[5,6]
>
> Lastly, decreasing $CMRO_2$ is an important overarching management principle in order to limit underlying brain injury.[7] Targeting a normal serum glucose level and normal temperature can assist in reducing $CMRO_2$ by minimizing stresses that make the brain more metabolically active.[5,6]
>
> Avoidance of fever is essential, with a goal temperature range of 36–37.5°C.[5] Further $CMRO_2$ reduction can be accomplished by keeping patients well sedated and often on neuromuscular blocking agents while intubated.
>
> Up to this point, the initial strategies discussed have primarily targeted reducing the ICP side of the CPP equation. There are also ways to augment MAP to target optimal CPP; firstly, by ensuring adequate intravascular volume, and, secondly, by using vasoactive medications that primarily increase vascular tone, such as norepinephrine or phenylephrine. It is generally recommended to target a MAP near the 90–95th percentile for age and height.[5] It is imperative to avoid hypotension, which can lead to a reduction in CPP and CBF, which predisposes the brain to ischaemia and infarction.

> **⊕ Clinical tip** Hyperventilation
>
> Controlled mild hyperventilation ($paCO_2$ 30–35 mmHg) is a management strategy that can be considered for refractory increased ICP in an emergency where the patient is at risk of impending herniation and surgery is planned. It is not part of routine initial management given the risk of ischaemia and stroke.[4,9]

➕ **Clinical tip** Mannitol

Recommended mannitol dosing ranges are a bolus dose of 0.5–1 g/kg intravenously and maintenance dosing of 0.25 g/kg every 6 hours. Clinicians should use discretion when administering mannitol and consider simultaneous normal saline fluid bolus administration so as to maintain intravascular volume. Monitoring serum osmolality (≤320 mOsm/L) is crucial to avoid mannitol-induced nephrotoxicity.

❝ Expert comment Hyperosmolar therapy

Hyperosmolar therapy works by creating an osmolar gradient across an intact membrane; in this case, the blood–brain barrier (BBB). This allows for the movement of water out of brain tissue and into the intravascular space where it can be resorbed into the systemic venous circulation. The two major pharmacological therapies that have been used traditionally in the management of cerebral oedema are mannitol and hypertonic saline. It is likely that these agents function in regions of the brain where the BBB remains intact, as opposed to where the primary brain injury has occurred, thus allowing for overall global removal of excess brain tissue oedema.[10]

Mannitol decreases ICP by both its rheological and osmolar properties. Mannitol's rheological properties work by reducing blood viscosity, thereby reducing CBV. This effect has a quick onset of action, but is transient. However, the osmotic effect of mannitol persists for a longer period of time but has a slower onset of action.[10]

The side effects of mannitol include hypotension and nephrotoxicity. Hypotension can counteract mannitol's beneficial effect of reducing the ICP by decreasing the CPP. The underlying mechanism of nephrotoxicity is poorly understood but is thought to be a combination of dehydration, resultant tubular necrosis, and exacerbation of any underlying chronic kidney injuries.[10]

Hypertonic saline (3%, 7.5%, 23%) has also been used as an osmolar agent for intracranial hypertension management. The BBB is more impermeable to hypertonic saline than mannitol owing to its higher capillary reflection coefficient (1 vs 0.9). Therefore, hypertonic saline has the ability to create a stronger osmotic gradient.[10] In contrast to mannitol, hypertonic saline expands intravascular volume and thus has an added beneficial effect on CPP by improving MAP. Hypertonic saline may be administered intravenously as a bolus dose or continuous infusion. Given its hypertonicity and risk of peripheral vein necrosis, central venous access is the preferred route of administration.[5,6]

The side effects of hypertonic saline are minimal, but complications include acute renal failure and haematological abnormalities. Acute respiratory distress may develop once serum sodium approximates 170 mEq/L (mmol/L).[11] Caution must be taken when weaning continuous hypertonic saline infusions to avoid acute, precipitous drops in sodium, which can lead to hyponatraemia, rebound cerebral oedema, and seizures. Rapid rise in sodium during the initiation of continuous infusions carries a risk of developing central pontine myelinolysis.

Increasingly, hypertonic saline has become the preferred osmotherapy for paediatric intensivists because of its favourable reflection coefficient and ability to increase intravascular volume. However, one must consider that as vasogenic oedema worsens, the BBB becomes increasingly disrupted, which reduces the potential and effectiveness of hypertonic saline to function as a potent osmotic agent.[10] Clear evidence supporting the use of one osmolar agent over another for the management of cerebral oedema in TBI continues to be lacking.[12] The decision to use either agent remains at the discretion of the caring physician.

➕ **Clinical tip** Hypertonic saline

Bolus doses of 3% saline are usually given in 1–3 mL/kg aliquots, which will raise the serum sodium level by 1–3 mEq/L (mmol/L). A central line is the preferred route of administration for hypertonic saline, especially as a continuous infusion. Continuous infusions of 3% saline can be initiated at 1–2 mEq/kg/h (mmol/kg/h), but clinicians should refer to their specific institutional pharmacy guidelines to address further titrations and continue to monitor frequent serum sodium values to target a goal sodium level of 140–155 mEq/L (mmol/L). It is preferable to keep the serum sodium level at < 160 mEq/L (mmol/L).

✔ Evidence base Nutritional support

Early, optimal nutrition is indicated for patients with severe TBI. This intervention has been correlated with decreased mortality and improved long-term outcomes in both paediatric and adult populations.[5,6] The current guidelines recommend initiating nutrition with titration to goal caloric requirements within 5–7 days after injury.[5,6] Adult guidelines support the use of enteral feeds using the small bowel in intubated patients, to reduce the risk of aspiration pneumonia further.[6]

Recent evidence suggests that early initiation of enteral feeding, i.e. within 48 hours of injury, may further improve outcomes, as demonstrated by an improvement in Glasgow Outcome Scales in a small paediatric cohort study before and after the initiation of early enteral feeding.[13]

Back to the case

The subdural haematoma was evacuated, and an EVD was placed for ongoing CSF drainage and intermittent ICP monitoring. Arterial and central venous lines were placed by the anaesthesiologist in the operating suite. The child was brought to the

Paediatric Intensive Care Unit (PICU) postoperatively for ongoing management. Vital signs on arrival to the PICU were as follows: temperature, 37.5°C; HR, 72 bpm; BP, 135/85 mmHg; RR, 20 breaths per minute (assisted); SpO_2, 100% on FiO_2 0.30 via conventional mechanical ventilation. He was well sedated with morphine, midazolam infusions and muscle relaxed with a vecuronium infusion. He was not on any vasoactive infusions. The nurse transduced his ICP monitor, which read 25 mmHg with a good waveform.

> ✪ **Learning point** Neurological monitoring
>
> ICP monitoring in patients with severe TBI is recommended for those who meet the criteria of a GCS <9 after initial resuscitation and have an abnormal CT scan with salvageable injuries.[5,6] ICP monitoring can be conducted by a variety of devices placed by a neurosurgeon. The accuracy and precision of ICP monitoring are dependent on the anatomical location of monitor placement. The gold-standard approach is to place an EVD in the lateral ventricles, which is externally attached to a pressure transducer, using gravity to properly zero at the level of the tragus in a 30-degree head-up position for an accurate reading.[14]
>
> Other ICP monitors include catheter-tipped microtransducers, which can be placed in a variety of locations, including the ventricles, subdural space, and intraparenchymal space (e.g. Camino ICP Bolt (Camino Laboratories, San Diego, CA, USA); Codman Microsensor (Johnson & Johnson Professional, Raynam, MA, USA)).[14] These monitors do not have the added capability of draining CSF and may result in unreliable ICP measurements as the calibration may drift by ± 2 mmHg/day. Complications of ICP monitors include risk of infection (especially EVDs), bleeding, CSF overdrainage (EVD), and technical equipment malfunctions.[14]

> ✔ **Evidence base** Intracranial pressure monitoring and outcome
>
> A challenge of ICP monitoring includes its unclear relationship with patient outcomes in severe TBI. Several observational studies favour decreased mortality rates in patients with severe TBI and ICP monitors, but in addition to having no control group comparisons, the presence of an ICP monitor was also associated with increased morbidities, including longer Intensive Care Unit (ICU) stays, longer overall hospital duration, and increased ventilator days.[15] One large randomized trial aimed to evaluate the treatment efficacy and outcomes in patients with severe TBI (≥ 13 years) by ICP monitor-targeted therapy of <20 mmHg. It failed to demonstrate a significant difference in mortality and functional neurological outcomes (at 3 and 6 months) between patients in the ICP-monitor targeted therapy group and patients in the group with treatment based on clinical or cranial imaging findings suggestive of elevated ICP.[8] Other recent studies also continue to demonstrate that the use of ICP monitoring in patients with severe TBI is variable, despite guideline recommendations for use.[5,6]

> ❝ **Expert comment** Advanced neuromonitoring
>
> Advanced neuromonitoring modalities remain in their infancy, but are exciting opportunities for ongoing development and future neurocritical care application. A few small studies examined the use of localized brain tissue monitoring oxygenation and cerebral microdialysis of glutamate to determine what target thresholds may be related to outcomes.[4] According to one adult study, partial pressure brain tissue oxygen (PbO_2) values <15 mmHg for long durations (>30 minutes) appeared to be associated with higher mortality rates.[3]
>
> Additional modalities that non-invasively measure information related to CBF and CPP, such as transcranial Doppler ultrasound and cerebral near-infrared spectroscopy, are lacking in evidence to support routine use. Transcranial Doppler ultrasound has been used to identify cerebral vasospasm in severe TBI by measuring blood flow velocities at various points in the cardiac cycle in the location of the middle cerebral artery.[16] Higher flow velocities are associated with narrowed vessel lumens, and

thus are used as a proxy to define the degree of vasospasm and to identify areas of brain tissue prone to ischaemia that may become infarcted if left untreated. Several recent studies have used adult criteria to define cerebral vasospasm in children with severe TBI, citing the presence of vasospasm in these children to be ~30–60%.[16,17] Further research and characterization of blood flow velocities through similar vessels in children is needed to both validate adult findings and establish paediatric definitions of vasospasm.

✅ Evidence base Seizure monitoring and antiepileptic drug prophylaxis

Seizures can occur after severe TBI; however, current guidelines do not recommend the routine use of prophylactic antiepileptic drugs (AEDs) given limited data to support use.[5] Children are known to have lower seizure thresholds than adults, especially infants, and, as such, more often have continuous EEG (cEEG) monitoring applied.

A group of investigators conducted a survey to establish current practices regarding the use of cEEG monitoring, AED medication prophylaxis, and treatment.[18] The majority of PICUs had the capability of performing cEEG but used it less than one-third of the time for patients with severe TBI.[18] Prophylactic AED use appeared to occur more frequently than the use of cEEG monitoring.[18,19] The use of cEEG monitoring increased for patients who were considered at highest risk of developing post-traumatic seizures, namely infants who were suspected of suffering non-accidental head trauma, or infants and children with subdural haemorrhages.[19,20] The majority of seizures observed on cEEG were subclinical, making it difficult to determine what the clinical impact on long-term neurological outcomes might be.[20] All clinical seizures were treated universally with AEDs, with specific agents varying across clinical settings.[18,19] More data are needed to define how AED use and cEEG monitoring can be best done for children with severe TBI to optimize long-term outcomes.

Back to the case

The patient's ICP improved after a sedation bolus and a bolus of hypertonic saline (3%). Intermittent hypertonic saline doses were needed in the last few hours. Several hours passed. The bedside nurse notified us that the ICP monitor is reporting a sustained rise in ICP of 30 mmHg with a good waveform. She has given additional boluses of sedative medications with no change. There have been no other changes in the patient's vital signs. The etCO$_2$ value was 38 mmHg and the last sodium level was 152 mEq/L (mmol/L) after multiple 3% saline boluses. The nurse asked what to do next to treat the persistently elevated ICP.

➕ Learning point Management of refractory intracranial hypertension in traumatic brain injury: second-tier therapies

For paediatric patients with severe TBI and ongoing elevated ICP despite optimization of the first-tier therapies, several second-tier therapies can be considered. Most of these therapies lack sufficient evidence to make strong recommendations regarding management that affect outcomes. The therapies that will be discussed individually include barbiturate therapy, controlled hyperventilation, controlled mild hypothermia, decompressive craniectomy, and lumbar CSF drainage.[5,6] These therapies have the theoretical possibility of either targeting a reduction in ICP or a reduction in CMRO$_2$.

💬 Expert comment Discussion of second-tier therapies in the management of refractory intracranial hypertension: part 1

Barbiturate therapy

Barbiturates (e.g. pentobarbital) decrease ICP by decreasing the CMRO$_2$. The lowest dose of medication that reduces the ICP to an acceptable range (<20 mmHg) should be used in order to prevent the occurrence of unwarranted medication side effects. Barbiturates are negative inotropes and can result in hypotension, decreased cardiac output, or poor systemic perfusion. Vasoactive infusions may be needed if high doses of barbiturates are needed to control elevated ICP. Typically, patients who have elevated ICP despite maximal doses of barbiturates have poor outcomes.[21] Some small retrospective studies suggest that control of ICP with barbiturate therapy may result in acceptable long-term outcomes in both adults and children. Hence, it continues to remain a potential therapy for refractory ICP.[21]

Controlled hyperventilation

Several decades ago, hyperventilation was considered a first-tier therapy in the management of elevated ICP in TBI owing to its quick effect on cerebral vasculature and CBV reduction. It became less favourable since patients with sustained hypocarbia (paCO$_2$ <25mmHg) were found to have worse outcomes, likely owing to the effects of hypoperfusion and resultant ischaemia resulting in permanent neurological deficits.[9] One study reviewing a cohort of paediatric patients with severe TBI found all patients to have decreased CBF post-injury, which was worsened by lower $paCO_2$ level ($paCO_2$ <25mmHg or 3.3 kPa) and corresponded with increased areas of regional brain tissue ischaemia versus children with normocarbia ($paCO_2$ >35mmHg).[5,6]

Therapeutic hypothermia

Several studies in animal models and newborns with hypoxic–ischaemic encephalopathy have demonstrated potential mortality benefits from therapeutic hypothermia initiated within 24–48 hours post-injury; however, these effects have not been reproduced in TBI.[22,23] Given that recent studies in both adults and children with severe TBI have failed to demonstrate a mortality benefit,[22,23] the most recent guidelines[7] recommend routine avoidance of therapeutic hypothermia prophylactically for paediatric patients with a TBI. However, they continue to recommend it as a potential therapy for those patients with refractory intracranial hypertension and no contraindications to hypothermia. The current guidelines[5] suggest the use of moderate hypothermia (32–33°C) initiated for 48 hours, while also recommending that patients are not rewarmed any faster than 0.5°C per hour in order to avoid rewarming complications, such as hypotension.

Further investigation regarding the use of therapeutic hypothermia as management for refractory increased intracranial hypertension is needed, as several recent studies have demonstrated conflicting data and significant confounding variables regarding its application and use.[24] For now, it continues to remain a second-tier therapy to consider for refractory increased ICP at the discretion of the caring clinician.

> **⊘ Evidence base**   Hypothermia in traumatic brain injury
>
> A recent meta-analysis reviewing paediatric TBI hypothermia trials suggested that, based on the heterogeneity of studies and related variance in definitions of hypothermia, rates of rewarming, and other variables, there may be no difference in mortality between paediatric patients with a TBI who are treated with hypothermia versus those treated with normothermia.[24] Further analysis of trials included in this study suggested that in patients treated with hypothermia, there may be a greater relative risk of death than in those who were normothermic.[24] However, given the low-quality data and study heterogeneity, more research is needed to better characterize the role and risk of hypothermia in paediatric patients with a severe TBI.

Back to the case

The patient's periodic elevated ICP spikes were treated with intermittent bolus doses of intravenous pentobarbital. Within 3 days of initiating this refractory therapy, the patient's ICP trend improved and his ICP monitor was removed by the neurosurgery team. In the subsequent days, the PICU team was able to de-escalate the medical management that had been initiated for elevated ICP. The patient was successfully extubated on day 7 of his hospitalization.

> **ⓕ Expert comment**   Discussion of second-tier therapies in the management of refractory intracranial hypertension: part 2
>
> **Decompressive craniectomy**
>
> In an effort to allow more volume for the brain to swell and thereby reduce ICP, decompressive craniectomy has been considered as a strategy to manage intracranial hypertension in patients with a severe TBI. This surgical procedure involves temporary removal of part of the skull and may involve opening the underlying dura mater. Patients undergo future cranial reconstruction using either the portion of the bone that was removed or another type of synthetic implant once recovered.[25]

> **➕ Clinical tip**   Barbiturates
>
> Barbiturate medications are often used as either intermittent dosing or continuous infusion to achieve a deep level of sedation. Patients should be placed on cEEG monitoring, as many patients require medication titration to burst suppression for adequate control of refractory elevated ICP.[21]

Restoring CPP by surgically enlarging the intracranial space is the primary goal and rationale for performing this procedure.

Several studies to date have investigated the role of decompressive craniectomy and its ability to reduce elevated ICP, decrease length of hospital stay, and improve overall mortality and 6-month functional neurological outcomes.[25,26] A few studies have investigated the impact of performing this surgery 'early' (i.e. within 24 hours post-injury) as opposed to 'late', reserving it as a strategy for management of refractory increased ICP.[25] Consistent with other second-tier therapies described, sufficient evidence-base is lacking to define a clear consensus on the benefit of this therapy in both paediatric and adult patients.[5,6]

⊘ Evidence base RESCUEicp trial

A group of TBI researchers recently published the results of their trial, which randomized patients aged 10–65 years with refractory elevated ICP (defined as >25 mmHg for 12 hours post-medical management of injury), to either undergo decompressive craniectomy or continue to receive ongoing medical care.[26] In contrast to the prior adult study,[25] their findings showed a reduction in overall 6-month mortality in the group of patients who underwent decompressive craniectomy.[26] However, that group had a higher incidence of more severe neurological disability and vegetative states in those who survived to 6 months. Patients with moderate-to-good functional neurological outcome scores at 6 months were similar between the two groups.[26] Thus, although this trial demonstrates an improvement in mortality in those patients undergoing decompressive craniectomy for refractory elevated ICP, families and healthcare providers will need to consider the patient's quality of life versus quantity of life when counselling families on this option.

⊕ Expert comment (continued)

Both sets of current guidelines[5,6] advise that there may be a role for decompressive craniectomy in the management of refractory increased ICP in severe TBI, but that it is not recommended to improve patient outcomes. In summary, decompressive craniectomy has been associated with lowering ICP values and decreasing length of ICU stay, but more data are needed to provide stronger recommendations regarding the timing and use of decompressive craniectomy as a management strategy for severe TBI.[5,6,25,26]

Back to the case

After extubation, the patient was able to follow verbal commands appropriately but continued to have difficulty with executive functioning, cognitive processing and memory, and emotional lability. He was discharged from the hospital to an acute inpatient rehabilitation facility within a week of extubation for both physical and neurocognitive rehabilitation. His first follow-up outpatient neurology appointment was scheduled for 1 month after discharge.

Discussion

Unsurprisingly, severe TBI has been associated with the poorest outcomes in children, often resulting in permanent brain damage or death. The main focus has been placed on initial injury prevention. However, the aims of early interventions that may prevent ongoing secondary injuries are important, too. The overall management strategies for prevention of secondary injuries are optimization of CPP and reduction of $CMRO_2$. A stepwise approach for control of intracranial hypertension, as suggested earlier and summarized in Table 7.1, forms the basis of management in severe TBI in the PICU.

Table 7.1 Summary of management strategies for severe traumatic brain injury

First-tier therapies	Second-tier therapies
Neurosurgical consult for emergency surgery or ICP monitor/EVD placement	Barbiturate therapy
Target SpO$_2$ 95–100%	Controlled hyperventilation (paCO$_2$ 30–35 mmHg (4.0–4.7 kPa))
Target pH 7.35–7.40	Controlled hypothermia (32–33°C)
Target paCO$_2$ 35–40 mmHg (4.7–5.3 kPa)	Decompressive craniectomy
Head of bed 30° upright	
Target normal serum glucose (80–180 mg/dL)	
Target temperature 36–37.5°C	
Target MAP 90–95th % for age/height	
Target serum sodium 140–155 mEq/L (mmol/L)	
Hyperosmolar therapy	
Sedation and/or muscle relaxants	

ICP, intracranial pressure; EVD, external ventricular drain; SpO$_2$, peripheral capillary oxygen saturation; paCO$_2$, partial pressure of paCO$_2$; MAP, mean arterial pressure.

A final word from the expert

Severe TBI remains a leading cause of major morbidity and mortality in critically ill children who have suffered head trauma. Insufficient high-quality evidence continues to bedevil the idea of promoting one single best management strategy for children with severe TBI given the heterogeneity of the underlying disease process. What can be taken away from this discussion is the concept that 'time is brain', and that close intensive care monitoring and early, stepwise medical and surgical interventions are key to managing these patients in order to optimize CPP and minimize secondary insults. Future directions should focus on advanced monitoring strategies or therapies that may be associated with both improved short- and long-term neurocognitive outcomes, as optimizing children's quality of life and ability to mature as functional adults are vital.

References

1. Taylor CA, Bell JM, Breiding MJ, et al. Traumatic brain injury-related emergency department visits, hospitalizations, and deaths—United States, 2007 and 2013. *MMWR Surveill. Summ.* 2017;66:1–16.
2. Teasdale G, Jennet B, Murray L, et al. Glasgow Coma Scale: to sum or not to sum? *Lancet* 1983;2:678.
3. Mokri B. The Monro–Kellie hypothesis: applications in CSF volume depletion. *Neurology* 2001;56:1746–8.
4. Udomphorn Y, Armstead WM, Vavilala MS. Cerebral blood flow and autoregulation after pediatric traumatic brain injury. *Pediatr. Neurol.* 2008;38:225–34.
5. Kochanek PM, Carney N, Adelson PD, et al. Guidelines for the acute medical management of severe traumatic brain injury in infants, children, and adolescents—second edition. *Pediatr. Crit. Care Med.* 2012;13(suppl. 1):S1–82.
6. Carney N, Totten AM, O'Reilly C, et al. Guidelines for the management of severe traumatic brain injury, fourth edition. *Neurosurgery* 2017;80:6–15.

7. Verweij BH, Amelink GJ, Muizelaar JP. Current concepts of cerebral oxygen transport and energy metabolism after severe traumatic brain injury. *Prog. Brain Res.* 2007;161:111–24.

8. Chestnut RM, Temkin, N, Carney N, et al. A trial of intracranial-pressure monitoring in traumatic brain injury. *N. Engl. J. Med.* 2012;367:2471–81.

9. Skippen P, Seear M, Poskitt K, et al. Effect of hyperventilation on regional cerebral blood flow in head-injured children. *Crit. Care Med.* 1997;25:1402–9.

10. Tasker RC. Pre- and postoperative management of the neurosurgical patient. In: Cohen AJ (ed.) *Pediatric Neurosurgery: Tricks of the Trade*, 1st edition. New York: Thieme Medical Publishers; 2016, pp. 30–50.

11. Gonda DD, Meltzer HS, Crawford JR, et al. Complications associated with prolonged hypertonic saline therapy in children with elevated intracranial pressure. *Pediatr. Crit. Care Med.* 2013;14:610–20.

12. Kamel H, Navi BB, Nakagawa K, et al. Hypertonic saline versus mannitol for the treatment of elevated intracranial pressure: a meta-analysis of randomized clinical trials. *Crit. Care Med.* 2011;39:554–59.

13. Chiang YH, Chao DP, Chu SF, et al. Early enteral nutrition and clinical outcomes of severe traumatic brain injury patients in acute stage: a multi-center cohort study. *J. Neurotrauma* 2012;29:75–80.

14. Riordan M, Chin L. Intracranial pressure monitors. *Atlas Oral Maxillofacial Surg. Clin. N. Am.* 2015;23:147–50.

15. Alkhoury F, Kyriakides TC. Intracranial pressure monitoring in children with severe traumatic brain injury. *JAMA Surg.* 2014;149:544–48.

16. LaRovere KL, O'Brien NF, Tasker RC. Current opinion and use of transcranial Doppler ultrasonography in traumatic brain injury in the pediatric intensive care unit. *J. Neurotrauma* 2016;33:2015–114.

17. O'Brien NF, Maa T, Yeates KO. The epidemiology of vasospasm in children with moderate-to-severe traumatic brain injury. *Crit. Care Med.* 2014;43:674–85.

18. Kurz JE, Poloyac SM, Abend NS, et al. Variation in anticonvulsant selection and electroencephalographic monitoring following severe traumatic brain injury in children—understanding resource availability in sites participating in a comparative effectiveness study. *Pediatr. Crit. Care Med.* 2016;17:649–57.

19. Ruzas CM, DeWitt PE, Bennett KS, et al. EEG monitoring and antiepileptic drugs in children with severe TBI. *Neurocrit. Care* 2017;26:256–66.

20. O'Neill BR, Handler MH, Tong S, et al. Incidence of seizures on continuous EEG monitoring following traumatic brain injury in children. *J. Neurosurg. Pediatr.* 2015;16:167–76.

21. Roberts I, Sydeham E. Barbiturates for acute traumatic brain injury. *Cochrane Database Syst. Rev.* 2012;12:CD000033.

22. Hutchinson JS, Ward RE, Lacroix J, et al. Hypothermia therapy after traumatic brain injury in children. *N. Engl. J. Med.* 2008;358:2447–56.

23. Adelson PD, Wisniewski SR, Beca J, et al. Comparison of hypothermia and normothermia after severe traumatic brain injury in children (Cool Kids): a phase 3, randomised controlled trial. *Lancet Neurol.* 2013;12:546–53.

24. Tasker RC, Vonberg FW, Ulano ED, et al. Updating evidence for using hypothermia in pediatric severe traumatic brain injury: conventional and Bayesian meta-analytic perspectives. *Pediatr. Crit. Care Med.* 2017;18:355–62.

25. Cooper DJ, Rosenfeld JV, Murray L, et al. Decompressive craniectomy in diffuse traumatic brain injury. *N. Engl. J. Med.* 2011;364:1493–502.

26. Hutchinson PJ, Kolias AG, Timofeev EA, et al. Trial of decompressive craniectomy for traumatic intracranial hypertension. *N. Engl. J. Med.* 2016;375:1119–30.

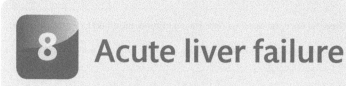

8 Acute liver failure

Andrew Jones

Expert commentary by Akash Deep

Case history

A previously healthy 11-year-old boy presented to his local Accident and Emergency (A&E) with a 2-week history of lethargy, diarrhoea, and vomiting. In the 5 days preceding presentation, he had become increasingly icteric, with abdominal distension and pale stools.

On assessment in A&E, he was maintaining his own airway and was breathing comfortably in air. He was warm and vasodilated, with a central and peripheral capillary refill time of less than 2 seconds. His heart rate was 90 beats per minute, he was in sinus rhythm, and a cuff blood pressure from the right arm was 118/55. His abdomen was distended but non-tender with hepatosplenomegaly. He was obviously jaundiced. His neurological status was of concern—he was sleepy, confused, and disorientated in time and place, with incomprehensible speech.

A panel of routine blood tests was performed. Of note, total bilirubin was 514 μmol/L, aspartate aminotransferase was 11,001 U/L, alkaline phosphatase (ALP) was 25 IU/L, platelet count was 43×10^9/L, and his international normalized ratio (INR) was >9.

The diagnostic criteria were met for paediatric acute liver failure (PALF). After discussion with the regional retrieval service he was intubated following a rapid sequence induction and was transferred safely to a Paediatric Intensive Care Unit (PICU) in a national paediatric liver unit.

> **Learning point** Grading hepatic encephalopathy in the child
>
> Hepatic encephalopathy (HE) is classified into four grades using a modification of the West Haven criteria (Table 8.1).[1] After the initial clinical assessment, the child should be regularly reassessed for progression of symptoms and signs. Encephalopathy is rare in the younger child, and more challenging to grade accurately. Modified criteria exist for children under 4 years of age.

Table 8.1 Grades of hepatic encephalopathy (West Haven criteria, modified to include children under 4 years of age)

		Grade			
		I	II	III	IV
Symptoms	≥4 years	Periods of lethargy, euphoria; reversal of day–night sleeping; may be alert	Drowsiness, inappropriate behaviour, agitation, wide mood swings, disorientation	Stupor but arousable, confused, incoherent speech	Coma
					IVa responds to noxious stimuli
	<4 years	Inconsolable crying, inattention to tasks, child is not acting like self to parents		Stupor, somnolence, combativeness	**IVb** no response
Signs	≥4 years	Trouble drawing figures, performing mental tasks	Asterixis, fetor hepaticus, incontinence	Asterixis, hyper-reflexia, extensor reflexes, rigidity	Areflexia, no asterixis, flaccidity
	<4 years	Normal or hyper-reflexic. Other neurological signs are difficult to test			
EEG	≥4 years	Normal	Generalized slowing, θ waves	Markedly abnormal, triphasic waves	Markedly abnormal bilateral slowing, δ waves, electrocortical silence
	<4 years	Difficult to test and interpret			

EEG, electroencephalogram.
Source: data from Conn HO. Quantifying the severity of hepatic encephalopathy. In: Conn HO, Bircher J [Eds] Hepatic encephalopathy: syndromes and therapies, pp. 13–26, Copyright (1994) Medi-Ed Press.

> **❝ Expert comment** Defining acute liver failure
>
> Acute liver failure (ALF) has now replaced previous terms such as fulminant hepatic failure or fulminant hepatitis.[2] The definition used in adults stipulates the onset of HE and coagulopathy within 8 weeks of the onset of symptoms in a patient with a previously healthy liver. These adult descriptions are, however, inappropriate for defining ALF in children:
>
> 1. ALF in children may present without clinical evidence of HE. Furthermore, HE can be difficult to recognize and diagnose in children.
> 2. ALF can present in neonates, rendering the 8-week onset time obsolete.
> 3. Uncorrectable coagulopathy is the essential, consistent, reliable finding in children with ALF, with or without encephalopathy. In adults, deranged coagulation, without encephalopathy with evidence of hepatitis is termed *acute liver injury*, not ALF.
> 4. ALF may be the first manifestation of an underlying unrecognized metabolic problem, which is usually associated with a variable degree of chronic liver injury, such as Wilson's disease (WD), inborn errors of metabolism, and Reye syndrome. ALF in children may reveal an underlying chronic liver disease.
>
> Paediatric ALF is thus best described as a clinical syndrome associated with massive necrosis of liver cells or sudden, severe impairment of liver function, with or without HE developing in an individual with no recognized chronic liver disease. The Pediatric Acute Liver Failure Study Group used the following criteria:[3]
>
> 1. No evidence of a known chronic liver disease.
> 2. Biochemical evidence of acute liver injury.
> 3. Hepatic-based coagulopathy that is not corrected by parenteral administration of vitamin K:
>   ○ HE must be present if the uncorrected prothrombin time (PT) or international normalized ratio (INR) is between 15 and 19.9 seconds or 1.5 to 1.9, respectively;
>   ○ HE was not required if the PT or INR was ≥20 seconds or 2.0, respectively.

Some authors have subclassified ALF into distinct groups: hyperacute liver failure; acute liver failure; and subacute liver failure. The rapidity of onset provides a clinician with valuable clues about probable aetiology and may predict outcome. In brief, a short interval between symptoms or jaundice and encephalopathy (like acetaminophen-induced ALF and some hepatitis A aetiologies) is associated with the high risk of brain oedema and greater possibility of spontaneous recovery, whereas a long interval is associated with a lower frequency of brain oedema but lower survival.

The term 'acute-on-chronic liver failure' is used widely in adults; however, there is no clear consensus on its definition. It is generally used to indicate rapid deterioration of a pre-existent chronic liver disease, which has high short-term mortality.

💠 **Learning point**   Resuscitation and retrieval of the child with ALF

Optimal early intensive care management will help to maximize the chance of recovery of native liver function or post-transplant survival. The aim should be to stabilize and transfer early before the onset of uncontrolled bleeding or rapidly deteriorating encephalopathy.

In addition to normal intensive care measures, the following specific management points should be considered.

Airway and breathing

Consider intubation if >grade 1 encephalopathy (to facilitate neuroprotection), fluid refractory shock, or pulmonary oedema. Avoid induction agents that cause hypotension (propofol and thiopentone). If encephalopathic give 3 mL/kg 2.7% hypertonic saline pre-induction. Aim for an SpO_2 of >96%. Use the minimum peak inspiratory pressure for an end-tidal CO_2 of 4–5 kPa.

Circulation

Use standard fluid resuscitation with 20 mL/kg aliquots. A central line will be needed. The first-line vasoactive drug is noradrenaline (norepinephrine). If cardiac function is poor, add adrenaline (epinephrine) or dopamine. Consider 2 mg/kg intravenous (IV) hydrocortisone for refractory shock. For vasoplegia refractory to noradrenaline, consider vasopressin or its synthetic analogue terlipressin. If encephalopathic, target a mean arterial pressure of >70 mmHg if >4 years old, >60 mmHg if <4 years old, and >50 mmHg if <1 year old.

Fluids

Avoid hypotonic fluids and restrict to 60% maintenance. Place a urinary catheter. Target a blood glucose of 4–7 mmol/L. If persistently hypoglycaemic increase the glucose concentration.

Neurology

Use morphine/fentanyl and midazolam for analgesia/sedation. Treat seizures with IV phenytoin. If hypertensive, bradycardic, or there are pupillary abnormalities, assume raised intracranial pressure (ICP) and treat with 2.7% sodium chloride (3 mL/kg) and/or mannitol (0.5 mg/kg). Note that fixed, dilated pupils may be reversible.

Haematology

Correct coagulation with vitamin K 1 mg/kg IV (up to a maximum of 10 mg), fresh frozen plasma (FFP) 10 mL/kg, cryoprecipitate 5 mL/kg, and platelets 15 mL/kg. Consider recombinant factor VIIa 80 µg/kg if there is persistent, uncontrolled bleeding. Ensure fibrinogen >1 g/L. If there is gastrointestinal bleeding (likely variceal) give an IV proton pump inhibitor, octreotide 1 µg/kg bolus followed by an infusion at 1–3 µg/kg/hour.

Renal

Acute kidney injury (AKI) may occur due to shock or hepatorenal syndrome. Maintain a urine output of >1 mL/kg/hour. Use furosemide if necessary. Correct dyselectrolytaemia.

Case history (continued)

Following an uneventful transfer by the regional retrieval service, the patient was stabilized by the paediatric intensive care team and reviewed by the paediatric liver consultant. A number of investigations were sent to try and determine the cause of his ALF.

✪ Learning point Diagnostic work-up in acute liver failure

The aetiology of ALF is age and region dependent, with viral hepatitis probably the most common identifiable cause in all age groups worldwide. ALF can be classified into seven categories: metabolic; infective; toxic; autoimmune; malignancy-induced; vascular-induced; and indeterminate (see Table 8.2). In infants, metabolic disease is the most frequent cause of ALF, whereas in children, viral hepatitis (in developing countries) or drug-induced ALF (in North America and the UK) is most frequently seen.[4] ALF of indeterminate cause is frequently observed: 40% of ALF in patients younger than 3 years of age and 60% in those aged 3 years and older. A full diagnostic work-up is described in Table 8.3.

Table 8.2 Aetiologies of acute liver failure by age

	Infectious disease	Cardiovascular	Drugs/toxins	Metabolic/immune
Infant	HSV Echovirus Hepatitis B Measles HHV6 VZV	Birth asphyxia Myocarditis CHD Cardiac surgery	Valproate TMP/SMX Paracetamol	Galactosaemia Tyrosinaemia Fatty acid defects Mitochondrial disease Haemochromatosis HFI
Child	Hepatitis A, B, C, D, E Leptospirosis EBV Dengue fever	Cardiomyopathy Budd–Chiari syndrome Myocarditis	Rifampicin TMP/SMX Valproate Halothane Paracetamol	Autoimmune disease Wilson's disease Leukaemia Haemophagocytic syndrome Mitochondrial disease
Adolescent	Hepatitis A, B, C, D, E Dengue fever	Heart failure Heat stroke Shock	Acetaminophen MAO inhibitor Tetracycline Mushroom poisoning	Wilson's disease Autoimmune disease Fatty liver of pregnancy Neimann–Pick type C

HSV, herpes simplex virus; HHV, human herpesvirus; VZV, varicella zoster virus; CHD, congenital heart disease; TMP, trimethoprim; SMX, sulfamethoxazole; HFI, hereditary fructose intolerance; EBV, Epstein–Barr virus; MAO, monoamine oxidase.
Source: Adapted from *Journal of Pediatric Critical Care*, 4(3), Dhaliwal MS, Raghunathan V, Mohan N, et al., Acute liver failure in children—a constant challenge for the treating intensivist, pp. 37–51, Copyright (2016), *Journal of Pediatric Critical Care*.

Table 8.3 Specific diagnostic tests to evaluate the aetiology of acute liver failure

Cause	Test
Hepatitis A infection	Anti-HAV antibody (IgM)
Hepatitis B infection	HbsAg, Anti-core antibody (HbcAb IgM)
Hepatitis D infection	Anti-hepatitis D virus antibody (IgM)
Hepatitis C infection	Anti-hepatitis C virus antibody (IgM)
Other infections	HSV-1, HSV-2; CMV; EBV; VZV; echovirus; parvovirus B19; malaria; dengue; leptospirosis
Autoimmune hepatitis	Autoantibodies ANA, ASMA, anti-LKM1, immunoglobulins IgG
Haemophagocytic Lymphohistiocytosis	Bone marrow aspiration (typical cells), raised ferritin , raised TGs, low/absent NK cell activity
Neonatal haemochromatosis/ congenital allo-immune hepatitis	Buccal mucosal biopsy, raised ferritin, high transferrin saturation, MRI abdomen (siderosis in liver and pancreas)
Veno-occlusive disease/ Malignancies	Doppler ultrasonography/venography imaging (CT/MRI) and histology
Toxicology screen and drug panel	Acetaminophen (paracetamol), opiates, barbiturates, cocaine, alcohol
Metabolic liver disease	
Galactosaemia	Galactose-1-phosphate uridyl transferase assay (provided child has not received blood transfusion in last 3 months)
Tyrosinaemia	Urinary succinylacetone
Wilson's disease	Urinary copper (>100 µg/day), Kayser–Fleischer ring, Coombs negative haemolytic anaemia, low serum ceruloplasmin (<10 mg/dL)
Urea cycle defect	Plasma aminoacidogram, Orotic acid estimation in urine (OTC deficiency)
Fatty acid oxidation defect	Carnitine–acyl carnitine profile
Mitochondrial hepatopathies	Muscle and liver biopsies for quantitative assay of respiratory chain enzymes, tandem mass spectroscopy, DNA (e.g. POLG)

HAV, hepatitis A virus; HbsAg, surface antigen of hepatitis B virus; HBcAb, hepatitis B core antibody; HSV, herpes simplex virus; CMV, cytomegalovirus; EBV, Epstein–Barr virus; VZV, varicella zoster virus; ANA, antinuclear antibody; ASMA, anti-smooth muscle antibody; LKMI, liver kidney macrosomal type 1; TG, triglyceride; NK, natural killer; MRI, magnetic resonance imaging; CT, computed tomography; OTC, ornithine transcarbamylase; POLG, polymerase gamma.
Source: Adapted from *Journal of Pediatric Critical Care*, 4(3), Dhaliwal MS, Raghunathan V, Mohan N, et al., Acute liver failure in children—a constant challenge for the treating intensivist, pp. 37–51, Copyright (2016), *Journal of Pediatric Critical Care*.

> **⊕ Clinical tip** The other organs
>
> As well as searching for a cause of the liver failure, it is also important to assess all major organ systems and look for evidence of sepsis, as described in Table 8.4.
>
> **Table 8.4 Investigation of other organ systems**
>
> | Systems | Investigations |
> |---|---|
> | **Haematological** | Complete blood cell count with platelets PT–INR, aPTT fibrinogen, D-dimer, blood group, cross-match |
> | **Electrolytes** | Blood glucose, lactate, ammonia, serum osmolarity. Blood gas with pH, sodium, potassium, calcium, magnesium, bicarbonate, creatinine |
> | **Sepsis** | CRP/procalcitonin, urinalysis and microscopic analysis, blood cultures, urine cultures, tracheal cultures (if intubated) |
> | **Imaging and other testing** | Chest radiograph, electrocardiogram, abdominal ultrasound with Doppler study of the liver |
> | **CNS** | Neuroimaging, EEG, BIS, ICP monitor |
>
> CNS, central nervous system; PT, prothrombin time; INR, international normalized ratio; aPTT, activated partial thromboplastin time; CRP, C-reactive protein; EEG, electroencephalogram; BIS, bispectral index; ICP, intracranial pressure.
> *Source:* Adapted from *Journal of Pediatric Critical Care*, 4(3), Dhaliwal MS, Raghunathan V, Mohan N, et al., Acute liver failure in children—a constant challenge for the treating intensivist, pp. 37–51, Copyright (2016), *Journal of Pediatric Critical Care*.

Case history (continued)

Repeat liver function tests in the PICU showed that his bilirubin had increased to 649 µmol/L, with a persistently high alanine aminotransferase but a low ALP of 20 IU/L. WD was suspected because of low ALP. Blood tests for ceruloplasmin and copper were sent. An ophthalmology consult was requested for slit-lamp examination. His coagulopathy was profound, with an INR > 9 and thrombocytopenia. A multidisciplinary team meeting, which included hepatologists, liver surgeons, and intensivists, was arranged. He was super-urgently listed for a liver transplant.

> **✪ Learning point** Wilson's disease
>
> The diagnosis of WD as a cause of ALF requires special consideration. Regardless of aetiology, low ceruloplasmin levels are not an uncommon finding in ALF. Kayser–Fleischer rings are not consistently present and acquiring a serum copper level can take days to weeks.
>
> In this case a low ALP of 20 IU/L serves as a pointer that WD could be the cause. The mechanism of a low ALP in WD is uncertain, but there is a well-established link, particularly in ALF. In addition, there is blood film evidence of haemolysis but with a negative Coomb's test, and a low uric acid level of 3 mg/dL—both findings consistent with a diagnosis of WD.
>
> To provide further evidence, the ratio of serum ALP (IU/L) to total bilirubin (mg/dL) can be calculated. A ratio of less than 4 has a sensitivity of 94% and specificity of 96% for WD.[5] In this case, the ratio is 0.5. ALF due to WD is invariably fatal without liver transplantation.

Case history (continued)

During the first 24 hours of admission, the patient developed severe multiorgan failure. Ventilation was complicated by a pulmonary haemorrhage. He required high-frequency oscillatory ventilation with a mean airway pressure of 24, fraction of inspired oxygen of 1.0 and 20 parts per million of inhaled nitric oxide.

His coagulation profile was very deranged. The PT and activated partial thromboplastin time were both greater then > 180 seconds, INR was > 9, and fibrinogen was 0.4 g/L. The platelet count was persistently < 50 × 10^9/L. In response to the bleeding he was transfused initially with FFP, cryoprecipitate, and platelets, and then Factor VII concentrate. The degree of vasoplegic shock necessitated three high-dose vasoactive infusions—adrenaline, noradrenaline, and vasopressin—and IV hydrocortisone.

> **❝ Expert comment** Principles of management
>
> The principles of managing ALF can be distilled into the following three imperatives:
>
> 1. Monitor and support the patient and organ systems.
> 2. Identify and treat complications.
> 3. Maximize the chances of spontaneous recovery and maintain optimal clinical condition for best post-transplant survival.
>
> Although these principles appear straightforward, their practical applications are more complex. Owing to the rapidity of the illness and potentially devastating course, the patient requires close observation in a suitable facility, where mechanical ventilation, rapid availability of blood products, ICP monitoring (if deemed beneficial), and renal replacement therapy (RRT) are available. Typically, this level of support warrants referral to transplant centre where emergency liver transplantation may be lifesaving.

> **Learning point** Coagulation
>
> Overt bleeding is uncommon in patients with PALF and this reflects a balanced haemostatic defect. The loss of hepatic synthesis of procoagulant factors is compensated by the loss of hepatically derived anticoagulants (protein C/S or antithrombin III).[6] Despite a profound elevation in INR, there can be minimal disturbance of global haemostasis. It is therefore recommended that correction of coagulopathy in patients with PALF should not be pursued in the absence of overt bleeding. In addition, administration of FFP will interfere with the evaluation of the PT/INR, which is essential for assessing disease progression and for prognostication.
>
> An exception to the rule of routine non-correction is when an invasive procedure is planned, such as placement of a central venous catheter or ICP monitor, or if a patient is undergoing liver transplant. In these cases, the procedure can be performed under cover of FFP, cryoprecipitate, and platelets. Reasonable targets would be to correct the INR to 1.5, fibrinogen to 1 g/L, and platelet count to 50 × 10^9/L.
>
> If FFP and cryoprecipitate fail to adequately normalize PT/INR, the use of recombinant factor VII (40 µg/kg) can be considered but would normally require a discussion with haematology team.

Case history (continued)

A reverse jugular venous catheter was placed and a transcranial Doppler (TCD) scan was performed. The information from the jugular venous catheter showed an increased jugular venous oxygen saturation (SjvO$_2$) of 80% suggesting hyperaemia. A decision was taken to insert an ICP monitor. After further correction of coagulation, the monitor was inserted by the neurosurgical team. The initial ICP reading was 48 mmHg. Full neuroprotective measures were instituted, including a thiopentone infusion (with continuous electroencephalogram (EEG) monitoring). The ICP decreased to < 20 mmHg.

> **Learning point** Neuromonitoring
>
> HE brain oedema and raised ICP due to multiple synergistic factors, most notably hyperammonaemia, is a significant cause of morbidity and mortality in PALF. For all children with ALF requiring ventilation, multimodal neuromonitoring should be commenced on admission to PICU. The information should help inform the need for escalation of neuroprotective measures and may prompt ICP monitor insertion.
>
> - SjVO$_2$[7]—Blood from the cerebral venous sinuses drains into the internal jugular vein. Monitoring of oxygen saturation in the jugular bulb gives an estimate of the balance of global oxygen supply versus demand ratio and hence of cerebral metabolism. Insert a reverse jugular venous line—preferably on the right side—and take blood gases from this line every 2 hours to compare with a paired arterial sample. The difference between the two will give the cerebral oxygen extraction.
>
> High and low jugular venous saturations are equally associated with poor outcome.
>
> Reduced SjVO$_2$—or a saturation difference of >40%—is seen in the following clinical scenarios: cerebral vasoconstriction (e.g. due to hyperventilation and hypocarbia); hypoxaemia; anaemia; diminished cerebral perfusion pressure; inappropriately high cerebral perfusion pressure (CPP); vasoconstriction induced by exogenous vasoconstrictor; and seizures. Elevated SjVO$_2$—or a saturation difference <20%—is seen in hyperaemia, vasodilatation (e.g. due to hypoventilation and hypercarbia), and brain death.
>
> - TCD—intermittent readings to be taken once or twice daily in all age groups. The temporal window is most commonly used. TCD is a simple and non-invasive method of quantifying flow velocities in the basal cerebral arteries (most commonly the middle cerebral artery). The two parameters of interest are the pulsatility index (PI) and mean flow velocity. Increased PI indicates decreased cerebral flow; similarly, decreased PI indicates increased cerebral blood flow or ischaemia. The normal PI is 0.8–1.2. Increased mean velocity can mean increased cerebral blood flow, but could also represent vasospasm or vessel stenosis.
> - EEG monitoring—if the patient is receiving a thiopentone infusion continuous EEG monitoring is mandatory to look for burst suppression and allow titration of the dose.
> - Neuroimaging (computed tomography scan)—rarely performed as moving an unstable child with raised ICP and high INR to the radiology suite is high risk.

➕ **Clinical tip** Neuroprotection

Full neuroprotection should be commenced in all ventilated patients with PALF:[8]

- head of bed raised at 30 degrees;
- neck in neutral position;
- sedation (opiates and benzodiazepines administered judiciously);
- use of fentanyl boluses or propofol pre-procedure/pre-suctioning;
- active surveillance for seizures and consider antiseizure prophylaxis with phenytoin if clinical or EEG evidence of seizures;
- aggressive temperature control aiming for normothermia (36–37°C);
- ammonia scavenging strategy (continuous veno-venous haemofiltration (CVVH));
- mechanical ventilation to normal pH and partial pressure of CO_2 (4.5–5.2 kpa);
- normoglycaemia (4–8 mmol/L);
- blood pressure targets—target mean arterial pressures of >70 mmHg if >4 years of age, >60 mmHg if <4 years, and >50 mmHg if <1 year of age.

🕮 **Expert comment** Intracranial pressure monitoring

Most of the monitoring devices discussed in the neuromonitoring section are either intermittent and/or provide surrogate information allowing inferences about ICP. Ideally, a form of continuous and direct monitoring would be used. ICP monitors ('bolts') give a continuous reading of the ICP, and would, in theory, allow titration of neuroprotective measures.[9,10]

However, inserting a bolt in a coagulopathic patient is risky, and there is no robust evidence suggesting a benefit to patient outcome to the insertion of an ICP bolt. A lack of consensus over therapeutic goals has done little to promote the role of ICP monitoring in ALF. The issues are even more complicated in small children where skulls are thin and fontanelles open. In general, bolts are not inserted in children aged <5 years. As there can be life-threatening consequences, it is imperative that a proper risk assessment is done before an ICP bolt is inserted. Therefore, before undertaking such a procedure, it is vital to assess the risk for developing raised ICP.

A suggested risk stratification algorithm might take into account:

- pupillary abnormality;
- persistent hyperammonaemia;
- abnormal SjO_2, or abnormal differential;
- abnormal PI and/or mean flow velocity on TCD.

Only after considering all these factors—the age, the clinical condition of the child, and consultation with other teams—should a bolt be inserted.

Case history (continued)

His ammonia level was 211 μmol/L, and he had grade 3 encephalopathy prior to intubation. Once the ICP bolt was inserted and full neuroprotection was underway, a dual lumen catheter was inserted and CVVH was commenced.

➕ **Clinical tip** Intracranial pressure targets

Goals of therapy

- Maintain an ICP of <20 mmHg.
- Maintain a CPP of >50 mmHg for children aged <4 years, >55 mmHg for children aged 4–10 years, and >60 mmHg for children older than 10 years.

➕ **Learning point** Renal/liver replacement therapy

Extracorporeal continuous RRT (CRRT) can serve a dual purpose in ALF. AKI is common (incidence varies from 30% to 85% depending on aetiology). ALF results in a sepsis-like hyperdynamic circulation with vasoplegia due to release of endogenous vasodilators. The drop in systemic vascular resistance, and consequent drop in blood pressure, compromises renal perfusion and can cause acute tubular necrosis. As well as providing necessary kidney support, CRRT also provides a detoxification mechanism, correcting hyperammonaemia, hyperlactataemia, and other metabolic disturbances.

The indications for starting CRRT in ALF are as follows:

- metabolic abnormalities (sodium <130 mEq/L; high/increasing lactate, despite optimizing fluid therapy, persistent metabolic acidosis);
- HE grade 3–4;
- ammonia >150 μmol/l and uncontrolled, or an absolute value >200 μmol/L—insert dual lumen catheter when serum ammonia reaches 100 μmol/L;
- renal dysfunction (oligoanuria, hyperkalaemia, fluid overload).

There is no single absolute for initiation of CRRT—seek expert advice before a decision to start CRRT is made.

Other systems exist specifically to perform 'liver dialysis'. In the Molecular Adsorbent Recirculation System (MARS®), the patient's blood is dialysed against 20% human albumin solution across a highly permeable membrane. Albumin scavenges protein-bound substances normally cleared by the liver and is then recycled though adsorbent charcoal columns with regeneration of albumin binding sites. Single-pass albumin dialysis works on a similar principle and uses a standard CVVH system. However, the albumin-rich dialysate is not recycled but discarded after a single pass.

High-volume plasma exchange (HVP) may also have a role, with patient plasma removed and replaced with FFP. This technique removes water-soluble and protein-bound toxins, decreases ammonia and bilirubin, and restores clotting factors. Larsen et al. published the first randomized controlled trial comparing HVP to standard medical therapy in adults with ALF, and demonstrated improved liver transplant-free survival.[11] [12] In a paediatric study by Ide et al.,[12] a combination of CVVH and plasma exchange was used to treat 17 infants with ALF until a donor graft became available. All the children survived to PICU discharge.

🄲 Expert comment   Kidney injury in acute liver failure

AKI in ALF is multifactorial. The most common causes include sepsis, hypovolaemia, direct nephrotoxicity, and acute tubular necrosis. Sepsis and the related inflammatory response can contribute to significant vasomotor changes, which can compromise renal perfusion. There is upregulation of endothelin receptor (ET-A) in renal epithelial cells during liver failure, and animal studies have shown that adding bosentan, an endothelin receptor antagonist, can improve creatinine clearance in liver failure by improving renal perfusion.

Direct nephrotoxicity and acute tubular necrosis can be multifactorial. In paracetamol overdose this can be due to antioxidant (glutathione) depletion. Ischaemia secondary to poor perfusion and toxins can cause loss of cellular integrity in proximal tubules and induce apoptosis. Studies show that as the severity of AKI worsens, as defined in Risk, Injury, Failure, Loss, and End-stage kidney disease (RIFLE)[13] criteria or Acute Kidney Injury Network (AKIN)[14] classification, the prognosis also worsens. Acute-on-chronic decompensation of liver disease with accompanying organ failure significantly increases the risk of mortality. Early intervention in the form of RRT is advised to prevent AKI associated electrolyte and haemodynamic changes as it increases the incidence of cerebral oedema in liver failure.

✚ **Clinical tip** Continuous veno-venous haemofiltration settings

Different units may employ different modalities of extracorporeal detoxification for ALF. Here we suggest how to start CVVH for a patient with ALF. Table 8.5 provides a summary based on the Aqualine S system.

Table 8.5 Running continuous veno-venous haemofiltration

Weight of child (kg)	<5	5–15	15–30	>30
Vascath size (Fr)	6.5	8–10	11.5	11.5–13.5
Length available (mm)	75	90–120	125–160	160–195
Filter size	HF03	HF03	HF07+	HF07+
Aqualine size	Aqualine S	Aqualine S	Aqualine S	Aqualine S
Blood flow rate (mL/min)	50–80	100	150	200
Predilution rate (mL/kg/h)	60	60	60	60 (max. 3000 mL)
Priming volume (mL)	96	96	118	159

If a child weighs <10 kg then prime the circuit with blood (except if immediately post-liver transplant, or those at risk of graft-versus-host disease or haemolytic disease). Blood flow should start at half of the desired blood flow rate. Electively change the complete circuit every 24 hours for 3 days. If the activated clotting time is <180 seconds, consider anticoagulation with epoprostenol or heparin.

★ **Learning point** Treating the cause

The cornerstone of management of ALF is supportive treatment, with a view to recovery of native liver function or liver transplant. However, some causes do have a specific treatment, which can be instituted in conjunction with the paediatric liver physicians (Table 8.6).

Table 8.6 Treating the cause of acute liver failure

Cause	Treatment
Acetaminophen poisoning	Activated charcoal 1 g/kg orally N-acetylcysteine IV
HSV	Aciclovir IV
Neonatal haemochromatosis	IV immunoglobulin Exchange transfusion Deferoxamine, selenium, N-acetylcysteine, tocopherol
Mushroom poisoning	Penicillin G, silymarin
Hepatitis B	Interferon-α2b for children >1 year of age and older Lamivudine or entecavir for children > 2 years of age and older
Autoimmune hepatitis	Methyl prednisolone IV Azathioprine may be added to steroids.

IV, intravenous; HSV, herpes simplex virus.
Source: Adapted from *Chest*, 138(1), Davison DL, Chawla LS, Selassie L, et al., Femoral-based central venous oxygen saturation is not a reliable substitute for subclavian/internal jugular-based central venous oxygen saturation in patients who are critically ill, pp. 76–83, Copyright (2010), with permission from The American College of Chest Physicians. Published by Elsevier Inc. All rights reserved.

Case history (continued)

After four days on the PICU a suitable liver became available. The CVVH was ceased and the patient was trialled successfully on conventional ventilation. He was taken to theatre for an orthotopic liver transplant. The graft—a whole liver—was of relatively small size and was harvested from a beating-heart donor. Reperfusion of the organ was smooth and the child was re-admitted to the PICU after surgery.

✪ Learning point Types of liver transplant

Whole livers for transplantation into children are limited, and so the majority will receive a technical variant graft.[15] The graft variants include:

- Whole liver—from either a donor after brain death, or a non-beating-heart donor. Occasionally in children, abdominal wall closure may not be possible owing to the size of the donor organ. This problem can be solved by use of a silastic silo.
- Reduced size—a whole liver from an adult cadaveric donor is reduced to an appropriate size on the back table in the operating theatre. With aggressive reduction, transplanting a liver from a donor 12 times the size has been described.
- Living related liver transplantation—a left lobectomy is performed on the healthy donor during which segments two and three are separated from the remaining liver, and then transplanted to the recipient.
- Split-liver transplantation—a whole liver from a cadaveric donor is divided into two sections along the round ligament, leaving vascular structures for both portions intact. The left lateral segment (segments 2 and 3) is appropriate for transplantation into child, and the remainder can be transplanted into an adult.

---

❻ Expert comment Liver regeneration

It is useful to think of the natural course of ALF in terms of four outcomes:

- survival with native liver;
- survival with transplanted liver;
- death with native liver;
- death with transplanted liver.

Liver transplantation, although often the only treatment option, is far from a perfect cure (see Learning point 'Complications post-transplant'). Clearly, survival with native liver is more desirable. The ability of the liver to regenerate is well described. In the ancient Greek myth, Prometheus, having angered Zeus, was chained to Mount Caucasus where an eagle feasted daily upon his liver. The liver regenerated as quickly as it was consumed, condemning Prometheus to eternal torment. This unique property of the liver provides interesting avenues of research, and the focus of management of ALF is moving away from liver transplantation to liver regeneration.

One alternative strategy to orthotopic liver transplantation is auxiliary transplantation. In this process a partial donor liver—placed next to the native liver—acts as temporary support. On return of native liver function the immunosuppression is halted and the graft is allowed to atrophy. Lifelong immunosuppression is avoided.

Another technique to promote liver recovery is the transplantation of hepatocytes. Hepatocytes are isolated from unused donor livers and transplanted to the recipient intravenously or intraperitoneally. The donor cells then engraft, function, and participate in the regenerative process. This process subjects the patient to considerably less physiological stress than whole-organ transplantation, and the consequences of rejection are much less severe. In the future donor cells may be derived from pluripotent stem cells.[16]

> ⭐ **Learning point** Complications post-transplant
>
> Transplant may be the most appropriate treatment for PALF, and it is tempting for doctor and family alike to think of it as a cure. However, it must be understood that the child is effectively swapping one disease for another, and must endure lifelong immunosuppression with its attendant complications.
>
> The short-term complications of liver transplant include bleeding; graft dysfunction or failure; biliary leak; biliary duct stricture; hepatic artery thrombosis; portal vein thrombosis; and hyperacute or acute rejection.
>
> The later complications include infection due to immunosuppression; hypertension; renal failure; chronic rejection; disease recurrence; diabetes mellitus; post-transplant lymphoproliferative disease; and malignancy.

Case history (continued)

He remained well postoperatively, with rapidly improving gas exchange and a rapidly reducing requirement for vasoactive drugs. He was started on immunosuppression with tacrolimus. Ultrasound of the graft remained satisfactory. He was extubated 4 days later, and was discharged from hospital after another 2 weeks. He continues to do very well with regular follow-up with the liver team. Histopathology of the explanted liver confirmed WD.

Table 8.7 King's College Hospital (KCH) and Clichy liver transplantation criteria for fulminant hepatic failure

King's College criteria[21,22]	
ALF secondary to acetaminophen (paracetamol) overdose	pH <7.30 (irrespective of encephalopathy grade), following volume resuscitation >24 h post-overdose Or HE III–IV, PT >100 seconds (INR >6.5), and Serum creatinine >300 µmol/L (3.4 mg/dL) Or The extended KCH criteria Serum lactate >3.5 mmol/L after early resuscitation Serum Lactate >3.0 mmol/L 24 h post-overdose and adequate volume resuscitation
ALF with other causes	PT >100 seconds (INR >6.5) (irrespective of encephalopathy grade), Or any three of the following (irrespective of encephalopathy grade) Age <10 or >40 years Non-A, non-B hepatitis or drug-induced origin Duration of jaundice before encephalopathy over 7 days Serum bilirubin >300 µmol/L (17.6 mg/dL) Prothrombin time >50 seconds (INR >3.5)
Clichy criteria[23]	
Presence of confusion or coma (stage III–IV HE) associated with:	
Factor V level lower than 20% of normal in patients aged <30 years	
Factor V level lower than 30% of normal in patients aged >30 years	

ALF, acute liver failure; HE, hepatic encephalopathy; PT, prothrombin time; INR, international normalized ratio.

Source: Data from *J Hepatol*, 53(3), McPhail MJ, Wendon JA, Bernal W, Meta-analysis of performance of King's College Hospital Criteria in prediction of outcome in non-paracetamol-induced acute liver failure, pp. 492–9, Copyright (2010), European Association for the Study of the Liver. Published by Elsevier Ireland Ltd; *Aliment Pharmacol Ther*, 31(10), Craig DG, Ford AC, Hayes PC, et al., Systematic review: Prognostic tests of paracetamol-induced acute liver failure, pp. 1064-76, Copyright (2010), Blackwell Publishing Ltd; *Hepatology*, 6(4), Bernau J, Goudeau A, Poynard T, et al., Multivariate analysis of prognostic factors in fulminant hepatitis B, pp. 648–51, Copyright (1986), American Association for the Study of Liver Diseases.

Table 8.8 Wilson's disease index

Score	Bilirubin (mg/dL)	Aspartate transaminase (U/L)	INR	White cell count (10^9/L)	Albumin (g/L)
0	<5.8	<100	<1.29	0–6.7	>45
1	5.9–8.8	100–150	1.3–1.6	6.8–8.3	34–44
2	8.9–11.7	151–300	1.7–1.9	8.4–10.3	25–33
3	11.8–17.5	301–400	2.0–2.4	10.4–15.3	21–24
4	>17.5	>401	>2.5	>15.4	<20

INR, international normalized ratio.
Source: Reproduced from *Liver Transpl*, 11(4), Dhawan A, Taylor RM, Cheeseman P, et al., Wilson's disease in children: 37-year experience and revised King's score for liver transplantation, pp. 441–448, Copyright (2005), with permission from American Association for the Study of Liver Diseases.

Discussion

Liver transplantation in ALF

Emergency liver transplantation remains the only treatment for some children with a poor prognosis from ALF. There may be no more significant a management decision than whether a patient with ALF should be listed for a liver transplant, or be given more time for spontaneous recovery. Unnecessary transplant introduces the need for lifelong immunosuppression therapy and the inevitability of long-term metabolic complications, while if the transplant is delayed, a window of opportunity may be missed. This decision to transplant or to wait remains fraught with uncertainty, although a number prognostic scores have been described.

The most commonly used transplantation criteria are those developed at King's College in London (Table 8.7) and Beaujon's Hospital in Paris.[17,18] However, in children, these criteria have a poor negative predictive value. A study in non-paracetamol-induced ALF in children found that an INR > 4, bilirubin > 13.74 mg/dL, age < 2 years, and a white blood cell count > 9 × 10^9/L are associated with poor outcome without liver transplantation. The group recommends using an INR > 4 or factor V concentration of < 25% as the best-available criteria for listing for liver transplant in the present era.[19] In conjunction with clinical judgement, this scoring system assists decision-making.

In children, aetiology is also a critical determinant of outcome. Fulminant WD and indeterminate PALF carry the worst prognosis and require emergency liver transplantation, whereas hepatitis A and paracetamol-induced ALF have a good chance of spontaneous recovery without transplantation. A scoring system has been developed in paediatric WD to predict mortality: the WD index (Table 8.8).[20] It can be helpful in identifying which children with PALF warrant transplantation. It has five parameters, with a score of 11 or more indicating the need for transplant.

Liver transplantation may be contraindicated in up to 20% of cases, such as metastatic malignant disease, lymphohistiocytosis, and systemic metabolic or mitochondrial respiratory chain disorders. Other contraindications are uncontrolled sepsis, fixed dilated pupils, and severe respiratory failure.

A final word from the expert

Acute liver failure in children is one of the deadliest conditions in critical care to treat, and owing to its relative rarity and propensity to rapidly deteriorate into multiorgan failure, perhaps one of the most intimidating to the treating intensivist. However, by prompt recognition of the problem and institution of basic intensive care measures, the native liver can be preserved, or the child can be optimized for transplant.

References

1. Conn HO. Quantifying the severity of hepatic encephalopathy. In: Conn HO, Bircher J (eds) *Hepatic Encephalopathy: Syndromes and Therapies*. Bloomington, IN: Medi-ed Press; 1994, pp. 13–26.
2. Lee WM, Stravitz RT, Larson AM. Introduction to the revised American Association for the Study of Liver Diseases Position Paper on acute liver failure 2011. *Hepatology* 2012;55:965–7.
3. Squires Jr RH, Shneider BL, Bucuvalas J, et al. Acute liver failure in children: the first 348 patients in the pediatric acute liver failure study group. *J. Pediatr.* 2006;148:652–8.
4. Durand P, Debray D, Mandel R, et al. Acute liver failure in infancy: a 14-year experience of a pediatric liver transplantation center. *J. Pediatr.* 2001;139:871–6.
5. Korman JD, Volenberg I, Balko J, et al. Screening for Wilson disease in acute liver failure by serum testing: a comparison of currently used tests. *Hepatology* 2008;48:1167–74.
6. Agarwal B, Wright G, Gatt A, et al. Evaluation of coagulation abnormalities in acute liver failure. *J. Hepatol.* 2012;57:780–6.
7. Sheinberg M, Kanter MJ, Robertson CS, Constant CF, Narayan RK, Grossman RG. Continuous monitoring of jugular venous oxygen saturation in head injured patients. *J. Neurosurg.* 1992;76:212–71.
8. Mazzola C, Adelson D. Critical care management of head trauma in children. *Crit. Care Med.* 2002;30:S393–401.
9. Vaquero J, Fontana RJ, Larson AM, et al. Complications and use of intracranial pressure monitoring in patients with acute liver failure and severe encephalopathy. *Liver Transpl.* 2005;11:1581–9.
10. Bernal W, Hall C, Karvellas CJ, et al. Arterial ammonia and clinical risk factors for encephalopathy and intracranial hypertension in acute liver failure. *Hepatology* 2007;46:1844–52.
11. Larsen FS, Schmidt LE, Bernsmeier C, et al. High-volume plasma exchange in patients with acute liver failure: an open randomised controlled trial. *J. Hepatol.* 2016;64:69–78.
12. Ide K, Muguruma T, Shinohara M, et al. Continuous veno-venous hemodiafiltration and plasma exchange in infantile acute liver failure. *Pediatr. Crit. Care Med.* 2015;16:e268–74.
13. Akcan-Arikan A, Zappitelli M, Loftis LL, et al. Modified RIFLE criteria in critically ill children with acute kidney injury. *Kidney Int.* 2007;71:1028–35.
14. Kavaz A, Ozcakar ZB, Kendirli T. Acute kidney injury in paediatric intensive care unit: comparison of the pRIFLE and AKIN criteria. *Acta Paediatr.* 2012;101:e126–9.
15. Spada M, Riva S, Maggiore G, et al. Pediatric liver transplantation. *World J. Gastroenterol.* 2009;15:648–74.
16. Forbes SJ, Gupta S, Dhawan A. Cell therapy for liver disease: from liver transplantation to cell therapy. *J. Hepatol.* 2015;62(1 Suppl.):S157–69.
17. O'Grady JG, Alexander GJ, Hayllar KM, et al. Early indicators of prognosis in fulminant hepatic failure. *Gastroenterology* 1989;97:439–45.
18. Bernuau J, Goudeau A, Poynard T, et al. Multivariate analysis of prognostic factors in fulminant hepatitis B. *Hepatology* 1986;6:648–51.

19. Shanmugam NP, Dhawan A. Selection criteria for liver transplantation in paediatric acute liver failure: the saga continues. *Pediatr. Transplant.* 2011;15:5–6.
20. Dhawan A, Taylor RM, Cheeseman P, De Silva P, Katsiyiannakis L, Mieli-Vergani G. Wilson's disease in children: 37-year experience and revised King's score for liver transplantation. *Liver Transpl* 2005;11:441–8.
21. McPhail MJ, Wendon JA, Bernal W. Meta-analysis of performance of King's College Hospital Criteria in prediction of outcome in non-paracetamol-induced acute liver failure. *J. Hepatol.* 2010;53:492–9.
22. Craig DG, Ford AC, Hayes PC, et al. Systematic review: prognostic tests of paracetamol-induced acute liver failure. *Aliment. Pharmacol. Ther.* 2010;31:1064–76.
23. Bernuau J, Goudeau A, Poynard T, et al. Multivariate analysis of prognostic factors in fulminant hepatitis B. *Hepatology* 1986;6:648–51.

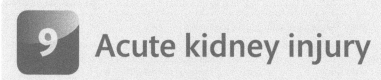

9 Acute kidney injury

Reshma Bholah

ⓘ **Expert commentary** by Timothy E. Bunchman

Case history

A 10-year-old boy with history of acute lymphoblastic leukaemia, in the consolidation phase of chemotherapy, presented to the Emergency Department (ED) with a fever of 39.5°C. He was also hypotensive, with a blood pressure (BP) of 80/35, and tachycardic with a heart rate of 135 beats per minute. His most recent weight was 30 kg. Work-up included a complete blood count (CBC), basic metabolic panel (BMP), hepatic panel, blood cultures, and a urine culture. His white blood cell (WBC) count was 0.5×10^9/L, with an absolute neutrophil count of 0.2×10^9/L, creatinine of 2.1 mg/dL (186 µmol/L), potassium of 6.1 mmol/L, and a lactate of 5.7 mmol/L.

In the ED, he received a fluid bolus of 20 mL/kg of normal saline, 2 mEq/kg of sodium bicarbonate, and was administered vancomycin and cefepime. He was admitted to the Paediatric Intensive Care Unit (PICU) for intubation owing to acute respiratory failure and further fluid resuscitation. Over the following 12 hours, the child's urine output was < 150 mL and with continued low BPs, was started on norepinephrine, titrating to goal mean arterial pressure of 70 mmHg. His weight increased by 1.5 kg.

> ✪ **Learning point** Definition of acute kidney injury
>
> Acute kidney injury (AKI), previously known as acute renal failure, is the condition where there is a decline in kidney function by a change in serum creatinine from baseline or change in urine output, from oliguria to anuric renal failure. The terminology changed when it was noted that acute renal failure was really an event secondary to kidney injury, be it primary or secondary, leading to changes in the structure or function of the kidneys. To date, numerous classification systems have been adopted to define AKI; however, these rely on the late findings of creatinine change and decline in urine output. Therefore, identification of new biomarkers of early kidney injury are under investigation with the goal of understanding and altering the course of early AKI.

Case history (continued)

Twenty-four hours after admission, he remained oliguric at < 0.3 mL/kg/hour with a positive fluid balance of 2.7 L. Ventilator settings escalated, with a positive end expiratory pressure of 8 cmH₂O and fraction of inspired oxygen of 60%. Blood cultures grew Gram-negative rods within the first 24 hours of admission and a repeat CBC revealed a dropping WBC, haemoglobin, and platelet count. Repeat BMP was significant, with a potassium level of 5.7 mmol/L, a calcium level of 7.2 mg/dL, and a creatinine level of 3.1 mg/dL. Albumin was 2.3 g/dL and lactate was 3.7 mmol/L. His baseline creatinine was 0.7 mg/dL. Nephrology was consulted for consideration of renal replacement therapy (RRT).

⊙ **Learning point** Diagnosis of acute kidney injury

AKI is present in at least one-third of hospitalized paediatric patients and is associated with higher morbidity and mortality.[1] Inconsistent and unstandardized definitions of paediatric AKI have hindered adequate estimations of prevalence. Hence, a concerted effort to develop a paediatric-specific classification system was undertaken to allow for consistent diagnosis and improvement in management for prevention of sequelae. The RIFLE classification (Risk for renal dysfunction, Injury to the kidney, Failure of kidney function, Loss of kidney function and End-stage renal disease), which had been proposed for critically ill adults by the Acute Dialysis Quality Initiative group in 2004,[2] has been modified for the paediatric population. These modified RIFLE criteria were coined the paediatric-modified RIFLE criteria (pRIFLE) in 2007.[3] From thereon, two other classification systems have defined AKI by expanding on the pRIFLE classification, these being the Acute Kidney Injury Network's (AKIN) definition in 2007 and the Kidney Disease Improving Global Outcomes (KDIGO) classification in 2012. The latter has attempted to put together the collective classifications from RIFLE, pRIFLE, and AKIN criteria.

pRIFLE criteria

The pRIFLE criteria take into consideration either or both a decrease in estimated creatinine clearance (eCCL), as well as declines in urine output, as seen in Table 9.1.

Table 9.1 pRIFLE classification of acute kidney injury

Stage	eCCL	Urine output
1: Risk	eCCL decrease by 25%	<0.5 mL/kg/h for 8 h
2: Injury	eCCL decrease by 50%	<0.5 ml/kg/h for 16 h
3: Failure	eCCL decrease by 75%	<0.3 mL/kg/h for 24 h OR anuria for 12 h
Loss	Persistent failure >4 weeks OR eCCL <35 mL/min/1.73 m^2	
End stage	End-stage renal disease (persistent failure >3 months)	

pRIFLE, paediatric-modified Risk for renal dysfunction, Injury to the kidney, Failure of kidney function, Loss of kidney function and End-stage renal disease; eCCL, estimated creatinine clearance
Source: Adapted from *Kidney Int.*, 71(10), Akcan-Arikan A, Zappitelli M, Loftis LL, et al., Modified RIFLE criteria in critically ill children with acute kidney injury, pp. 1028–35, Copyright (2007), with permission from International Society of Nephrology. Published by Elsevier Inc. All rights reserved.

AKIN criteria

The AKIN classification was a modification of the pRIFLE criteria, by adding the criterion of a 0.3 mg/dL increase in serum creatinine over a 48-hour period to stage 1 AKI. Table 9.2 shows the AKIN classification of AKI.

Table 9.2 AKIN classification of acute kidney injury

Stage	Serum creatinine	Urine output
1	Increase in serum creatinine of ≥0.3 mg/dL (≥26.5 µmol/L) over a 48 h period OR increase to ≥1.5 to 2-fold from baseline	<0.5 mL/kg/h for >6 h
2	Increase in serum creatinine to >2 to 3-fold from baseline	<0.5 mL/kg/h for >12 h
3	Increase in serum creatinine to >3-fold from baseline OR serum creatinine of ≥4.0 mg/dL (≥354 µmol/L) with an acute increase of at least 0.5 mg/dL (44 µmol/L)	<0.3 mL/kg/h for 24 h OR anuria for 12 h

AKIN, Acute Kidney Injury Network.
Source: Adapted from *Crit Care*, 11(2), Mehta RL, Kellum JA, Shah SV, et al., Acute Kidney Injury Network: report of an initiative to improve outcomes in acute kidney injury, pp. R31, Copyright (2007), with permission from Springer Nature.

KDIGO criteria

The KDIGO classification of AKI combines aspects of the RIFLE, pRIFLE, and AKIN classifications, as show in Table 9.3.

Table 9.3 KDIGO classification of acute kidney injury

Stage	Serum creatinine	Urine output
1	1.5–1.9 times baseline OR ≥0.3 mg/dL (≥26.5 μmol/L) increase	<0.5 mL/kg/h for 6–12 h
2	2.0–2.9 times baseline	<0.5 mL/kg/h for ≥12 h
3	3.0 times baseline OR initiation of RRT OR in patients <18 years, decrease in eGFR to <35 mL/min/1.73 m²	<0.3 mL/kg/h for ≥24 h OR anuria for ≥12 h

KDIGO, Kidney Disease Improving Global Outcomes; RRT, renal replacement therapy; eGFR, estimated glomerular filtration rate.

Source: Adapted from *Kidney Int. Suppl.*, 2(1), Summary of Recommendation Statements, pp. 8–12, Copyright (2012), with permission from International Society of Nephrology. Published by Elsevier Inc. All rights reserved.

⊗ Learning point Role of biomarkers

Serum creatinine, although widely used to diagnose AKI, remains an insensitive marker to detect early kidney injury. As a result, urinary and plasma biomarkers have been under study. Alge and Arthur provide a thorough review of AKI biomarkers in the adult population,[4] while a multitude of paediatric studies have studied similar biomarkers.[5,6] They include neutrophil gelatinase-associated lipocalin (NGAL), kidney injury molecule 1 (KIM-1), interleukin (IL)-18, liver-type fatty acid-binding protein, neutrophil elastase 2 (Ela-2), beta-2 microglobulin (β2M), matrix metalloproteinase (MMP)-8, tissue inhibitor of metalloproteinase (TIMP)-2, insulin-like growth factor binding protein (IGFBP)-7, and cystatin C (CysC). While serum creatinine or CysC represent functional damage to the kidney, the other biomarkers represent structural damage.

Urinary NGAL

Urinary NGAL is elevated in patients with AKI in the emergency care setting, using pRIFLE, and early after cardiac surgery before a rise in serum creatinine.

Urinary KIM-1 and β2M

Urinary KIM-1 and β2M are elevated in patients with AKI in the emergency care setting, using pRIFLE.

Urinary IL-18

Urinary IL-18 is elevated early after cardiac surgery before a rise in serum creatinine.

Plasma NGAL

Plasma NGAL shows good predictability of AKI in the general PICU population, but it is also elevated in septic patients without AKI.[7]

Serum CysC

Serum CysC shows good predictability of AKI in the general PICU population. It is more accurate as it is not elevated in sepsis, unlike plasma NGAL. Early postoperative CysC concentrations are also predictive of AKI development in children undergoing cardiac surgery.

Urinary TIMP-2 and IGFBP-7

The product of urinary TIMP-2 and IGFBP-7 ([TIMP-2]*[IGFBP-7]) has been used to diagnose AKI. It is elevated in neonatal and paediatric sepsis and is a good predictor of mortality—this remains to be validated.

⑰ Expert comment Biomarkers

Over the past decade, multiple biomarkers to predict AKI have emerged. Common biomarkers include urinary NGAL and serum CysC, while less common ones are urinary KIM-1, IL-18, plasma MMP-8, and Ela-2, among others. Research suggests that the combination of biomarkers used over different time points may be more predictive of AKI than when used alone in one snapshot. As most of these are research tools, these tests are likely to be developed for clinical use in the near future.

Others

Basu et al. have developed a renal angina index (RAI)[8] to improve the prediction of AKI in critically ill children. This looks into risk factors for AKI, including Intensive Care Unit (ICU) admissions, history of solid organ or bone marrow transplantation, and intubation with use of vasopressors alongside the percentage of fluid overload, which confers added risk for AKI. The incorporation of plasma NGAL, MMP-8, and Ela-2 with the RAI improved diagnosis of severe AKI.

Back to our case …

Our patient presented with a urine output < 0.5 mL/kg/h over the first 12 hours, putting him at AKI stage 1, based on pRIFLE and AKIN, and AKI stage 2 based on the KDIGO classification. When considering his AKI classification based on serum creatinine changes, he presented at AKI stage 2 using pRIFLE and AKIN classifications, and AKI stage 3 using the KDIGO classification. Based on further decline in urine output and further rise in serum creatinine at 24 hours after PICU admission, his staging changed to AKI stage 3 based on all three classification systems.

⊕ Learning point Aetiology of acute kidney injury

With the advances in treatments of congenital heart diseases, oncological disorders, and liver dysfunction, as well as advents in intensive care management, the causes of AKI have shifted from primary renal disorders to a vast array of aetiologies. However, one has to consider demographics when evaluating for causes of AKI as these continue to be region-specific. For instance, in sub-Saharan Africa, sepsis, glomerular-based diseases, and nephrotoxins, including haemoglobinuria due to malaria, are the top three causes of AKI.[9] In contrast, the causes of AKI in South India included acute glomerulonephritis and infection, with tropical diseases such as dengue, cholera, scrub typhus, enteric fever, tuberculosis, malaria, and leptospirosis.[10] Of note, in the 1990s, haemolytic uraemic syndrome was a major contributor to AKI in the Indian subcontinent, showing how perhaps dynamic changes in healthcare delivery can change the epidemiology and aetiology of disease processes. A national US cohort identified liver disease, respiratory failure, shock, sepsis, and coagulation disorders to be associated with AKI in children older than 1 month, while those in their first month of life had congenital heart disease and postoperative complications as added factors associated with AKI.[11] This delineation of congenital heart diseases associated with and causing AKI in neonates and young children has been described in multiple studies.[12,13]

AKI can be subclassified into three categories, namely pre-renal, intrarenal, and postrenal injury. Pre-renal failure involves decreased perfusion to the kidney; intrarenal or intrinsic renal injury involves processes that affect the renal vasculature, tubules, interstitium or glomeruli; and postrenal injury occurs with obstructive processes to the urinary system. As this has been well reviewed in previous publications, please refer to Geary's *Comprehensive Pediatric Nephrology* (Chapter 39, Table 39-3) for a comprehensive list of the causes of AKI.

⑰ Expert comment Diagnosis

The diagnosis of AKI has changed dramatically over time. The various classification systems rely on serum creatinine, which is a poor indicator of glomerular filtration rate in children due to variable muscle mass. Patients often have other comorbidities, including pre-existing underlying unrecognized chronic kidney disease (CKD). The combination of haemodynamic compromise, sepsis, endotoxin, and underlying unrecognized CKD are multiple factors that may result in kidney failure. Regardless of the classification used, this child has deterioration that will require further intervention.

Back to our case …

Our patient presented in septic shock with sepsis-induced AKI (SAKI). The aetiology of SAKI is not only a result of decreased effective circulating volume from sepsis, but also of inflammatory mediators that cause tubular damage.[14] His history of chemotherapy conferred an added risk for kidney injury compounding the current AKI event. One also needs to consider pigment nephropathy from haemolysis as a result of sepsis as another potential cause of AKI. The use of vancomycin requires renal dosage adjustments in the face of a change in kidney function.

Often, the aetiology of AKI is multifactorial, and the use of biomarkers may be helpful in diagnosis and recognition, but interventions need to be considered. What is the optimal blood pressure? What is the optimal colloid oncotic pressure? What is the optimal osmotic pressure?

Over a decade ago, Bellomo et al. identified that the use of intravenous (IV) dopamine does not impact upon urine output or recovery of renal function.[15] There has been a paradigm shift of using renal-based norepinephrine. Variable data suggest that norepinephrine may be renal-sparing and may promote better renal perfusion.

There is a variation of opinion on the adjustment and definition of an optimal oncotic pressure, which can be measured by a surrogate marker serum albumin. There is some suggestion that an albumin >2.5–3 g/dL would be optimal to maintain intravascular volume, but this is debatable.

✪ Learning point Modalities of renal replacement therapy

Four modalities are utilized for the treatment of kidney failure, including peritoneal dialysis (PD), haemodialysis (HD), and continuous RRT (CRRT), as well as slow low-efficiency dialysis (SLED). A systematic comparison of which modality leads to the best outcome has not occurred to date and is unlikely to occur in the future. Table 9.4 delineates the specifics of these different modes of RRT.

✪ Learning point Peritoneal dialysis

PD is commonly used worldwide for AKI. Access for this modality can be a non-cuffed or cuffed catheter, placed percutaneously or surgically at bedside. A low volume of PD solution at roughly 10 mL/kg/pass is often used as frequently as every hour. The decision for a high glucose (4.25%) or a low glucose (1.5%) PD solution is determined by the ultrafiltration requirements of the patient. A higher glucose concentration will result in more ultrafiltration and lower concentration will result in less ultrafiltration. Solute clearance, such as urea and potassium, will be affected by volume, frequency, and duration of dwell time. Therefore, in low-volume PD, 10 mL/kg/pass every hour may give less solute clearance per hour but will result in overall better clearance if done 24 hours a day. As time allows and as wound healing occurs the volume can be slowly increased to a maximum of 40 mL/kg/pass. As one increases the volume in the abdomen, some pulmonary impairment may be noted with a degree of transient hypoxia. Further increase of volume will potentiate the risk of nutritional losses with significant loss of amino acids and albumin over time. In essence, PD can be done easily at bedside and will result in adequate solute clearance and ultrafiltration in the vast majority of patients.

✪ Learning point Haemodialysis

HD is used throughout the world and is divided into standard and high flux. Standard HD is done in most patients, while high-flux dialysis is often used in situations of intoxications or in very hypermetabolic states. Access for HD can be a non-cuffed or a cuffed catheter with preferable placement in the right internal jugular (IJ) vein. HD requires an extracorporeal circuit, the volume of which should be <10% of the intravascular blood volume of the patient to preclude haemodynamic compromise. If the circuit is >10% blood volume and haemodynamic compromise exists in the patient then one should consider blood priming.

In classic HD the blood flow rate is 3–5 mL/kg/min and the dialysate flow rate is somewhere between 500 and 800 mL/min for clearance. The goal of HD is solute clearance, which can often be easily obtained over 3–4 hours and ultrafiltration if haemodynamic stability is present. HD may have some degree of hypothermia associated with it, especially in smaller children, so an increase in the temperature of the HD bath may be in order. In the vast majority of patients on HD, anticoagulation can be achieved with heparin or it can be done without anticoagulation. This decision can be made at bedside based on the haemodynamics and the natural anticoagulation profile of the patient.

➕ Clinical tip Blood prime

Blood priming can result in hyperkalaemia, metabolic acidosis, and hypocalcaemia due to the components and the constituents of the blood. Attention to this transient problem is needed to avoid any complications from the blood transfusion.

✚ Clinical tip Low phosphate on continuous renal replacement therapy

Most dialysate and convective baths are low in phosphate, and thus the need for attention to phosphate supplementation. Phosphate can be supplemented via addition to the convection or the diffusion bath, by adding it to enteral nutrition or through an IV infusion.

★ Learning point Continuous renal replacement therapy

CRRT is often used as either convection (continuous veno-venous haemofiltration (CVVH)) or diffusion (continuous veno-venous haemodiafiltration (CVVHD)). This has become the preference for PICU-based RRT over the last two decades. The CRRT modality allows for better haemodynamic stability, as shown in Table 9.4. It is only inferior to HD in terms of rate of solute clearance, but the continuous nature of CRRT makes up for this deficit. CRRT requires trained nursing staff at bedside to maintain the circuit. Access for CRRT is similar to that for HD, preferably in the right IJ vein. Patients are often ventilated when they are on CRRT, not because of CRRT, but because of the severity of the illness. In a classic prescription the blood flow rate would range from 3 to 5 mL/kg/min, but it is often access based. Higher blood flow rates are not unreasonable as long as the risk of severe osmolar shifts is not present. Replacement fluid or diffusion fluid can run between 2000 and 3000 mL/1.73m^2/h or roughly 30–60 mL/kg/h. This will result in adequate clearance in the vast majority of patients. A successful circuit is often dependent on systemic or circuit-limited anticoagulation. Heparin is the standard used worldwide, with many alternatively using citrate or prostacyclin, both of which have been described as effective and safe. Protocols for anticoagulation with heparin, citrate, and prostacyclin are available at http://www.pcrrt.com.

Often the goal of CRRT is ultrafiltration without compromising haemodynamic stability. Net ultrafiltration of roughly 1–2 mL/kg/h can be achieved in a 24-hour time period. Hourly assessment of volume status is important in order to maintain the goal for net fluid loss. Solute clearance needs to be looked at very closely. Concurrently, a discussion between nutrition services and dialytic services is needed to ensure adequate clearance and avoidance of electrolyte disturbances based upon electrolyte components of nutrition and the dialysate/replacement fluid.

★ Learning point Slow low-efficiency dialysis

SLED has been commonly used in the adult world, while a single paper from Taiwan has described a series of 14 children who underwent SLED.[16] SLED machines are essentially an adapted HD machine. As opposed to CRRT, the dialysis solutions for SLED are made on-line, similar to HD. The SLED blood flow rate and access options are similar to CRRT and HD. The contrast between CRRT, HD, and SLED is that SLED dialysate flow rate is roughly 100 mL/min or 6 L/h (Table 9.4). This will allow for a less adequate clearance than HD but more clearance than CRRT per minute of time. SLED is often used for 6–8 hours a day; therefore, it is a hybrid between CRRT and HD.

✚ Clinical tip Thermic control on continuous renal replacement therapy

The CRRT circuit, much as the extracorporeal membrane oxygenation (ECMO) circuit, can provide a cooling effect on patients. So one should be mindful that the absence of a fever while on this modality does not equate a lack of infection if there are signs to suggest so clinically. Most machines available worldwide have some degree of thermic control, but it is often inadequate in some patients. Therefore, attention to thermic control and the use of overhead warmers may be necessary in patients.

Back to our case ...

Our patient had a positive fluid balance of 2.7 L, had a lactic acidosis, hyperkalaemia, was oliguric, and given his requirement for pressor agents to achieve adequate haemodynamic status, dialysis was needed to correct his electrolyte imbalances and fluid overload. CRRT was initiated since, as discussed, this modality of dialysis allows for less fluctuation in haemodynamics and confers the ability to titrate fluid removal based on a patient's blood pressure parameters. He was given vancomycin and cefepime for broad coverage of antimicrobials; vancomycin levels were measured while on CRRT to allow for optimal dosing of the medication. He had marked clinical improvement within 48 hours of antibiotic therapy. His blood culture grew *Pseudomonas aeruginosa*, prompting tailoring of antibiotic therapy to cefepime.

Table 9.4 Modalities of renal replacement therapy (RRT)

Modality	Continuous RRT	SLED	HD (standard or HF)	PD
Blood flow rate	3–5 mL/kg/min access dependent	3–5 mL/kg/min access dependent	3–5 mL/kg/min access dependent	10–20 mL/kg/pass
Dialysate flow rate	0–4 L/h	6 L/h	30–50 L/h	0.5–2 L/h
Convective flow rate	0–4 L/h	0	0	0
Anticoagulation	Heparin, prostacyclin, or citrate	Heparin or citrate	Heparin or none	None
Thermic control	Yes	Yes	Yes	Partial
Ultrafiltration control	Yes	Yes	Yes	Partial
Solutions	Industry made	On-line production	On-line production	Industry made
Medication clearance	Continuous	Intermittent	Intermittent	Continuous
Nutritional clearance	Continuous	Intermittent	Intermittent	Continuous
Haemodynamic stability	++++	++	+	+++
Solute clearance	+++	++	++++	+

SLED, slow low-efficiency dialysis; HD, haemodialysis; HF, haemofiltration; PD, peritoneal dialysis.

> **★ Learning point** Medication clearance
>
> Medication clearance is a consideration in these modalities and attention should be paid to adjustment at the bedside, especially at the start of RRT. Medication clearance is often related to protein binding, volume of distribution, as well as molecular weight, and is highest on HD, especially with high-flux modalities. Clearance is least in PD because of limited diffusion of medications across the peritoneal membrane. Clearance on CRRT is relatively common, with sedatives and vasoactive agents such as norepinephrine, dopamine, dobutamine, and epinephrine being easily cleared on CRRT owing to their low molecular weight, no protein binding, and limited volume of distribution.
>
> Antibiotics such as vancomycin and aminoglycosides can be easily managed in patients on RRT as kinetics can be determined. Antibiotics whose kinetics cannot be measured, such as meropenem and the cephalosporins, should be given at the end of a HD or SLED session, and interval dosing should depend on residual kidney function, as well as the timing of the next RRT session. With CRRT or PD, medications should be scheduled with regular intervals. If one is on vancomycin or aminoglycosides, one can look at the relative clearance of those medications and to have the 'best guess' of how to adjust other medications.

> **➕ Clinical tip** Nutrition
>
> Nutrition needs to be considered in all modalities. PD removes amino acids and immunoglobulins and thus a higher protein intake may be necessary. HD and SLED have a neutral impact on nutrition, whereas CRRT will remove amino acids, trace elements, and vitamins, making supplementation necessary.

> **❝ Expert comment** Advantages of continuous renal replacement therapy
>
> If one looks at haemodynamic stability, CRRT and probably PD maintain better haemodynamic stability over time. However, if one looks at solute clearance, HD is clearly superior as a modality. In this clinical scenario, the child is haemodynamically compromised and needs solute clearance. Therefore, if available, CRRT would be the optimal form of dialysis. Vascular access is an important and primary consideration when one starts considering RRT. Research by Hackbarth et al. has suggested the optimal location and size of access.[18] A dialysis catheter should be placed in the right IJ vein for optimal blood flow rates. Unpublished data by our group suggest that convection would give a better clearance of cytokines and inflammatory mediators than diffusion. Clearance of low molecular weight and low protein-bound molecules such as citrate or blood urea nitrogen (BUN) does not change whether one is doing convection (CVVH) or diffusion (CVVHD). Medication dosing while on RRT needs to be considered owing to rapid clearance of certain medications on CRRT, and attention to detail on adjustment of vasopressor agents is necessary. Data by Maxvold et al. suggest that nutrition needs to be considered early in the course of RRT and optimized with target protein loads of 3–4 g/kg/day.[19]

> **❝ Expert comment** Drug toxicity
>
> Chemotherapy and interventions need to be considered with variable AKI. This septic child has been placed on vancomycin and cefepime. These medications need to be looked at from both a toxicity and dosing point of view. Recent unpublished data by our group identified that in paediatrics, the combination of piperacillin–tazobactam and vancomycin is more nephrotoxic than either medication alone. This has been corroborated in the adult literature.[17] Hence, drug toxicity as an additive impact upon AKI needs to be considered.

Back to our case …

Our patient's degree of fluid overload was < 10%, based on his body weight of 30 kg. Our patient's creatinine eventually plateaued at 1.1 mg/dL, where his prior baseline was 0.7 mg/dL. This indicates progressive kidney injury from multiple hits; past use of chemotherapeutic agents likely led to renal damage, which was compounded by the current SAKI. He did not have evidence of haemolysis on labs to consider pigment nephropathy as an added cause of AKI. This leaves this child with CKD, which will have to be monitored periodically for progression of a decline in renal function.

Discussion

Prognosis of AKI and recent advances

Several poor prognostic factors for AKI have been described in the literature to include oliguric/anuric renal failure, the need for dialysis, the use of vasopressors, age < 1 year, and multiorgan systems failure.[12] The paediatric critical care literature describes SAKI as an independent risk factor for death in a multinational cohort of critically ill children with severe sepsis.[20] It is now well known that fluid overload confers an added mortality to those with AKI, with fluid overload also being an independent risk factor for cause of mortality.[21] The impact of fluid overload on AKI in different categories of patients, including neonates, children undergoing cardiac surgery or ECMO, and in the general PICU population, has been well reviewed by Selewski and Goldstein.[21] The timing of initiation of CRRT relative to degree of fluid overload has also been studied, with 10–20% of fluid overload conferring a risk factor for mortality in these patients.[21]

The AWARE study (Assessment of Worldwide Acute Kidney Injury, Renal Angina, and Epidemiology) is a multinational prospective study that assessed the epidemiology of AKI in the critically ill paediatric population.[1] AKI was defined using KDIGO guidelines, with severe AKI denoted as stage 2 or 3. They found AKI to present in 26.9% of paediatric patients in the ICU, with severe AKI developing in 11.6% of the patients. Severe AKI was an independent risk factor for death and maximum stages of AKI conferred an increased risk for death.[1] Their primary outcome of 28-day mortality in the ICU setting was 3.4%, and was comparable to prior studies in paediatric critical care.[22] Additionally, AKI progressed in staging within the first week of diagnosis and organ transplantation, including bone marrow transplantation, was associated with severe AKI.[1] When comparing the diagnosis of AKI using plasma creatinine or urine output, the use of plasma creatinine only would have led to missed diagnoses of AKI,[1] and, as previously demonstrated, mortality is higher with oliguric/anuric renal failure.[12]

Some medications have been studied in the setting of AKI and fluid overload, in particular to improve urine output in such children. Adenosine leads to renal vasoconstriction, and aminophylline and theophylline are methylxanthine adenosine receptor inhibitors, which naturally cause the opposite effect. Jenik et al. conducted a randomized controlled trial (RCT) in 2000 and found that prophylactic theophylline reduced AKI in asphyxiated newborns.[23] However, in a RCT in 2016 of 144 children post-congenital heart surgery, no such preventive effects of AKI were noted with aminophylline use.[24] The KDIGO guidelines suggest giving a single dose of theophylline in severely asphyxiated neonates who are at high risk of AKI. The largest RCT to date in 159 neonates with perinatal asphyxia from India showed that a single dose of theophylline given within the first hour after birth increased creatinine clearance and lowered rates of AKI in treatment versus a control group (15% vs 49%).[25]

A final word from the expert

It is generally thought that patients do not die from kidney failure but from the underlying insults that led to renal failure. Therefore, prognosis is often related to underlying pre-existing CKD, recovery from the precipitating factor, which in this case was sepsis, and from secondary insults such as nephrotoxic medications.

Lane et al.[26] identified fluid overload as an independent risk factor of death in AKI. However, strategies to manage fluid overload have not been well established and there is no cut-off point to initiate CRRT based on the percentage of fluid overload. Ronco et al.[27] suggest that patients with a pre-CRRT BUN >18 mmol/L had a worse prognosis than those with a lower BUN at initiation. Based on these studies, perhaps fluid overload >10% and BUN >18 mmol/L could guide the decision to initiate RRT.[26]

Over the past two decades, numerous milestones have been achieved in paediatric AKI. The association of fluid overload with poor outcomes, better definitions for paediatric AKI, and the study of urinary and serum biomarkers have already changed the landscape of paediatric AKI research. This will allow us to expand on our understanding of the aetiology and implement targeted interventions to improve the outcomes of paediatric AKI.

References

1. Kaddourah A, Basu RK, Bagshaw SM, Goldstein SL, AWARE Investigators. Epidemiology of acute kidney injury in critically ill children and young adults. *N. Engl. J. Med.* 2017;376:11–20.
2. Bellomo R, Ronco C, Kellum JA, Mehta RL, Palevsky P. Acute renal failure—definition, outcome measures, animal models, fluid therapy and information technology needs: the Second International Consensus Conference of the Acute Dialysis Quality Initiative (ADQI) Group. *Crit. Care.* 2004;8:R204.
3. Akcan Arikan A, Zappitelli M, Loftis LL, Washburn KK, Jefferson LS, Goldstein SL. Modified RIFLE criteria in critically ill children with acute kidney injury. *Kidney Int.* 2007;71:1028–35.
4. Alge JL, Arthur JM. Biomarkers of AKI: a review of mechanistic relevance and potential therapeutic implications. *Clin. J. Am. Soc. Nephrol.* 2015;10:147–55.
5. Basu RK, Wang Y, Wong HR, Chawla LS, Wheeler DS, Goldstein SL. Incorporation of bio-markers with the renal angina index for prediction of severe AKI in critically ill children. *Clin. J. Am. Soc. Nephrol.* 2014;9:654–62.
6. Parikh CR, Devarajan P, Zappitelli M, et al. Postoperative biomarkers predict acute kidney injury and poor outcomes after pediatric cardiac surgery. *J. Am. Soc. Nephrol.* 2011;22:1737–47.
7. Di Nardo M, Ficarella A, Ricci Z, et al. Impact of severe sepsis on serum and urinary bio-markers of acute kidney injury in critically ill children: an observational study. *Blood Purif.* 2013;35:172–6.
8. Basu RK, Zappitelli M, Brunner L, et al. Derivation and validation of the renal angina index to improve the prediction of acute kidney injury in critically ill children. *Kidney Int.* 2014;85:659–67.

9. Olowu WA, Niang A, Osafo C, et al. Outcomes of acute kidney injury in children and adults in sub-Saharan Africa: a systematic review. *Lancet Glob. Health.* 2016;4:e242–50.

10. Krishnamurthy S, Mondal N, Narayanan P, Biswal N, Srinivasan S, Soundravally R. Incidence and etiology of acute kidney injury in Southern India. *Indian J. Pediatr.* 2013;80:183–9.

11. Sutherland SM, Ji J, Sheikhi FH, et al. AKI in hospitalized children: epidemiology and clinical associations in a national cohort. *Clin. J. Am. Soc. Nephrol.* 2013;8:1661–9.

12. Hui-Stickle S, Brewer ED, Goldstein SL. Pediatric ARF epidemiology at a tertiary care center from 1999 to 2001. *Am. J. Kidney Dis.* 2005;45:96–101.

13. Morgan CJ, Zappitelli M, Robertson CMT, et al. Risk factors for and outcomes of acute kidney injury in neonates undergoing complex cardiac surgery. *J. Pediatr.* 2013;162:120–7.e1.

14. Martensson J, Bellomo R. Sepsis-induced acute kidney injury. *Crit. Care Clin.* 2015;31:649–60.

15. Bellomo R, Chapman M, Finfer S, Hickling K, Myburgh J. Low-dose dopamine in patients with early renal dysfunction: a placebo-controlled randomised trial. Australian and New Zealand Intensive Care Society (ANZICS) Clinical Trials Group. *Lancet* 2000;356:2139–43.

16. Lee C-Y, Yeh H-C, Lin C-Y. Treatment of critically ill children with kidney injury by sustained low-efficiency daily diafiltration. *Pediatr. Nephrol.* 2012;27:2301–9.

17. Burgess LD, Drew RH. Comparison of the incidence of vancomycin-induced nephrotoxicity in hospitalized patients with and without concomitant piperacillin-tazobactam. *Pharmacotherapy* 2014;34:670–6.

18. Hackbarth R, Bunchman TE, Chua AN, et al. The effect of vascular access location and size on circuit survival in pediatric continuous renal replacement therapy: a report from the PPCRRT registry. *Int. J. Artif. Organs* 2007;30:1116–21.

19. Maxvold NJ, Smoyer WE, Custer JR, Bunchman TE. Amino acid loss and nitrogen balance in critically ill children with acute renal failure: a prospective comparison between classic hemofiltration and hemofiltration with dialysis. *Crit. Care Med.* 2000;28:1161–5.

20. Fitzgerald JC, Basu R, Akcan-Arikan A, et al. Acute kidney injury in pediatric severe sepsis, an independent risk factor for death and new disability. *Crit. Care Med.* 2016;44:2241–50.

21. Selewski DT, Goldstein SL. The role of fluid overload in the prediction of outcome in acute kidney injury. *Pediatr. Nephrol.* 2018;33:13–24.

22. Pollack MM, Holubkov R, Funai T, et al. The Pediatric Risk of Mortality Score: update 2015. *Pediatr. Crit. Care Med.* 2016;17:2–9.

23. Jenik AG, Ceriani Cernadas JM, Gorenstein A, et al. A randomized, double-blind, placebo-controlled trial of the effects of prophylactic theophylline on renal function in term neonates with perinatal asphyxia. *Pediatrics* 2000;105:E45.

24. Axelrod DM, Sutherland SM, Anglemyer A, Grimm PC, Roth SJ. A double-blinded, randomized, placebo-controlled clinical trial of aminophylline to prevent acute kidney injury in children following congenital heart surgery with cardiopulmonary bypass. *Pediatr. Crit. Care Med.* 2016;17:135–43.

25. Raina A, Pandita A, Harish R, Yachha M, Jamwal A. Treating perinatal asphyxia with theophylline at birth helps to reduce the severity of renal dysfunction in term neonates. *Acta Paediatr.* 2016;105:e448–51.

26. Lane PH, Mauer SM, Blazar BR, Ramsay NK, Kashtan CE. Outcome of dialysis for acute renal failure in pediatric bone marrow transplant patients. *Bone Marrow Transplant* 1994;13:613–17.

27. Ronco C, Bellomo R, Homel P, et al. Effects of different doses on continuous veno-venous haemofiltration on outcomes of acute renal failure: a prospective randomised trial. *Lancet* 2000;356:26–30.

Difficult airway in the Paediatric Intensive Care Unit

Elizabeth O'Donohoe and Thomas Breen

ⓘ **Expert commentary** by Fiona Reynolds

Case history

A 5-month-old boy presented to the Emergency Department (ED) with difficulty in breathing. His parents reported a 2-day history of cough, raised temperature, and poor appetite. He had developed an audible wheeze and his parents were worried as they felt he was becoming more unwell and breathless, despite regular paracetamol and ibuprofen. Following a discussion and follow-up call with the out-of-hours general practitioner, his parents had been advised to take him to hospital. Clinical examination in the ED demonstrated nasal flaring and intercostal recession, with audible bilateral wheeze and scattered crepitations. He was tachypnoeic, tachycardic, and hypoxic (peripheral capillary oxygen saturation (SpO_2) 88%). His weight was 5.2 kg. An initial diagnosis was made of respiratory failure secondary to bronchiolitis.

Further enquiry revealed an uncomplicated antenatal history and a spontaneous vaginal delivery at 38 weeks' gestation. At birth he was noted to have an isolated cleft palate and micrognathia. He was diagnosed with Pierre Robin sequence (PRS) and scheduled to have a cleft palate repair at 9 months. He was successfully breastfed and was gaining weight and achieving milestones appropriately. His parents described noisy breathing at night, and, as a result, they generally positioned him prone to sleep, which significantly improved his symptoms. Nasogastric tube feeding and airway support with a nasopharyngeal prong had been discussed with them shortly after his birth, but he had not required either to date. There was no other past medical history of note, no allergies, and he had not previously required a general anaesthetic. There was no family history of anaesthetic complications or congenital abnormalities. His last breastfeed was approximately 5 hours previously.

He had a peripheral intravenous (IV) cannula inserted uneventfully in the ED and routine blood tests were taken, along with blood cultures, and a nasopharyngeal aspirate was sent for viral polymerase chain reaction. A chest radiograph showed clear lung fields.

⊕ **Clinical tip** Signs of airway compromise in children

- Snoring (e.g. from pharyngeal obstruction).
- Drooling (e.g. secondary to epiglottitis).
- Gurgling (e.g. from secretions).
- Hoarseness (e.g. secondary to laryngeal oedema or vocal cord paralysis).
- Inspiratory stridor (e.g. secondary to croup).
- Tracheal tug.
- Paradoxical chest wall movement.

IV maintenance fluid was commenced, he was kept nil by mouth and received oxygen (O_2) therapy at 2 L/min via nasal cannulae, which was well tolerated. He was trialled on bronchodilator therapy to determine responsiveness, and was allocated a bed on the children's ward. His case was later discussed with the Paediatric Intensive Care Unit (PICU) registrar to alert her to the possibility of an admission for nasal continuous positive airway pressure (CPAP) if he did not respond to conservative management. He did not require antibiotics. Over the following 6 hours, his oxygen saturation started to fall and he became more lethargic. A capillary blood gas demonstrated a rising partial pressure of carbon dioxide (pCO_2). He was admitted to PICU for high-flow O_2 via nasal cannulae. But, after no improvement, a decision was taken to intubate him in order to provide mechanical ventilatory support.

⭐ **Learning point** Indications for intubation

It can be very stressful being faced with a child who requires intubation for airway, respiratory, and/or cardiovascular support. In all cases, the priority is to oxygenate and ventilate the patient and not primarily to secure the airway. The safety of the patient remains paramount, and even in the emergency setting, appropriate steps should be taken to optimize success. In many cases the decision to intubate is made following a multidisciplinary discussion.

Indications for intubation

- Airway compromise:
  ○ obstruction (acute or insidious);
  ○ failed extubation.
- Breathing difficulties:
  ○ acute/chronic respiratory failure (hypoxaemia or hypercarbia);
  ○ upper or lower respiratory tract infection;
  ○ neuromuscular disease;
  ○ recurrent apnoeas.
- Cardiovascular compromise:
  ○ congenital cardiac disease;
  ○ acquired cardiac/cardiovascular disease.
- Neurological compromise:
  ○ reduced Glasgow Coma Scale and at-risk airway;
  ○ residual anaesthetic drugs;
  ○ seizure control/respiratory depression following antiseizure medication.
- Procedural:
  ○ for investigations (e.g. computed tomography (CT)/magnetic resonance imaging (MRI), lumbar puncture);
  ○ for procedures (e.g. chest drain insertion, central venous access);
  ○ for emergency surgery (e.g. laparotomy, cranial decompression, post-tonsillectomy bleeding, trauma).
- Other:
  ○ for pain control;
  ○ for transfer;
  ○ in anticipation of worsening airway compromise (e.g. burns/anaphylaxis).

In view of the child's history of PRS and cleft palate, it was recognized that he was at high risk of being a difficult intubation. The PICU registrar discussed her intubation plan with the on-call PICU consultant, who was still in the hospital. As it was now out-of-hours, the anaesthetic registrar on call was called and the ear, nose, and throat (ENT) team (on site) was informed of the events in case emergency front-of-neck access was required. The on-call anaesthetic consultant was also informed. Multidisciplinary discussion confirmed that anticipated difficult intubation was likely, and that difficult bag valve mask (BVM) ventilation was also a possibility.

✪ Learning point   The paediatric airway and respiratory physiology

The airway anatomy and respiratory physiology of neonates and infants predisposes them to airway compromise; it is therefore important to recognize and manage these differences appropriately, in order to optimize successful intubation in a young, and likely physiologically compromised, child. Some important clinical consequences of these differences are outlined below:

Anatomical considerations

* Compared with adults and older children, the young child's head is large, with a prominent occiput, small mouth, and short neck see Figure 10.1. As a result, positioning may be difficult, and airway obstruction more common at induction as the neck is flexed when lying flat.
* The tongue is relatively large and the larynx is high and anterior, at the level of C3–4 (compared to C4–5 in adults). The epiglottis is long and U-shaped, and often sits or flops posteriorly across the glottic opening; it is for this reason that straight-blade laryngoscopes are sometimes used to intubate infants up to the age of 6 months. Curved-blade Macintosh laryngoscopes and video-laryngoscopes can also be used, especially when an airway is predicted to be difficult.
* Neonates are preferential nasal breathers and their narrow nasal passages can be easily blocked by secretions or the mucosa damaged by a nasogastric tube or a nasally placed endotracheal tube (ETT) sited without due care.
* The paediatric airway epithelium is susceptible to trauma. It is suggested that an audible leak around the ETT at a pressure of 20 cmH₂O can help to prevent subglottic oedema and potential post-extubation stridor and stenosis.
* Traditional teaching is to use an uncuffed ETT in children under the age of 6 years due to concerns about airway trauma, but appropriately-sized cuffed ETTs are now more widely available, are not associated with greater airway trauma than uncuffed ETTs, and are preferable where higher pressure ventilation is required. The ETT must be inserted to the correct length and should be taped securely so as to prevent dislodgement with head movement, or an accidental endobronchial intubation.

✚ Clinical tip   Positioning

A roll under the shoulders may be required to keep the head in a 'neutral' position (i.e. midline, with the neck neither flexed nor extended), and gentle external laryngeal pressure may help to visualize the glottis. The 'sniffing the morning air' position (i.e. midline, with slight neck extension) used for adults may be helpful in older children.

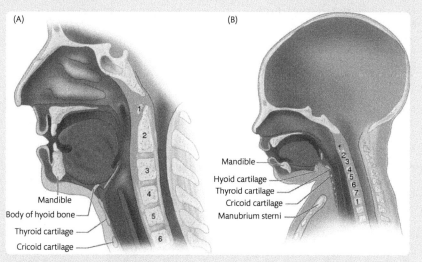

Figure 10.1 The anatomy of the (A) adult and (B) paediatric airway.
Source: Reproduced from Butterworth JF, Mackey DC, Wasnick JD, Morgan and Mikhail's Clinical Anesthesiology, 6th Edition, Copyright (2018), with permission from McGraw-Hill.

Physiological considerations

- Neonates and infants have limited respiratory reserve compared to adults. Ventilation is primarily diaphragmatic and therefore gas in the stomach following BVM ventilation can 'splint' the diaphragm and prevent adequate gas exchange, as well as increase the possibility of aspiration. Infants and young children cannot increase their lung capacity to the same extent as adults, and may therefore require a higher respiratory rate to achieve adequate minute ventilation. There is an increased tendency for airway closure at the end of expiration and resultant alveolar collapse.
- Apnoeas are common in premature infants.
- Hypoxia can develop quickly following induction of anaesthesia due to an increased metabolic rate, a low functional residual capacity, an increased risk of apnoea, difficulty in pre-oxygenating, and where mask ventilation is difficult.

It was agreed that, as the patient was already in the PICU, the procedure should be performed there in the presence of anaesthetic support. The Difficult Airway Trolley was set up at the patient's bedside, and all equipment checked. As per the Difficult Airway Society (DAS) guidelines, plans A–D were discussed at a pre-induction multidisciplinary team brief, which included the PICU consultant and registrar, the anaesthetic registrar and operating department practitioner from theatre, the nurse looking after the patient, and the nurse in charge of the PICU. The PICU consultant explained the sequence of events to the parents, who went to wait in the relatives' room.

⊕ **Learning point** Recognition of the difficult paediatric airway

For the purposes of their Practice Guidelines, the American Society of Anesthesiologists defines a difficult airway as 'the clinical situation in which a conventionally trained anesthesiologist experiences difficulty with facemask ventilation, tracheal intubation, or both'.[1] The anatomical and physiological differences discussed above can present a further challenge in an already stressful clinical environment. Although the incidence of difficult airway management or difficult intubation in the general paediatric population is unknown, it is widely acknowledged to be lower than in adult practice. Importantly, however, the presence of a congenital or acquired condition involving the airway significantly increases this risk. Therefore, as with adults, a good pre-operative assessment and adequate preparation is the key to successfully managing a difficult airway in a child.

Congenital abnormalities associated with a hypoplastic mandible are typically associated with difficult intubation, those with midface hypoplasia with difficult BVM ventilation, and those with macroglossia both difficult BVM ventilation and difficult intubation. In some instances (e.g. PRS) the airway difficulty can improve as the child grows; in other conditions (e.g. Treacher Collins syndrome or the mucopolysaccharidoses) this is not the case, and, in fact, the airway may become more difficult to manage with age.

It is also important to remember that many congenital syndromes involve multiple organ systems. It is essential that associated cardiac or cranial pathology is identified and planned for carefully, as alterations in physiology related to these systems may reduce the time to hypoxia or collapse at induction. If difficult airway management or IV access is anticipated, a two-clinician technique should be considered prior to starting the intubation. It will almost certainly be necessary to notify and involve an anaesthetist.

Common causes of upper airway obstruction in children

- Congenital:
  - ○ Choanal atresia
  - ○ Craniofacial malformations
    - PRS
    - Treacher Collins syndrome
    - Goldenhar syndrome
    - mid-facial hypoplasia
  - ○ Macroglossia
    - Trisomy 21
    - Beckwith-Wiedemann syndrome
    - mucopolysaccharidoses
  - ○ Laryngeal abnormalities
    - laryngomalacia
    - laryngeal web
    - laryngeal cleft
    - vocal cord palsy
    - subglottic stenosis
    - haemangioma
    - cysts
  - ○ Tracheal abnormalities
    - tracheomalacia
    - tracheal stenosis
    - vascular rings
  - ○ Neck abnormalities
    - Klippel Feil syndrome

- Acquired:
  - ○ Physical obstruction
    - foreign body
    - adenotonsillar hypertrophy
    - trauma
    - thermal or chemical burns
    - angioedema
    - anaphylaxis
    - post-intubation oedema
    - postoperative oedema
    - laryngeal or subglottic stenosis
    - tumours
    - papillomas
    - cysts
    - lymph nodes
    - radiotherapy
  - ○ Infection
    - epiglotittis
    - croup
    - bacterial tracheitis
    - quinsy
    - retropharyngeal abscess
    - Ludwig's angina
    - diphtheria
  - ○ Neurogenic
    - depressed consciousness
    - vocal cord palsy.

SpO_2, electrocardiogram (ECG), and blood pressure (BP) monitoring were already attached, and an arterial line transducer was prepared for use post-intubation. In-line end-tidal CO_2 ($etCO_2$) monitoring was attached to the Ayre's T-piece circuit for use during pre-oxygenation and then transferred to the closed ventilation circuit after intubation. Drugs at appropriate doses for weight were drawn up (including extra syringes in case of spillage or extravasation), cannula patency checked, and two fluid boluses of 10 mL/kg each were prepared. An emergency intubation checklist was completed (see Expert comment) and each person present was designated a role; the PICU consultant would attempt intubation, followed by the anaesthetist in case of difficulty.

⭐ **Learning point** Assessment of the paediatric airway

As with assessment of any system, essential information about the airway can be gathered by taking a thorough history, carrying out a physical examination, and reviewing investigations if appropriate and available.

Important factors to note in the history:

- Previous airway problems or airway surgery.
- Previous intubation and ventilation—an effort should be made to review the anaesthetic chart to assess ease of BVM ventilation, grade of intubation, and size and length of ETT used. Requirement for airway adjuncts and any difficulties encountered should also be noted.
- Previous respiratory problems, e.g. asthma, noisy breathing, change of voice, recurrent croup, snoring, and obstructive sleep apnoea.

- Current respiratory reserve, e.g. intercurrent respiratory tract infection, exercise tolerance compared to peer group, feeding problems (particularly for infants), and added airway sounds (e.g. stridor).
- Previous cardiac surgery or repair of trachea-oesophageal fistula, which increases the likelihood of tracheomalacia.

Pre-intubation examination should include assessment of the severity of respiratory distress, evidence of hypoxaemia (pulse oximetry, cyanosis), and the presence of inspiratory or expiratory stridor. It is useful to assess the patency of the nasal airway if nasal intubation is to be carried out. Airway examination should also assess:

- mouth opening and size of the tongue;
- examination of the teeth (particularly those that are loose/protruding);
- mandibular size and neck mobility;
- presence of any soft-tissue masses around the airway, such as a cystic hygroma.

In an emergency it is unlikely that there will be time for investigations. If time permits, however, some or all of the following may provide useful additional information:

- a nasendoscopy to visualize the larynx;
- a plain chest X-ray, and a lateral view if indicated;
- arterial blood gases to assess severity and progression of respiratory distress;
- respiratory function tests to help differentiate between extra-thoracic and intra-thoracic obstruction;
- further imaging including ultrasound scan, CT or MRI of the head and/or neck;
- a flexible bronchoscopy to visualise the lower airways;
- a sleep study to assess severity of sleep apnoea, or overnight pulse oximetry.

The nasal prongs were removed and full pre-oxygenation was attempted via a tight-fitting facemask and T-piece circuit. IV induction was performed with fentanyl 2 µg/kg and ketamine 2 mg/kg; rocuronium 1 mg/kg was used for neuromuscular blockade. Both oxygenation and ventilation were found to be easy with the use of CPAP and an oropharyngeal airway. Using a Miller blade, a grade III laryngeal view was achieved on first attempt. The cleft palate was also identified but did not appear to be the cause of the poor view. Following withdrawal of the laryngoscope, further oxygenation, re-positioning with a shoulder roll, and external laryngeal manipulation, this view was not improved. A third attempt using a video-laryngoscope (a Glidescope) revealed a grade II view and a size 3.5 cuffed ETT was placed successfully at a length of 10 cm at the lips. SpO_2 did not drop below 92% and the patient remained haemodynamically stable throughout.

☆ **Learning point** Choice of drugs for PICU rapid sequence induction

It is vital that the clinician performing the induction of anaesthesia is familiar with the drugs being used, including the indications, anticipated side effects, and risks. Dosing in children is based on weight, but much smaller doses of induction agent may be required in haemodynamically compromised children. In all cases, the appropriate choice of agent will depend on the clinical circumstances.

Induction agents

- Ketamine.

Ketamine is the most cardiostable induction agent, and is also a strong analgesic. It results in a tachycardia and maintains systemic vascular resistance (SVR). It can, however, lead to a reduction in cardiac output if not used with caution. Historically, there were concerns that ketamine might increase intracranial pressure and it was therefore avoided in traumatic brain injury, but these concerns have

❝ Expert comment Assess and anticipate

Taking a thorough clinical history and completing a full assessment of the airway aids recognition of the difficult airway and anticipation of the likely nature of the difficulty. Appropriate preparation can then be undertaken to mitigate against any problems encountered.

been largely dismissed, and it is now used widely by pre-hospital teams, paediatric critical care transport teams, and in the ED as a first-line induction agent.

Usual dosage 1–2 mg/kg (lower if shocked/ unstable).

- Propofol.

Propofol is the most commonly used induction agent for elective anaesthesia and therefore frequently chosen by anaesthetists owing to its familiarity. It causes a dose-related reduction in cardiac output, associated with a drop in SVR. It should be used with caution in emergency intubations in children, and is not recommended as a first-line agent for induction of anaesthesia in the shocked child.

Usual dosage for elective induction of anaesthesia 3–5 mg/kg (likely much lower in an emergency).

- Thiopentone.

Thiopentone causes significant veno-dilatation and dose-related reduction in cardiac output. Caution is necessary for use in any cardiovascularly compromised patients. Thiopentone was historically the first-line agent for induction of anaesthesia in status epilepticus, but now propofol (which also has antiepileptic properties) is usually used in preference, where available.

- Fentanyl

Fentanyl is a short-acting opioid analgesic, which is relatively cardiostable. It dampens the sympathetic response to direct laryngoscopy and reduces the dose of induction agent required. It is particularly useful in patients with cardiovascular instability though, as with all induction agents, should be administered with caution in the shocked patient.

Usual dosage 1–3 µg/kg

Neuromuscular blocking drugs (also commonly known as 'muscle relaxants' or agents inducing 'paralysis')

- Rocuronium.

Rocuronium is a fast-acting non-depolarzing neuromuscular blocker, with a medium duration of action of 30–40 minutes. It can be reversed immediately with Sugammadex.

Usual dosage for elective intubation 0.6 mg/kg (onset up to 120 seconds).

Usual dosage for rapid sequence induction (RSI) 1 mg/kg (onset within 60 seconds and usually less in children).

- Suxamethonium.

Suxamethonium is a depolarizing neuromuscular blocking agent classically used for RSI, but it is associated with considerable risks including hyperkalaemia ± malignant hyperthermia and suxamethonium apnoea. It can also be given intramuscularly (IM) but with a longer time to onset of effect.

Usual dosage 1–2 mg/kg (onset 45–60 seconds) IV (or 4mg/kg IM).

- Atracurium

Attacurium is a non-depolarizing neuromuscular blocking drug commonly used for elective anaesthesia procedures.

Usual dosage 0.5 mg/kg.

Emergency drugs

- Adrenaline, atropine, and IV resuscitation fluids—as per the Advanced Paediatric Life Support protocol.[2]
- Inotropes: consider starting an infusion pre-induction if the child is at risk of cardiovascular collapse or instability. In children without central access, inotropes may be infused via a peripheral vascular cannula at a more dilute concentration to help maintain cardiac output during induction of anaesthesia.

ⓘ Expert comment Managing the intubation process

The use of guidelines, algorithms and checklists at the preparation stage can aid the intubation process and prevent the omission of important steps. The DAS/Association of Paediatric Anaesthetists of Great Britain and Ireland (APAGBI) algorithm shown is an example of one such guide—see Figures 10.2 and 10.3.[3]

Two patent (checked and flushed) peripheral cannulae should be present, but one access site or even intra-osseous access may suffice in the emergency setting. Monitoring must be attached and the minimum standards set out by the Association of Anaesthetists of Great Britain and Ireland should be followed: ECG, BP, SpO_2, and $etCO_2$ measurement must be available.[4]

Positioning of and access to the child are two important considerations if intubation is to be successful and safe. Both age and technique-appropriate positioning are vital when approaching the difficult airway: the child should be positioned on a relatively hard bed or mattress that can be adjusted as required to seated, Trendelenberg (supine, with the feet elevated 15–30° higher than the head), and reverse Trendelenberg (supine, with head elevated 15–30° higher than the feet). Full 360° access to the patient is imperative.

The patient must be appropriately pre-oxygenated for at least 3 minutes with high-flow oxygen via a tight-fitting facemask attached to a T-piece circuit. In those who are hypoxic and with marked respiratory failure, apnoeic oxygenation can be considered as an adjunct to increase the time to desaturation post-induction. If deemed appropriate, gentle hand ventilation may be required after administration of muscle relaxant, taking care not to insufflate the stomach. It may be prudent to pass a naso- or orogastric tube prior to induction of anaesthesia. Gentle manual pressure over the stomach on the left upper quadrant may help reduce gastric insufflation but is not advised in the context of an acute abdomen or known full stomach. Following the administration of induction agents, some practitioners check that the patient can be hand-bagged prior to the administration of neuromuscular blocking agents. Others suggest that neuromuscular blocking agents can make a difficult manual ventilation easier, and therefore should be given in quick succession after induction, without checking for ease of manual ventilation.

Drug administration should be followed immediately by a saline flush, and the appropriate time allowed to pass prior to airway instrumentation.

The choice of laryngoscope will depend upon the skill and the experience of the operator and the age of the child. Neonatologists and those from a paediatric background may feel more comfortable using a straight Miller or Robertshaw blade for the intubation of the neonate or infant. Adult-trained anaesthetists will be competent in the use of a curved Macintosh blade. For the paediatric intensivist, understanding and mastery of both the straight and the curved blade are required. Successful endotracheal intubation must be confirmed by capnometry, visible chest movement, chest auscultation, and, if possible, by visualizing passage of the tracheal tube through the cords.

Choosing the right team to facilitate the intubation process is fundamental to a successful and safe procedure. Personnel required will include an intubator ± anaesthetist, a trained airway assistant, a drug administrator, and a runner or another member of staff for assistance. In most units, it is standard practice to ensure that the consultant and nurse in charge are aware of the intended procedure.

Once the ETT was firmly secured, a nasogastric tube was inserted and the stomach decompressed. Morphine and midazolam infusions were started. A chest radiograph confirmed appropriate ETT and gastric tube positioning.

ⓘ Expert comment Team brief

Before intubation is attempted a team briefing should be held with the relevant personnel, and the plan reviewed and explained in full to all involved. All present should introduce themselves and their role, and all equipment should be checked by the operator. Planning the management of a difficult airway must include the action to be taken if there is failure in any step of plans A, B, C, or D (see

Figure 10.2). For example, what to do if direct laryngoscopy fails, or how to proceed in a 'cannot intubate, cannot oxygenate' (CICO) or the 'cannot intubate, cannot ventilate' (CICV) situation. The difficult intubation should be managed in a safe environment where relevant expertise and equipment is available: this could be the intensive care unit, but in certain cases it may be more appropriate to transfer the patient to theatre. This may be particularly necessary in the presence of upper airway obstruction when a gas induction by an anaesthetist is often the preferred technique and early involvement of the ENT team may be required. If a tracheostomy is considered during the planning stage, the safest location for induction is on the theatre table itself. The anaesthetist, ENT surgeon, and scrub staff should be available with staff scrubbed and equipment open and ready to proceed expediently.

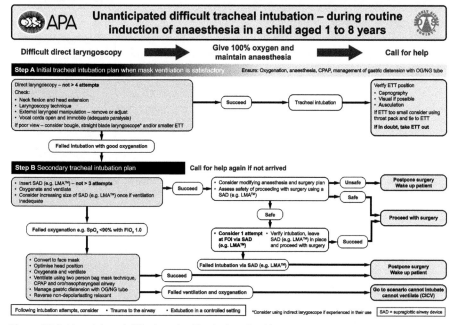

Figure 10.2 Unanticipated difficult tracheal intubation algorithm.
Source: Reproduced from Paediatric Airway Guidelines Group, Paediatric Difficult Airway Guidelines. Copyright (2012), Difficult Airway Society. Available from: https://www.das.uk.com/guidelines/paediatric-difficult-airway-guidelines

> ⊗ **Learning point** Cannot intubate, cannot ventilate
>
> If, despite planning or in an unanticipated situation, tracheal intubation fails and attempts to ventilate the child are also unsuccessful, this is a life-threatening medical emergency that needs urgent acknowledgement and intervention. Figure 10.3 sets out the UK DAS's CICV management algorithm,[3] which requires urgent front-of-neck access—ideally by an ENT surgeon. However, if no ENT surgeon is available then the most appropriately equipped personnel must take action. These cases are extremely rare in children, but they can occur in a range of environments—including pre-hospital and during elective cases, as well as in the PICU, and prompt action is vital.

> ⊘ **Evidence base** Airway management in the PICU
>
> Airway management in the paediatric population is generally straightforward but can occasionally be very difficult and result in significant morbidity, and indeed mortality, as evidenced by a large national audit published in the UK in 2011.[5] In elective anaesthetic practice, data have been

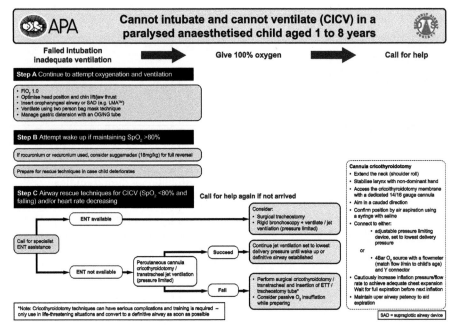

Figure 10.3 Cannot intubate and cannot ventilate (CICV) algorithm.

Source: Reproduced from Paediatric Airway Guidelines Group, Paediatric Difficult Airway Guidelines., Copyright (2012), Difficult Airway Society. Available from: https://www.das.uk.com/guidelines/paediatric-difficult-airway-guidelines

collected showing that in certain higher-risk groups, the incidence of difficulty in managing the airway is increased: difficult laryngoscopy in 4.7% of children with cleft lip and palate,[6] and difficult intubation in 1.25% of children undergoing cardiac surgery.[7] In a retrospective review of 11,219 paediatric anaesthesia procedures in the USA, the overall risk of difficult laryngoscopy was estimated to be 1.35%. Perhaps unsurprisingly, the risk was found to be higher in patients younger than 1 year, underweight children, and those with Mallampati score III and IV (an assessment of the airway used by anaesthetists to predict the ease of intubation).[8] A more recent large prospective cohort analysis showed that more than two attempts at direct laryngoscopy in children with difficult tracheal intubation is associated with a high failure rate and an increased incidence of complications. In their discussion, the authors postulate that limiting the number of direct laryngoscopy attempts with earlier transition to an indirect technique may enhance patient safety.[9] This is also reflected in the paediatric intubation guidelines published by the DAS in conjunction with the APAGBI.[3] A study from 2010 demonstrated that emergency paediatric endotracheal intubations were twice as likely to occur out of hours, and were associated with three times the risk of complications versus non-emergency intubations.[10] In PICUs specifically, difficult tracheal intubation was reported in 9% of all instances in a wide variety of units in the USA.[11] These cases were associated with pre-intubation signs of upper airway obstruction and a history of a difficult airway, and were also associated with significantly longer PICU admissions. Another retrospective study reported a significant rate of difficult intubation and mild-to-moderate intubation-related adverse events in emergency tracheal intubations on inpatient units and the ED in children performed by a paediatric anaesthetic emergency airway team. Difficult intubation was frequently observed in children with pre-existing airway and craniofacial abnormalities, and often required the use of an alternative airway device to successfully secure the airway.[12] This body of evidence demonstrates that emergency tracheal intubation in the paediatric population is associated with a degree of difficulty and morbidity.

> **Expert comment** Checklists and crisis resource management
>
> Checklists have become commonplace in high-pressure environments such as the ED and the ICU. They have been shown to improve outcomes across medical specialties, but particularly in these areas, as well as the operating theatre. Checklists play a fundamental role within military and pre-hospital medicine; allowing team members to reduce their cognitive load so they are less likely to make mistakes and miss important steps during stressful scenarios.
>
> The concept of crisis resource management was developed from emergency management in the aviation industry, and other high-risk environments such as oil rigs, where it is known as crew resource management (CRM). This more recent addition to training can help to improve outcomes in the PICU and includes learning to recognize when things have gone wrong, communicating, and reacting appropriately. It describes an effective form of leadership and management, promoting communication and assertiveness, and appropriate distribution of workload and resources.

Following 2 days of uneventful mechanical ventilation, the child was successfully extubated successfully onto nasal CPAP. He continued to make a good recovery in the PICU and was discharged to the ward on 2 L/min O_2 via nasal cannulae a further 24 hours later.

> **Expert comment** Fibreoptic intubation
>
> In managing the predicted or unanticipated difficult airway, a sound understanding and experience with the flexible fibreoptic scope is necessary. Use of this piece of equipment is considered the 'gold standard' for difficult intubations, although there are limitations to the technique:
>
> - The fibrescope is very versatile, allowing visualization of almost the entire airway via the nasal or oral route. However, significant training is required to achieve and maintain competence.
> - Setting up the fibrescope and screen can take some time, often negating its use in a true emergency. However, there is increasing availability of single-use scopes, which have a less complicated set-up.

> **Clinical tip** Fibreoptic intubation techniques in children
>
> Awake fibreoptic intubation is not usually feasible in the infant and small child, although in the competent older teenager it may be an option.
>
> For asleep fibreoptic intubations in adults either the nasal route or the oral route with a split airway (e.g. Berman) is used. If there are no airway adjuncts available to facilitate paediatric oral fibreoptic intubation, a larger nasopharyngeal airway can be used orally and cut along its length to allow removal prior to passage of the oral ETT.

> **Clinical tip** Fibreoptic intubation via a laryngeal mask airway
>
> In the patient with difficult mask ventilation, when an LMA is in use, a 'low-skill' fibreoptic technique can be used.
>
> - After preloading the fibrescope with an airway exchange catheter, it is passed down the LMA and through the cords until the carina is seen. The exchange catheter is then left in situ, through the cords into the trachea. The fibrescope is removed, and the catheter is used as a guide for the passage of an appropriately sized ETT, after which it can be removed.
> - In the smaller child a modified technique can be used. A soft-tipped guidewire is passed down the side port of the fibrescope. Again, the fibrescope is removed leaving the guidewire in situ in the trachea and an ETT is passed over it. If the wire is too flimsy, a more rigid catheter can be passed such as a nasogastric tube, and then exchanged for the ETT.

Discussion

Managing the child in PICU following difficult intubation

The management of a child in the PICU after a difficult intubation is particularly important. The clinical team often experiences a sense of relief, which can lead to the potential for a lull in activity. Those involved directly in the caregiving may require some direction to continue further treatment in a prompt and safe manner. The checklists mentioned previously can aid this process and keep the team focused. In addition to national clinical guidelines, other useful resources for ongoing management at this stage are available locally and regionally, for example from paediatric critical care transport team websites such as the South Thames Retrieval Service for Children (STRS).[13] The important goals of PICU management post-intubation are suggested below.

Immediate

- Start sedation and analgesia
- Order investigations and decide on ventilation strategy.
- Document procedure, including information regarding the difficult airway.

Medium term

- Set goals, e.g. clinical parameters for ventilation.
- Consider ventilation technique and indication, e.g. protective strategies, oscillation.
- Institute care bundles eg. for prevention of acute respiratory distress syndrome and ventilator-associated pneumonia
- Ensure ongoing medical/surgical management, e.g. management of sepsis.

Longer term

- Assess parameters indicating improvement ± weaning and extubation.
- Decide on extubation strategy.
- Complete 'airway alert' documentation for medical notes and for patient/carers.

There is variation in the use of drugs for sedation in the PICU and practice is often unit specific. Other factors, including duration of sedation and the age of the child, must be taken into consideration in drug choice. If time permits, the appropriate post-intubation sedation should be considered as part of the planning process. Ketamine and fentanyl, used at the time of intubation are significantly shorter-acting than rocuronium. Once the patient has been connected to the ventilator, adequate sedation must be administered. This usually takes the form of an opioid such as morphine administered as a weight-related infusion. In some cases, such as in neonates, this alone may be adequate, but the addition of a midazolam infusion is common practice. If there is a delay in connection of these infusions, intermittent bolus doses of fentanyl either alone or in conjunction with ketamine or midazolam can be administered. It may also be necessary to continue with neuromuscular blockade, depending on the clinical circumstances.

As with all high risk airway procedures, close monitoring of the patient is essential. A systems-based approach will help to prevent key issues being missed:

- A: Confirm position of ETT with etCO$_2$, chest auscultation and chest X-ray.
- B: Auscultate to assess chest pathology and for endobronchial intubation. Ventilator settings primarily to oxygenate, secondarily to target an appropriate PaCO$_2$.
- C: Clinical assessment of cardiovascular status, including capillary refill time, peripheral temperature, evidence of mottling, HR, and BP.
- D: If required, initiate neuroprotection with adequacy of sedation and neuromuscular blocking agents.
- E: Warming and temperature monitoring, glucose, pressure points, eye protection, and further investigations.

A final word from the expert

The unanticipated difficult airway is a potentially dangerous, and very stressful, scenario, particularly in the paediatric population. Most paediatric patients are looked after in non-specialist hospitals, where specialist paediatric services are neither necessary nor appropriate in many settings. To this end, and as previously mentioned, DAS and the APAGBI have produced guidelines for the management of the unanticipated difficult airway in children aged 1–8 years.[3] As well as guiding clinical practice, these provide a structure to facilitate the maintenance of paediatric airway skills, rehearse unexpected difficult airway scenarios, and teach good practice. There is currently minimal grade I evidence for the management of the difficult paediatric airway, and good practice is based on a pragmatic approach and expert opinion.

References

1. Apfelbaum JL, Hagberg C, Caplan RA, et al. Practice guidelines for management of the difficult airway: an updated report by the American Society of Anesthesiologists Task Force on Management of the Difficult Airway. *Anesthesiology* 2013;118:251–70.
2. Advanced Life Support Group. Advanced Paediatric Life Support (APLS) Course. Available from: http://www.alsg.org/en/files/PFactsheet.pdf (accessed 5 August 2020).
3. Paediatric Airway Guidelines Group. Paediatric Difficult Airway Guidelines. Available from: https://www.das.uk.com/guidelines/paediatric-difficult-airway-guidelines (accessed 5 August 2020).
4. Association of Anaesthetists of Great Britain and Ireland. Standards of monitoring during anaesthesia and recovery. Available from: https://www.aagbi.org/sites/default/files/Standards_of_monitoring_2015_0.pdf (accessed 5 August 2020).
5. Royal College of Anaesthetists and Difficult Airway Society. 4th National Audit Project. Major complications of airway management in the United Kingdom. 2011. Available from: https://www.rcoa.ac.uk/sites/default/files/documents/2019-09/NAP4%20Full%20Report.pdf (accessed 5 August 2020).
6. Xue FS, Zhang GH, Li P, et al. The clinical observation of difficult laryngoscopy and difficult intubation in infants with cleft lip and palate. *Pediatr. Anesth.* 2006;16:283–9.
7. Akpek EA, Mutlu H, Kayhan Z. Difficult intubation in pediatric cardiac anesthesia. *J. Cardiothorac. Vasc. Anesth.* 2004;18:610–12.

8. Heinrich S, Birkholz T, Ihmsen H, Irouschek A, Ackermann A, Schmidt J. Incidence and predictors of difficult laryngoscopy in 11,219 pediatric anesthesia procedures. *Pediatr. Anesth.* 2012;22:729–36.

9. Fiadjoe JE, Nishisaki A, Jagannathan N, et al. Airway management complications in children with difficult tracheal intubation from the Pediatric Difficult Intubation (PeDI) registry: a prospective cohort analysis. *Lancet Respir. Med.* 2016;4:37–48.

10. Carroll CL, Spinella PC, Corsi JM, Stoltz P, Zucker AR. Emergent endotracheal intubations in children: be careful if it's late when you intubate. *Pediatr. Crit. Care Med.* 2010;11:343–8.

11. Graciano AL, Tamburro R, Thompson AE, Fiadjoe J, Nadkarni VM, Nishisaki A. Incidence and associated factors of difficult tracheal intubations in pediatric ICUs: a report from National Emergency Airway Registry for Children (NEAR4KIDS). *Intensive Care Med.* 2014;40:1659–69.

12. Bai W, Golmirzaie K, Burke C, et al. Evaluation of emergency pediatric tracheal intubation by pediatric anesthesiologists on inpatient units and the emergency department. *Pediatr. Anesth.* 2016;26:384–91.

13. South Thames Retrieval Service. Clinical guidelines and drug calculator. Available from: https://www.evelinalondon.nhs.uk/our-services/hospital/south-thames-retrieval-service/clinical-guidelines.aspx (accessed 5 August 2020).

11 The stem cell transplant patient in the Paediatric Intensive Care Unit

Omer Aziz

ⓘ **Expert commentary** by Rachel Agbeko

Case history

A 15-year-old female was admitted to the Paediatric Intensive Care Unit (PICU) with acute hypoxic respiratory failure. She had a history of high-risk refractory acute lymphoblastic leukaemia for which she had received an allogeneic stem cell transplant (SCT) 46 days prior to PICU admission. Two weeks previously, the patient had been ad-mitted to the PICU with a history of febrile neutropenia, fluid overload, and was found via a nasopharyngeal aspirate to have respiratory syncytial virus (RSV). During the previous PICU admission, the patient received non-invasive ventilation for 48 hours and was subsequently discharged back to the ward.

✪ **Learning point** Stem cell transplant

SCT or bone marrow transplant refers to the replacement of a patient's bone marrow with progenitor cells that originate either from the same patient (autologous SCT) or are donated by another individual (allogeneic SCT). SCT was originally used for high-risk and refractory haematological malignancies. With an improving safety profile of SCT and better understanding of the molecular basis for many pathologies, the indications for SCT have vastly expanded to include non-malignant haematological disorders, non-haematological malignancies, immune deficiency disorders, inherited metabolic disorders, and autoimmune disorders.[1] SCT offers a treatment for conditions that would otherwise be fatal or incurable.

Allogeneic SCT can be subdivided according to the donor type, donor source, and degree of human leukocyte antigen (HLA) matching. The degree of HLA matching influences the risk of graft failure in the recipient and also potential complications post-SCT, such as graft-versus-host disease (GVHD). Autologous SCT can be divided according to the source of the progenitor cells (see Table 11.1)

Table 11.1 Type of stem cell transplant (SCT), donor source, donor type and possible human leukocyte antigen (HLA) matching

Type of SCT	Donor source	Donor type	HLA matching
Allogeneic	Bone marrow	Related	Fully matched
	Peripheral blood	Unrelated	Mismatched relative: • single antigen mismatch • haplo-identical related donor
	Umbilical		Unrelated: • fully matched • mismatched
Autologous	Bone marrow Peripheral blood	The patients is the donor	Fully matched as from the same patient

Prior to the donor stem cells being infused into the recipient, the recipient's own bone marrow and immune system need to be suppressed or ablated in a process termed 'conditioning'. The purpose of the conditioning regimen will be dependent upon the patient's underlying indication for SCT but may include destroying malignant disease, creating 'space' for the donor stem cells, and/or prevention of the recipient's immune system from attacking the donor stem cell. The conditioning regimen involves administration of highly toxic levels of chemotherapy and or radiotherapy, which would not be possible if replacement with donor stem cells were not available. The conditioning regimen may completely destroy the recipient's bone marrow function, i.e. myeloablative conditioning, or may be highly immunosuppressive but not destroy the recipient's bone marrow function, i.e. reduced-intensity conditioning.

⊕ Expert comment SCT patients needing the PICU

An estimated 15–44% of all paediatric patients having a SCT will have an unplanned PICU admission.[2] Risk factors for requiring PICU admission in the post-SCT patient include allogeneic SCT, mismatched SCT, umbilical donor as SCT, and also non-malignant indication for SCT.[3] The most common reason for post-SCT patients to be admitted to the PICU is respiratory failure.[3] Overall, the post-SCT patient population has one of the highest mortality rates in the PICU.[4] The management of the SCT patient in the PICU requires close collaboration between the intensivist, the bone marrow transplantation team, and the microbiologist, as the course and potential outcome of illness in the SCT patient is dependent upon his/her immune status, presence of SCT complications, and microbiological status.[5] Post-SCT patients requiring ventilation for respiratory support have a PICU mortality rate of between 42% and 75%,[3] with a mortality of up to 78% at 8 months.[6]

Case history (continued)

After the previous discharge from the PICU, she had an ongoing oxygen requirement, varying between 30% and 45% to maintain oxygen saturations of 92–95%. A computed tomography scan of the chest showed diffuse interstitial changes, suggestive of either of fungal infection or idiopathic pulmonary syndrome (IPS). Respiratory secretions re-isolated RSV; hence, the patient received a course of ribavirin and intravenous specific immunoglobulins. She had also developed a diffuse maculopapular rash affecting the perineum, which was diagnosed as grade 1 GVHD. The patient deteriorated over several hours, becoming ever more hypoxic, maintaining oxygen saturations of only 88% via a non-rebreather mask bag at 15 L/min oxygen flow, dyspnoeic, and hypercapnic, which prompted referral to the PICU.

Capillary blood gas prior to admission to the PICU

pH	7.10
$paCO_2$	11.8
pO_2	3.4
Base excess	−7.2
Bicarbonate	18.2
Lactate	4.2

✪ Learning point Infectious causes of respiratory failure in the post-stem cell transplant patient

The underlying causes of respiratory distress and failure in the post-SCT patient are multiple and can be broadly categorized into infectious and non-infectious. Multiple causes contributing to the respiratory failure may occur in the same post-SCT patient. The significantly impaired humoral and innate immunity in the post-SCT period explains some of the susceptibility of the post-SCT patient to respiratory infections. The susceptibility of the SCT patient to different organisms varies with the time from the SCT (Table 11.2), reflecting stages of the immune system reconstitution. It is essential that the SCT patient has the appropriate microbiological investigations and proactive screening, including cultures from bodily fluids, serological testing, and blood for polymerase chain reaction (PCR) for viruses (e.g. cytomegalovirus (CMV), RSV, herpes virus, Epstein–Barr virus, and adenovirus) and possible histological examination for *Pneumocystis jirovecii*, which would require bronchoalveolar lavage. RSV, which may cause a self-limiting illness in the majority of immunocompetent individuals, is associated with up to 50% mortality in the paediatric SCT patient.[7] Disseminated adenoviral infection is associated with nearly 100% mortality in the post-SCT patient.[7] Adenoviral infection has various different clinical presentations and may mimic other complications occurring in the SCT patient, such as GVHD.[7] The importance of identifying adenovirus lies in the risk of immunosuppressive treatment for GVHD, which would exacerbate any adenoviral infection. Most SCT units adopt a screening programme for adenovirus in SCT patients, using blood PCR, which also allows quantification of the viral load of any viraemia.[7] Use of direct immunofluorescence antigen allows for the rapid diagnosis of these viruses, whereas blood PCR for viral load may help guide escalation and response to treatment.

CMV pneumonia is the most common infection in the post-SCT patient, although CMV infection can affect any organ system.[8] More recently, the mortality associated with CMV infections has reduced with preventative strategies, including pre-emptive treatment (i.e. initiation of treatment on the first microbiological detection of the CMV prior to the onset of symptoms) and also prophylaxis.[8] The risk of CMV infection is related to the CMV status of the recipient and donor prior to the SCT; the lowest risk of CMV infection in the post-SCT patient is when both the donor and recipient are seronegative for CMV.[8] The greatest risk of CMV reactivation is in SCT patients who are seronegative for CMV and have a CMV seropositive donor.[8] If a pre-emptive rather than prophylaxis strategy is undertaken for CMV, then all haematopoietic SCT (HSCT) patients should have routine CMV serological testing until 100 days after HSCT.[6] For a comprehensive review of infections affecting post-SCT patients, see Wingard et al.[9]

Table 11.2 Likely organisms in relation to the time since the stem cell transplant

	Pre-Engraftment (Neutropenia) 0–30 Days	Early Engraftment (Impaired Cell Mediated Immunity) 30–100 Days	Late Engraftment (Impaired Cell Mediated & Humoral Immunity) > 100 Days
Viruses	Herpes Simplex Virus		
	Respiratory syncytial virus		
	Parainfluenza & Influenza		
	Human Metapneumovirus		
	Adenovirus		
	Rotavirus		
	Cytomegalovirus		
	Human herpesvirus 6		
	Epstein-Barr Virus		
	Polyoma viruses (BK & JC)		
			Varicella zoster
Gram Positive Bacteria	Staphylococcus epidermis, Staphylococcus aureus, viridians & streptococci		
			Streptococcus pneumoniae Haemophilus Influenzae
Gram Negative Bacteria	Escherichia coli, Klebsiella spp, Pseudomonas		
Fungi/Parasites	Candida Sp		
	Aspergillus Sp		
	Mucor Sp		
	Pneumocystis jirovecii		
	Toxoplasma gondii		

Source: Adapted from *Pediatr Clin N Am*, 60(3), Chima RS, Abulebda K, Jodele S, Advances in Critical Care of the Pediatric Hematopoietic Stem Cell Transplant Patient, pp. 689–707, Copyright (2013), with permission from Elsevier Inc.; *Immunol Res.*, 50(1), Coomes SM, Hubbard LLN, Moore BB, Impaired pulmonary immunity post-bone marrow transplant, pp. 78–86, Copyright (2011), with permission from Springer Nature.

Case history (continued)

On admission to the PICU the patient was intubated after a short trial of non-invasive ventilation owing to persistent hypoxia and respiratory acidosis. Oxygenation and ventilation remained difficult with conventional synchronized intermittent mandatory ventilation; therefore, high-frequency oscillatory ventilation (HFOV) was commenced, after which the patient's oxygen saturation and respiratory acidosis improved.

⭕ **Learning point** Non-infectious causes of respiratory failure in the post-stem cell transplant patient

The most common non-infectious causes of respiratory failure in the SCT patient include pulmonary oedema, alveolar haemorrhage, transplant-associated thrombotic microangiopathy (TA-TMA), GVHD, and pulmonary toxicity secondary to the conditioning regimen.[5]

TA-TMA is a well-recognized multisystem condition characterized by small-vessel endothelial injury.[10] Although most frequently affecting the kidneys, it can affect any organ system, including the heart, lungs, and brain.[10] The diagnosis of TA-TMA requires a high index of suspicion. Features of TA-TMA include microangiopathic anaemia with schistocytes, thrombocytopenia, and raised lactate dehydrogenase. It may be mistaken for other complications that occur in the post-SCT patient, such as GVHD, sepsis, or multiorgan failure.[10] The management of TA-TMA is mainly supportive, with removal of the trigger and aggressive control of hypertension,[10] although more specific treatment for TA-TMA has been suggested in the form of rituximab, defibrotide,[5] or, more recently, eculizumab.[10]

GVHD is, respectively, classified as acute or chronic, depending on presentation before or after 100 days after SCT. Acute GVHD is one of the major risk factors for SCT patients requiring PICU admission.[5] GVHD is characterized by the interaction between the immune cells from the graft and the recipient's antigens.[5] The conditioning regimen results in the release of pro-inflammatory mediators, as well as break down of the mucous membrane barrier, which, in turn, leads to the stimulation of the donor T cells by the recipient's antigen presenting cells. This leads to further stimulation of the inflammatory cascade and recruitment of further differentiated T cells, and thus damage to the recipient's tissue.[5] The clinical features of acute GVHD manifest predominantly in the skin, gastrointestinal system, and the liver.[5] The skin features can be an erythematous, maculopapular, bullous, or desquamating rash in sun-exposed areas, as well as classically involving the palms and soles.[5,11] Hepatic involvement is characterized by cholestasis, transaminitis, and right upper quadrant pain, whereas the main features of intestinal GVHD are that of abdominal pain and secretory diarrhoea, which may become bloody.[5,11] The diagnosis of GVHD is predominantly clinically based, bearing in mind the extensive differential diagnosis, such as drug reactions, infection, or veno-occlusive disease (VOD).[5] GVHD may be confirmed with skin and gastroenterology biopsy.[5] Acute GVHD may also affect the lungs and present with respiratory failure. The outcome of acute GVHD is related to the degree of its severity, which is dependent upon the degree to which the different organ systems are involved.[5] Acute GVHD is graded most commonly using the modified Seattle Glucksberg criteria.[12] Acute GVHD, as well as the subsequent treatment, renders the patient more immunocompromised and thus at even greater risk of infection. Acute GVHD may also affect other systems, including the eyes and pancreas.[5] The mortality associated with severe degrees of acute GVHD may be up to 95% at 5 years.[5,11] Chronic GVHD is a distinct pathological entity from acute GVHD. Whereas acute GVHD is a predominately an inflammatory process, chronic GVHD is not dissimilar to an autoimmune vasculitis with fibrotic changes.[13] The severe form of chronic GVHD is associated with a 5-year mortality of up to 50%.[13]

Close monitoring for and aggressive treatment of infection is essential because of the associated markedly increased risk of opportunistic infection. This is particularly so for severe skin GVHD, as it leads to break down of the mucosal membrane barrier. For gut GVHD, gut rest should be considered with appropriate attention to nutrition. Patients at risk of GVHD are commenced on GVHD prophylaxis, which is usually a calcineurin inhibitor or, occasionally, mycophenolate mofetil.

ⓘ Expert comment Graft-versus-host disease

On diagnosis of acute GVHD, prophylaxis in the form of a calcineurin inhibitor or mycophenolate mofetil is continued, or the dose increased. Steroids, either topical or systemic, may also be added. Severe gastrointestinal GVHD may require polyclonal antithymocyte globulins, leading to the elimination of T cells, which is further severely immunosuppressive. Evolving novel treatments for GVHD not responsive to first-line treatment include extracorporeal photopheresis (ECP), mesenchymal stem cell infusion, and T-cell suicide gene therapy. ECP involves leukapheresis and collection of peripheral mononuclear cells, which are then exposed to a photosensitizing agent followed by ultraviolet A.[14] The mononuclear cells are then re-infused in to the patient. This is then thought to set up an immune modulatory effect mediated via apoptosis.[14] ECP has been reported to be 50–100% effective in retrospective studies.[14] T-cell suicide gene therapy involves ex vivo modification of the donor T cells with a 'suicide gene', which can be activated in vivo should GVHD occur.[15] Mesenchymal stem cell infusion has also been suggested for the prophylaxis and treatment of acute GVHD. This involves infusion of mesenchymal stem cells, which are thought to have a immunomodulatory effect, through their inhibition of the cytotoxic effects of the immune system.[16]

Over the next week it was not possible to wean the HFOV, with hypoxia and or respiratory acidosis resulting each time it was attempted. The patient remained sedated and muscle relaxed. Broad-spectrum antimicrobials, including antibiotics, antivirals, and antifungals, continued to be given, although blood, urine, and respiratory cultures remained negative. In addition, a bronchoalveolar lavage specimen did not reveal any fungal elements or evidence of *P. jirovecii* infection. The patient continued to receive regular physiotherapy, DNAse treatment to aid secretion clearance, aggressive diuresis to maintain a negative fluid balance, prone positioning to aid lung recruitment, and an attempt to respiratory wean. Treatment included high-dose steroids and etanercept (in view of the possibility of IPS). Despite these measures it was not possible to significantly wean the ventilation.

✪ Learning point Idiopathic pulmonary syndrome

IPS is reported to occur in up to 25% of allogeneic SCT patients.[4] It is a distinct condition characterized by widespread radiological evidence of lung parenchymal changes and respiratory compromise in the absence of active infection or pulmonary oedema.[5] Risk factors for IPS include GVHD, allogeneic SCT, and HLA mismatch.[5] Radiological features of IPS may overlap with those of infection or other causes of respiratory failure. Hence, treatment of IPS will invariably be carried out in conjunction with treatment of other causes of respiratory failure. Treatment of IPS is largely supportive and had previously been based on giving high-dose steroids.[5] More recently, addition of the tumour necrosis factor-α-binding protein compound etanercept has been shown to improve survival of paediatric patients with IPS.[5]

✚ Clinical tip Differential diagnoses

Keep an open mind—consider secondary causes of respiratory failure, such as cardiac impairment. Several commonly used chemotherapy agents have cardiotoxic effects, of which the alkylating agent cyclophosphamide is the most commonly implicated.[11] Similarly, VOD and acute kidney injury (AKI), both of which will be discussed, may cause or contribute to respiratory failure in the post-SCT patient.

During the second week of PICU admission the patient went on to develop air leak, which was treated conservatively. Extracorporeal membrane oxygenation (ECMO) was considered; however, the overall consensus from the PICU team was that this patient was not a suitable candidate, as the likely outcome for a SCT patient on ECMO is very poor.

❝ Expert comment Mechanical ventilation in stem cell transplant patients

Internationally, there is variation in the proportion of post-SCT patients that require non-elective mechanical ventilation,[2] with some centres reporting up to 30% of paediatric patients post-SCT requiring mechanical ventilation.[5] The need for mechanical ventilation, due to respiratory failure, is one of the strongest predictors of mortality in the post-SCT patient admitted to the PICU.[4,5] Although the overall outcome of SCT patients admitted to the PICU has improved, SCT patients who require mechanical ventilation continue to have a poor prognosis.[2,4]

HFOV may be required for SCT patients if conventional ventilation fails or as part of a protective strategy. Similarly, addition of inhaled nitric oxide may be useful for patients with evidence of pulmonary hypertension and persistent hypoxia. Neither intervention has a solid evidence base in this particular patient cohort. Respiratory and or cardiovascular failure requiring extracorporeal support has an almost universally poor outcome.[17]

✔ Evidence base Role of non-invasive ventilation

It has been suggested that SCT patients managed only with non-invasive ventilation (NIV) have a better outcome than those requiring intubation.[3,18] However, there is some evidence to suggest post-SCT patients who fail NIV and require intubation have a poorer outcome than any of the SCT patients who require ventilatory support.[18] Hence, patients commenced on NIV require close monitoring and escalation to intubation if they fail to improve. Recent trial evidence in children with severe immunocompromise suggests that early initiation of NIV has no benefit and may be detrimental.[19]

✚ Clinical tip Fluid balance

One central tenet of managing the ventilated post-SCT patient is aggressive management of fluid overload. There are a number of factors that may contribute to fluid overload in the SCT patient, including fluid administration during the conditioning regimen, volume associated with the polypharmacy post-SCT, volume administrated during any resuscitation phase, capillary leak associated with sepsis, or endothelial dysfunction complications of the SCT such as VOD and AKI. Fluid management is mostly pursued by strict fluid balance control by means of diuretics. Early initiation of renal replacement therapy (RRT) might be considered, which, theoretically, would aid management of the respiratory failure.[4] However, attempts to pursue such a clinical trial were abandoned owing to the inability to recruit patients.

Case history (continued)

Ten days into the PICU stay the patient was commenced on noradrenaline infusion owing to persistent hypotension. A blood culture taken at this stage yielded *Escherichia coli* and a full blood count revealed a new-onset pancytopenia. The patient was commenced on meropenem and granulocyte colony-stimulating factor. The source of the *E. coli* was attributed to breakdown of skin and mucosal membrane around the perineum as a result of the GVHD.

Post-SCT patients are often commenced on prophylactic antimicrobials. Each unit should have their own guideline for antimicrobial prophylaxis post-SCT, which may typically involve the use of co-trimoxazole for prophylaxis against *P. jirovecii*, itraconazole or fluconazole as antifungal prophylaxis, and aciclovir for antiviral prophylaxis.[1] Some units adopt a reactive approach for the management of viral infections and hence may not use prophylactic antiviral therapy and only commence on positive microbiological sampling prior to the onset of symptoms, which has been shown to be equally effective as using prophylaxis.

❝ Expert comment Healthcare-associated infection

Measures to reduce the risk of healthcare-associated infection, such as effective hand washing, are vitally important in the SCT patient in the hospital setting given the high risk of the post-SCT patient to opportunistic infection. The SCT patient should be placed in isolation with a protective barrier—ideally with high-efficiency particulate air-filtered rooms—in order to reduce the risk of acquiring infection.

Suspected infection requires prompt treatment with broad-spectrum antimicrobials. The most appropriate antibiotic is dependent upon the local microbiology environment, current or previous sensitivities, likely organism based upon the timing of the SCT, and presence of complications from the SCT.

It is usual to commence broad-spectrum antibiotics, which may then be rationalized once an organism and the sensitivities are identified. There are limited specific treatments available for viral infections and, when available, there is a paucity of clinical trials to review their effectiveness.[8] Management remains largely supportive. Ribavirin is effective in the reduction of mortality of adult SCT patients who have RSV infection, and the addition of immunoglobulin may also have some benefit.[8] Ribavarin, with or without immunoglobulins, in the treatment of parainfluenza infection in the SCT patient, has variable results.[8] Given the high mortality associated with disseminated adenoviral infection, pre-emptive treatment with cidofovir may be considered to prevent disseminated infection. However, use of cidofovir is limited by its significant nephrotoxic side effects.[8] CMV is also treated on a pre-emptive basis, Local guidance will inform thresholds to treat in the absence of consensus on treatable CMV titres.[20] Treatment options for CMV include ganciclovir, valganciclovir, foscarnet, and cidofovir.[20] The latter is usually reserved for when other treatments are ineffective.[3]

> **⊕ Clinical tip** Healthcare-associated infection
>
> It is important to consider the possibility of central line or catheter-associated infections. If suspected, removal of lines/catheters should be considered if there is no prompt response to antibacterial therapy or the microorganism species is unlikely to be eradicated without removal of the central line.

> **Expert comment** Antifungal treatment
>
> Antifungal medications, in treatment rather than prophylaxis doses, should be commenced if there are ongoing concerns regarding sepsis despite broad-spectrum antibiotics, or if there is a strong clinical suspicion of fungal infection.[5]

Case history (continued)

The patient recovered from the *E. coli* sepsis, and inotropes were weaned and then stopped. However, it was still not possible to wean the ventilation. Furthermore, the patient developed AKI, with worsening renal function and then eventually oliguria, with metabolic, as well as respiratory, acidosis and increasing serum potassium.

At this stage there were discussions with the family regarding the poor prognosis. In view of the extensive burden of the patient's condition, as well as the burden of the highly invasive treatment, the family and the medical team agreed that continuing treatment was not in the best interests of this patient. Hence, withdrawal of mechanical ventilation was planned. The patient was extubated and she died in the presence of her family.

Discussion

Multiorgan failure in post-SCT patients

Although respiratory failure is the commonest reason for PICU admission in post-SCT patients, multiorgan failure is the dreaded complication, with an extremely poor prognosis, despite organ support.

AKI may occur in 33% of post-SCT paediatric patients.[22] AKI is often a result a combination of a number of different factors, including nephrotoxic medication, infection, and immune-mediated complications of the SCT such as TA-TMA, VOD, or GVHD.[22] AKI is also a part of multiorgan failure as a result of any aetiology. Addition of regular monitoring for proteinuria to renal function monitoring may also aid for the early diagnosis of TA-TMA.[10] Hypertension is also a salient feature of TA-TMA and should be considered in any SCT patient. There are many factors that may contribute to hypertension in the post-SCT patient such as the use of corticosteroids and a calcineurin inhibitor.[10] TA-TMA is to be considered, especially if the post-SCT patient requires more than one antihypertensive agent to control their blood pressure.[10]

Diligent attention to basic PICU management of fluid balance and appropriate dosing of potentially nephrotoxic medication is essential in the post-SCT patient. Renal failure is often an ominous sign in the SCT patient on the PICU. Historically, the need for RRT in the paediatric SCT patient was associated with an almost universal mortality. Although more recent evidence suggests that there is an improved outcome of SCT patients requiring RRT, the mortality remains significantly high,[4] particularly in the context of multiorgan failure.

Hepatic VOD may also contribute to AKI in the post-SCT patient. Hepatic VOD occurs as a result of sinusoidal damage caused by the conditioning regimen.[5] This leads to sloughing of the sinusoidal endothelium and thus obstruction of the hepatic circulation, leading to hepatic necrosis.[5] VOD presents as hepatomegaly, ascites, jaundice, and fluid overload.[5] Severe VOD associated with multiorgan failure is associated with an exceptionally high mortality rate. Defibrotide, an oligonucleotide, which is thought to have antithrombotic and anti-inflammatory action, is curative in paediatric VOD.[23] There is also evidence to suggest that defibrotide has a role in the prophylaxis for the prevention of VOD in high-risk groups.[23]

A final word from the expert

Allogeneic SCT patients have one of the poorest outcomes in the PICU, with a PICU mortality rate of 43%, as opposed to the overall PICU mortality rate of 3–5%.[4] This is a reflection of the complexity and also the frailty of the post-SCT patient, with limited physiological reserve and subject to a multitude of potential complications. Effective clinical management of the post-SCT patient in the PICU requires a multiprofessional and multidisciplinary approach, given the complexity of such patients. The patient and family are to be seen as partners in dialogue and decision-making, which may involve frank, yet considered, discussion regarding the outcome. At the centre of these discussions should be the patient's best interests and wishes. The appropriateness of escalating invasive treatment, in the context of a poor outcome, needs to be considered. Improving outcome in the critically ill paediatric SCT population remains a challenge, with interventions that may well lie out with the actual PICU environment, although informed by paediatric intensivists.

References

1. Bailey S, Skinner R. *Paediatric Haematology and Oncology (Oxford Specialist Handbooks in Paediatrics)*. Oxford: Oxford University Press; 2009.
2. van Gestel JPJ, Bollen CW, van der Tweel I, Boelens JJ, van Vught AJ. Intensive care unit mortality trends in children after hematopoietic stem cell transplantation: a meta-regression analysis. *Crit. Care Med.* 2008;36::2898–904.

3. Zinter MS, Dvorak CC, Spicer A, Cowan MJ, Sapru A. New insights into multicenter PICU mortality among pediatric hematopoietic stem cell transplant patients. *Crit. Care Med.* 2015; 43: 1986–94.

4. Balit CR, Horan R, Dorofaeff T, et al. Pediatric hematopoietic stem cell transplant and intensive care: have things changed? *Pediatr. Crit. Care Med.* 2016;17:e109–16.

5. Chima RS, Abulebda K, Jodele S. Advances in critical care of the pediatric hematopoietic stem cell transplant patient. *Pediatr. Clin. N. Am.* 2013;60:689–707.

6. Aspesberro F, Guthrie KA, Woolfrey AE, Brogan TV, Roberts JS. Outcome of pediatric hematopoietic stem cell transplant recipients requiring mechanical ventilation. *J. Intensive Care Med.* 2014;29:31–7.

7. Walls T, Shankar AG, Shingadia D. Adenovirus: an increasingly important pathogen in paediatric bone marrow transplant patients. *Lancet Infect. Dis.* 2003;3:79–86.

8. Ljungman P, Hakki M, Boeckh M. Cytomegalovirus in hematopoietic stem cell transplant recipients. *Hematol. Oncol. Clin. North Am.* 2011;25:151–169.

9. Wingard JR, Hsu J, Hiemenz JW. Hematopoietic stem cell transplantation: an overview of infection risks and epidemiology. *Hematol. Oncol. Clin. N. Am.* 2011;25:101–16.

10. Jodele S, Laskin BL, Dandoy CL, et al. A new paradigm: diagnosis and management of HSCT-associated thrombotic microangiopathy as multi-system endothelial injury. *Blood Rev.* 2015;29:191–204.

11. Munchel A, Chen A, Symons H, Emergent complications in the pediatric hematopoietic stem cell transplant patient. *Clin. Pediatr. Emerg. Med.* 2011;12:233–44.

12. Przepiorka D, Weisdorf D, Martin P, et al. 1994 Consensus Conference on Acute GVHD Grading. *Bone Marrow Transplant.* 1995;15:825–8.

13. Blazar BR, Murphy WJ, Abedi M. Advances in graft-versus-host disease biology and therapy. *Nat. Rev. Immunol.* 2012;12:443–58.

14. Weitz M, Strahm B, Meerpohl JJ, Schmidt M, Bassler D. Extracorporeal photopheresis versus standard treatment for acute graft-versus-host disease after haematopoietic stem cell transplanta-tion in paediatric patients. *Cochrane Database Syst. Rev.* 2015;12: CD009759.

15. Georgoudaki A, Sutlu T, Alici E. Suicide gene therapy for graft-versus-host disease. *Immunotherapy* 2010;2:521–37.

16. Amorin B, Algretti AP, Valim V, et al. Mesenchymal stem cell therapy and acute graft-versus-host disease: a review. *Hum. Cell.* 2014;27:137–50.

17. Di Nardo M, Locatelli F, Palmer K, et al. Extracorporeal membrane oxygenation in pediatric recipients of hematopoietic stem cell transplantation: an updated analysis of the Extracorporeal Life Support Organization experience. *Intensive Care Med.* 2014;40:754–6.

18. Rowan CM, Gertz SJ, McArthur J, et al. for the Investigators of the Pediatric Acute Lung Injury and Sepsis Network. Invasive mechanical ventilation and mortality in pediatric hematopoietic stem cell transplantation: a multicenter study. *Pediatr. Crit. Care Med.* 2016;17:294–302.

19. Peters MJ, Agbeko R, Davis P, et al. on behalf of the SCARF Study Investigators and the Pediatric Intensive Care Society Study Group (PICS-SG). Randomized study of early continuous positive airways pressure in acute respiratory failure in children with impaired immunity (SCARF). *Pediatr. Crit. Care Med.* 2018;19:939–48.

20. Emery V, Zuckerman M, Jackson G, et al. on behalf of the British Committee for Standards in Haematology, the British Society of Blood and Marrow Transplantation and the UK Virology Network Management of cytomegalovirus infection in haemopoietic stem cell transplantation. *Br. J. Haematol.* 2013;162:25–39.

21. Larcher V, Craig F, Bhogal K, Wilkinson D, Brieley J on behalf of the Royal College of Paediatrics and Child Health. Making decisions to limit treatment in life-limiting and life-threatening conditions in children: a framework for practice. *Arch. Dis. Child* 2015;100:s1–s23.

22. Didsbury ME, Mackie FE, Kennedy SE. A systematic review of acute kidney injury in pediatric allogeneic hematopoietic stem cell recipients. *Pediatr. Transplant.* 2015;19:460–70.

23. Dignan FL, Wynn RF, Hadzic N, et al.; Haemato-oncology Task Force of British Committee for Standards in Haematology; British Society for Blood and Marrow Transplantation. BCSH/BSBMT guideline: diagnosis and management of veno-occlusive disease (sinusoidal obstruction syndrome) following haematopoietic stem cell transplantation. *Br. J. Haematol.* 2013;163:444–57.

12 Ethical, legal, and end-of-life decision-making

Samiran Ray and Miriam R. Fine-Goulden

⏱ **Expert commentary** by Joe Brierley

Case history 1

A 15-year-old girl with relapsed acute lymphoblastic leukaemia is admitted to the Paediatric Intensive Care Unit (PICU). She was diagnosed 2 years previously and has had several courses of chemotherapy. Another course of chemotherapy treatment is possible but has a less than 1% chance of success. She had developed a chest infection 5 days previously and her parents had brought her to hospital. Over the course of the day, she has been deteriorating on the oncology ward and is admitted to the PICU for non-invasive ventilation (NIV). Her parents cannot bear the thought that she might be coming towards the end of her life. They tell you that they would like her to be intubated if she deteriorates on NIV and to undergo another round of chemotherapy. She has been intubated in the PICU twice before but now feels that she has had enough and does not want to be intubated if she gets any worse. She has stated very clearly that she does not want to undergo another round of chemotherapy with all of the associated side effects given the poor chances of success. She hates being in hospital and wants to go home. She says that she understands fully that she is going to die and that she would rather die than undergo the pain and discomfort of any further treatment.

> ✪ **Learning point** Ethics and decision-making
>
> 'Medical ethics' refers to the application of values and judgements to medical practice: working out what is morally acceptable within a society. Moral theories and ethical principles provide a framework to help develop ethical consensus and provide guidance on appropriate action. For the majority of our clinical practice, we follow the principles of medical ethics without much thought, but when there are choices to be made between two or more options where these principles come into conflict, decision-making is more challenging.

> ✪ **Learning point** The four principles of medical ethics
>
> Beauchamp and Childress formulated the now broadly accepted four principles of medical ethics in the 1970s:[1]
>
> ### 1. Respect for autonomy
>
> Autonomy is the ability to self-govern. To possess autonomy, a person must be able to have desires, to formulate options that can realize those desires, and be able to choose the most appropriate option. Autonomous actions should be intentional, fully understood, and devoid of controlling influences. To exercise autonomy, a person must be able to express their medical problem, understand the different treatment options and consent to the most appropriate one. In line with this principle, it would be unethical to treat someone against their wishes, fail to present available treatment options to them, or influence or disregard their consented option. For children, this might be the relative autonomy of a Gillick-competent child (see Learning point '"Gillick" competence and "Fraser" guidelines'), or the autonomy of parents to decide for their children, restricted by the need to act in the child's best interests.
>
> ### 2. Non-maleficence
>
> *Primum non nocere*—'above all, do no harm': harm being defined as against a person's interests. This would include causing pain or incapacity, but allowing death to occur may not always be against a person's interests: if a condition is unbearable such that the person suffering wishes to die, then continuing life-sustaining treatment may be both maleficent and counter to their autonomy. Non-maleficence could therefore be interpreted as not acting against a person's interests.

3. Beneficence

One of the fundamental aims in medicine is to act in a person's interests by promoting their welfare, i.e. ensuring their well-being or safety. Beneficence encompasses both the requirement to provide positive benefit, and utility ('usefulness'), in which benefits and risks are balanced to provide an overall positive result. An act of beneficence may involve an *overall reduction in risk*, for example in the case of vaccination or thrombo-prophylaxis.

4. Justice

This refers to the fair and consistent treatment of everyone within a population. In medical ethics, the principle mainly refers to *distributive justice*: the fair and equitable distribution of resources within a population. The fairness of distribution is based on specific principles, for example clinical need. The equity is based on treating individuals equally, i.e. people with the same clinical needs get the same care irrespective of their individual characteristics such as ability to pay, religious/racial group, or age.

✪ Learning point 'Gillick' competence and 'Fraser' guidelines

The term 'Gillick' competence arises from the outcome of a legal battle in England that was initiated by Mrs Victoria Gillick in 1982. She took her local health authority (West Norfolk and Wisbech Area) to court in an attempt to prevent doctors from providing contraceptive advice and treatment to people under the age of 16 years without the consent of their parents. The case eventually reached the House of Lords, where the Law Lords (including Lord Fraser) ruled against Mrs Gillick's claims:

> '... whether or not a child is capable of giving the necessary consent will depend on the child's maturity and understanding and the nature of the consent required. The child must be capable of making a reasonable assessment of the advantages and disadvantages of the treatment proposed, so the consent, if given, can be properly and fairly described as true consent'.[a]

The guidelines set out in Lord Fraser's judgement provide a set of criteria that relates specifically to doctors providing contraceptive advice or treatment.

The ruling on this case provides a legal basis to support young people under the age of 16 years consenting to medical advice or treatment if they are able to demonstrate that they can understand it and have sufficient maturity to appreciate what is involved. It also puts the rights of young people to make their own decisions over those of parental rights to prevent them from doing so in these particular cases.

It is very important to note, however, that this applies to *consent to* treatment and not *refusal of* treatment. In UK law, young people under the age of 18 *do not* have the right to veto treatments deemed to be in their best interests.

✚ Clinical tip Assessing Gillick competence

In practice, the concept of Gillick competence is important when it comes to making controversial treatment decisions. For a person to provide valid consent to medical treatment, they must be deemed competent to do so. Although in legal terms a young person is considered either competent or not, in reality there is a spectrum of competency, and while there are criteria for competence defined in law, there is no single 'test' that proves competence.

The legal responsibility for assessing competence to consent to medical treatment rests with doctors, but other health professionals may be able to do so, and all those with responsibilities to the young person (including non-health professionals, such as teachers and social workers) have an ethical duty to enhance the young person's competence. Clinical psychologists will often be involved, and legal advice should be obtained where disputes over competence cannot be successfully resolved.[2]

---

[a] Gillick vs. West Norfolk & Wisbck Area Health Authority [1984–6].

You talk to the girl and conclude that she is competent; however, she is under the age of 16 years and is attempting to refuse treatment. While her parents do accept that she is competent, they do not feel that they can allow her to refuse treatment, however small the chances of success, irrespective of the pain, distress, and discomfort it will cause her.

You discuss the situation with the girl's oncology consultant. She explains that the relapse is recent and believes that the girl's parents have been resistant to meeting the palliative care team because they feel that would signal that they are giving up on their daughter.

⓭ Expert comment Involving the palliative care team

Expert palliative care[b] should be provided to any child. The United Nations Convention of the Rights of the Child is clear in Article 12:

> Children have the right to say what they think should happen, when adults are making decisions that affect them, and to have their opinions taken into account.[c]

How can the parents vetoing palliative care involvement be consistent with Article 12? The parents need a clear discussion that emphasizes that palliative care referral is consistent with continuing aggressive treatment, albeit admitting the chance of cure is decreasing: it is not 'either/or'.

The 2015 Royal College of Paediatrics and Child Health (RCPCH) framework[3] envisages the withholding of further chemotherapy in this situation if the child decides this—supported by her family and the clinical team, but if there is disagreement, one of the usual mechanisms for resolution is recommended. These include: further discussion with the family and expert teams, second opinions, clinical ethics services, and finally, if necessary, the legal process. It is worth noting the 'key/lock' model of consent suggested by Lord Donaldson;[4] consent being provided when one of a number of *key-holders* opens the lock. Such key-holders include children over 16 years of age, the Gillick-competent child, those with parental responsibility, and, of course, the courts.

✪ Learning point Considering treatment limitation

The RCPCH in the UK published guidance in 2015 (updating previous documents from 1997 and 2004) to provide an ethical and legal framework for decision-making when considering limiting life-sustaining treatments in life-limiting and life-threatening conditions in children.[3]

The RCPCH lists three sets of circumstances in which treatment limitation can be considered where it is no longer in the child's best interests to continue, because treatments cannot provide overall benefit:

1. **When life is limited in quantity**—where treatment is unable or unlikely to prolong life significantly. These include *brainstem death* (see Case history 2), *imminent death* (where physiological deterioration is occurring irrespective of treatment), and *inevitable death* (where death is not immediately imminent but will follow and where prolonging life confers no overall benefit).
2. **When life is limited in quality**—where treatment may prolong life significantly but will not alleviate the burdens associated with illness or treatment itself. These include *burdens of treatments* (where treatments themselves provide pain and suffering, outweighing any potential or actual benefits), *burdens of the underlying condition* (in which the severity and impact of the child's underlying condition produces such pain and distress as to overcome any potential or actual

---

[b] The World Health Organization (WHO) defines palliative care as 'an approach that improves the quality of life of patients and their families facing the problems associated with life-threatening illness, through the prevention and relief of suffering by means of early identification and impeccable assessment and treatment of pain and other problems, physical, psychosocial and spiritual' (http://www.who.int/cancer/palliative/definition/en/).

[c] The UN Convention of the Rights of the Child, Article 12.

benefits in sustaining life), and *lack of ability to benefit* (where the severity of the child's condition renders it difficult or impossible for them to gain any benefit from continued life).

3. **Informed competent refusal of treatment**—where an older child who is deemed sufficiently competent and is supported by his/her parents and the clinical team, consents to the withdrawal or withholding of life-sustaining treatment (see Learning point 'Gillick competence and Fraser guidelines').

Similar guidance has been published in the USA—most recently in a policy statement from the American Academy of Pediatrics in 2017, based on the principles of the child's *best interests* and *balancing benefits and burdens* of treatment. In its process guidance, it discusses the roles of the physician; involving children and families; communicating resuscitation status; disagreements concerning forgoing life-sustaining medical treatment; interdisciplinary planning and consultation, and includes special situations, such as extreme prematurity and children with developmental disabilities.[5]

The oncology consultant has never seen a child survive a further course of chemotherapy at this stage, but there are reports in the medical literature of children surviving. It is now after 7pm and there is no one from the palliative care team available.

⚮ Expert comment Emergency legal advice

Effectively, the decision about whether to offer the chemotherapy itself remains with the oncology consultant. In this situation, it would then remain to be seen if the parents could persuade their daughter to allow therapy if they override her objection to it. If the consultant decides that, based on the child's (fully informed) view, the team would not insist on treatment, agreement should then be sought from the parents not to treat. Practical considerations include whether a second expert clinical opinion could be obtained at this stage (i.e. out of hours and when the child is deteriorating with respiratory failure). If agreement cannot be achieved, the courts are available 24 hours a day, although it is, of course, preferable to provide them with time to evaluate the evidence and hear from witnesses to enable the optimal decision-making process. In an emergency, while the presumption of sustaining life is wise, medical teams ought not to deliver treatment they do not consider to be in the patient's best interests. Any resuscitation measures required to enable more leisurely discussion of chemotherapy must be balanced by possible harms to the child. In cases like this, it is recommended to seek early legal advice, involvement of the entire multidisciplinary team, and senior hospital management.

Case history 2

A 4-month-old boy sustains a severe head injury after his mother trips and falls while carrying him down the stairs. He arrives in the Emergency Department unconscious after suffering a seizure, with a single fixed dilated pupil. He is intubated immediately, given a loading dose of phenytoin, and taken for an urgent computed tomography (CT) scan of his head. The CT scan reveals a large intracerebral haemorrhage with midline shift, so urgent transfer to a neurosurgical centre is arranged. The bleed is evacuated and he is returned to the PICU. The anaesthetist reports that the baby's heart rate and blood pressure were unstable in theatre and he has had a large volume of osmotherapy. On examination, he has fixed dilated pupils.

Neuromuscular blocking agents and sedation are discontinued, but overnight there is no spontaneous movement. In the morning he is on low-dose noradrenaline and minimal ventilation. A peripheral nerve stimulator ('train-of-four' monitor) is used to assess the level of neuromuscular blockade, which confirms that there is no persistent neuromuscular blocking effect. He continues to have fixed dilated pupils and there is no respiratory effort on the ventilator. You explain to his parents that it appears that his brain injury will not recover, and plan for brainstem death testing.

⊗ **Learning point** Brainstem death, death by neurological criteria, or brain death

The three terms are often used inter-changeably in literature. Death by neurological criteria or brain death may be the preferred terminology. However, brainstem death is still commonly mentioned in the literature in the UK and elsewhere. There is no legal definition of death. In 2008, the UK Academy of Medical Royal Colleges (AoMRC) published a code of practice for the diagnosis and confirmation of death, in which dying is described as 'a process rather than an event':

'Death entails the irreversible loss of those essential characteristics which are necessary to the existence of a living human person and, thus, the definition of death should be regarded as the irreversible loss of the capacity for consciousness, combined with irreversible loss of the capacity to breathe.'[6]

⊕ **Clinical tip** How to perform brainstem death tests

Figures 12.1 and 12.2 are reproduced from the 2008 AoMRC paper cited.[6]

APPENDIX 1

PROCEDURE FOR THE DIAGNOSIS AND CONFIRMATION OF CESSATION OF BRAIN-STEM FUNCTION BY NEUROLOGICAL TESTING OF BRAIN-STEM REFLEXES

Diagnosis is to be made by two doctors who have been registered for more than five years and are competent in the procedure. At least one should be a consultant. Testing should be undertaken by the doctors together and must always be performed completely and successfully on two occasions in total.

Patient Name: Unit No:

Pre-conditions

Are you satisfied that the patient suffers from a condition that has led to irreversible brain damage?

Specify the condition:

Dr A: Dr B:

Time of onset of unresponsive coma:

Dr A: Dr B:

Are you satisfied that potentially reversible causes for the patient's condition have been adequately excluded, in particular:

	DR A:	DR B:
DEPRESSANT DRUGS		
NEUROMUSCULAR BLOCKING DRUGS		
HYPOTHERMIA		
METABOLIC OR ENDOCRINE DISTURBANCES		

TESTS FOR ABSENCE OF BRAIN-STEM FUNCTION	1ST SET OF TESTS	2ND SET OF TESTS	1ST SET OF TESTS	2ND SET OF TESTS
DO THE PUPILS REACT TO LIGHT?				
ARE THERE CORNEAL REFLEXES?				
IS THERE EYE MOVEMENT ON CALORIC TESTING?				
ARE THERE MOTOR RESPONSES IN THE CRANIAL NERVE DISTRIBUTION IN RESPONSE TO STIMULATION OF FACE, LIMBS OR TRUNK?				
IS THE GAG REFLEX PRESENT?				
IS THERE A COUGH REFLEX?				
HAVE THE RECOMMENDATIONS CONCERNING TESTING FOR APNOEA BEEN FOLLOWED?				
WERE THERE ANY RESPIRATORY MOVEMENTS SEEN?				

Date and time of first set of tests:

Date and time of second set of tests:

Dr A Signature: Dr B Signature:

Status: Status:

22

A CODE OF PRACTICE FOR THE DIAGNOSIS AND CONFIRMATION OF DEATH

Figure 12.1 Procedure for the diagnosis and confirmation of cessation of brain-stem function by neurological testing of brain-stem reflexes.
Source: Reproduced from Academy of Medical Royal Colleges, A Code of Practice for the Diagnosis and Confirmation of Death, Copyright (2008), with permission from Academy of Medical Royal Colleges.

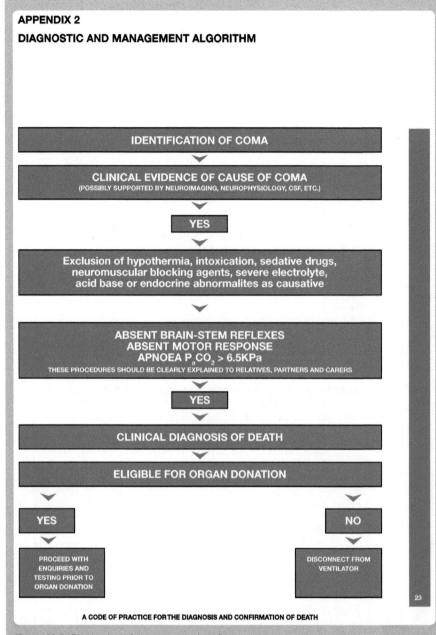

APPENDIX 2

DIAGNOSTIC AND MANAGEMENT ALGORITHM

IDENTIFICATION OF COMA

CLINICAL EVIDENCE OF CAUSE OF COMA
(POSSIBLY SUPPORTED BY NEUROIMAGING, NEUROPHYSIOLOGY, CSF, ETC.)

YES

Exclusion of hypothermia, intoxication, sedative drugs, neuromuscular blocking agents, severe electrolyte, acid base or endocrine abnormalites as causative

ABSENT BRAIN-STEM REFLEXES
ABSENT MOTOR RESPONSE
APNOEA P_aCO_2 > 6.5KPa
THESE PROCEDURES SHOULD BE CLEARLY EXPLAINED TO RELATIVES, PARTNERS AND CARERS

YES

CLINICAL DIAGNOSIS OF DEATH

ELIGIBLE FOR ORGAN DONATION

YES

NO

PROCEED WITH ENQUIRIES AND TESTING PRIOR TO ORGAN DONATION

DISCONNECT FROM VENTILATOR

23

A CODE OF PRACTICE FOR THE DIAGNOSIS AND CONFIRMATION OF DEATH

Figure 12.2 Diagnostic and management algorithm.
Source: Reproduced from Academy of Medical Royal Colleges, A Code of Practice for the Diagnosis and Confirmation of Death, Copyright (2008), with permission from Academy of Medical Royal Colleges

✚ **Clinical tip** Clinical examination in brainstem death[6-8]

Step 1

Brainstem function tests begin by the *identification of coma*, which is confirmed by the absence of eye opening or motor response to the application of a standardized painful stimulus, e.g. pressing on the supraorbital nerve or nail bed.

⊕ Clinical tip Identifying pharmacological and metabolic factors impacting assessment in brainstem death testing

Step 2

It is then vital to exclude the influence of any potentially *reversible effects of drugs or other physiological disturbances* for the patient's condition, which include the following:

Depressant drugs

Commonly used sedative, analgesic, and anticonvulsant drugs in the PICU, particularly opiates, benzodiazepines and barbiturates, may have prolonged effects—especially in critically unwell children with altered drug metabolism and excretion. These drugs must have been discontinued for a suitable period of time such that there is no evidence that the patient's state is due to any depressant drugs. If there is any uncertainty, specific drug assays—interpreted with expert pharmacological advice—may be useful.

Neuromuscular blocking drugs

The presence of peripheral reflexes and/or peripheral nerve stimulators may be used to demonstrate the cessation of effects of these drugs (if in doubt, see the Expert comment 'Ancillary tests in brainstem death testing').

Hypothermia

Brainstem reflexes are generally lost when the body's temperature falls below 28°C, and temperatures of 32–34°C may be associated with impaired consciousness; deficits that are potentially reversible. Core temperature is recommended to be >34°C at the time of brainstem testing.

Metabolic or endocrine disturbances

It is rare for metabolic or endocrine disturbances to be so severe as to be the cause of unresponsiveness, and cessation of brainstem function may, in fact, be the cause rather than the effect of any changes—for example, diabetes insipidus. It may also be detrimental to attempt to correct derangements too rapidly—for example, in the case of hyponatraemia, which could lead to central pontine myelinolysis. A sodium level within the range of 115–160 mmol/L is unlikely to be the cause of unresponsiveness, and it is not recommended to delay testing of brainstem reflexes until levels are within the accepted 'normal' range. Profound derangements of other electrolytes, including potassium, phosphate, and magnesium, may be associated with peripheral muscle weakness but would not be expected to contribute to brainstem dysfunction.

Blood glucose levels should be measured immediately prior to testing brainstem reflexes, and as severe hypoglycaemia may be associated with reduced responsiveness, should be treated if <3.0 mmol/L. Severe hyperglycaemia may be associated with unresponsiveness, at levels >20 mmol/L. Other endocrine abnormalities to be considered are thyroid (thyroid storm or myxoedema may lead to unresponsiveness and/or myopathy) and adrenal (Addisonian crises in severe cases leading to encephalopathy) if suggested by the history. These are, however, very rare in children and would not form part of routine assessment prior to brainstem death testing.

⊕ Clinical tip Tests for absence of brainstem function

Step 3

- Pupil response to bright light: pupils are fixed and do not respond to sharp changes in light intensity.
- Corneal reflexes: no response to light touch on edge of cornea with soft swab.
- Oculo-vestibular reflexes: elevate head to 30 degrees and ensure that there is clear access to the tympanic membrane. Inject ice water (at least 50 mL over 1 minute) and confirm no eye movement during or after the stimulus.
- Eye opening or motor response (grimacing) in the cranial nerve distribution in response to painful stimulation: apply deep pressure over both condyles at the level of the temporomandibular joint.
- Gag reflex: tested with laryngoscope and tongue-depressor/spatula to the posterior pharynx.
- No cough reflex: tested on deep tracheal suctioning.

Apnoea test

This challenges the respiratory centres in the medulla to respond to hypercarbia. To ensure adequate oxygenation and minimize the risk of cardiovascular complications, e.g. hypotension or cardiac arrhythmias, the patient should receive pre-oxygenation, be normothermic, and have systolic blood pressure optimized as far as possible:

- Pre-oxygenate (on ventilator) at fraction of inspired oxygen 1.0 for 10 minutes;
- Reduce the respiratory rate on the ventilator, allowing the end-tidal carbon dioxide (etCO$_2$) to rise;
- Once the etCO$_2$ is above 6 kPa check an arterial blood gas (ABG) to confirm partial pressure of carbon dioxide (paCO$_2$) and pH <7.40;
- Disconnect from the ventilator and insert an oxygen catheter into the airway, delivering oxygen at a rate of 6–8 L/min (to avoid desaturation);
- Observe for any signs of respiration (chest/abdominal wall movements) for 5 minutes and repeat a further ABG;
- If the PaCO$_2$ rises to ≥8 kPa (60 mmHg) (in neonates)/>6.5 kPa (50 mmHg) (in children/adults) or rises ≥ 2.7 kPa (20 mmHg) above baseline with no observed respiratory effort, this confirms apnoea (i.e. is compatible with a diagnosis of brainstem death).

---

❻ Expert comment Ancillary tests in brainstem death testing

Ancillary tests used in the investigation of brainstem function include tests of arterial blood flow (including four-vessel cerebral angiography and transcranial Doppler studies), brain tissue perfusion (such as positron emission tomography), and brain electrical activity (electroencephalograms and brainstem-evoked potentials). Owing to limitations in their reliability, in the UK these do not comprise part of the diagnosis of death by neurological criteria, which remains a clinical diagnosis based on neurological assessment. It is important to note that death by neurological criteria is not synonymous with the absence of *all* brain activity, rather it equates to the *irreversible loss of the capacity for consciousness along with the absence of brainstem function*. If some neurological activity is detected on ancillary testing, this is not, therefore, according to UK guidelines, incompatible with a clinical diagnosis of brainstem death. Having noted these important caveats, it is recognized that in certain special circumstances ancillary tests may be used by the clinician to assist in making the clinical diagnosis. These include:

1. Where comprehensive neurological examination is not possible (e.g. extensive facio-maxillary injuries).
2. Where a primary metabolic or pharmacological derangement cannot be ruled out.
3. In cases of high cervical cord injury.
4. Where an apnoea test cannot be completed owing to physiological instability.

Guidelines in the USA are similar, stating that:[8]

> … ancillary studies are not required to establish brain death and should not be viewed as a substitute for the neurologic examination. Ancillary studies may be used to assist the clinician in making the diagnosis of brain death 1) when components of the examination or apnea testing cannot be completed safely as a result of the underlying medical condition of the patient; 2) if there is uncertainty about the results of the neurologic examination; 3) if a medication effect may be present; or 4) to reduce the inter-examination observation period…. Ancillary studies may also be helpful for social reasons allowing family members to better comprehend the diagnosis of brain death.

However, according to US guidelines, if an ancillary test is performed and is equivocal or there is concern about its validity, the patient cannot be pronounced dead:[8]

> The patient should continue to be observed until brain death can be declared on clinical examination criteria and apnea testing or a follow-up ancillary study can be performed to assist with the determination of brain death. A waiting period of 24 hrs is recommended before further clinical re-evaluation or repeat ancillary study is performed. Supportive patient care should continue during this time period.

The European Society of Paediatric and Neonatal Intensive Care (ESPNIC) Standards for End of Life Care 2017 state that 'every child that may be potentially "brain-dead" should undergo appropriate brainstem death (BSD) testing, in accordance with national guidelines'.[9]

There are several complex clinical, social and legal aspects of brain death that vary significantly between countries and regions. The World Brain Death Project is an international collaboration between professional societies that has aimed to address some of these with the recent publication of a consensus document and recommendations for clinical standards and guidance.[10]

⊕ **Learning point** Children under the age of 2 months

In 2015, the RCPCH published updated recommendations regarding 'The diagnosis of death by neurological criteria (DNC) in infants less than two months old'.[11] The recommendations are that DNC in infants from 37 weeks' corrected gestation to 2 months post term is a *clinical diagnosis* with certain *preconditions*.

In addition to the preconditions detailed in the 2008 AoMRC's code of practice (discussed earlier), it is recommended that an additional precaution is taken in this age group:[11]

In post-asphyxiated infants, or those receiving intensive care after resuscitation, whether or not they have undergone therapeutic hypothermia, there should be a period of at least 24 hours of observation during which the preconditions necessary for the assessment for DNC should be present before clinical testing for DNC. If there are concerns about residual drug-induced sedation, then this period of observation may need to be extended.

In addition to the clinical examination criteria used to establish death in adults, children, and older infants, the recommendations are that:

'a stronger hypercarbic stimulus is used to establish respiratory unresponsiveness. Specifically there should be a clear rise in $PaCO_2$ levels of >2.7 kPa (20 mmHg) above a baseline of at least 5.3 kPa (40 mmHg) to >8.0 kPa (60 mmHg) with no respiratory response at that level'. And that 'the interval between tests need not be prolonged as stated in the 2008 AoMRC's Code of Practice'.[11]

With respect to ancillary tests, the recommendations state that these are neither required nor sufficiently robust to diagnose DNC in infants.

The brainstem function tests are completed, and they confirm the diagnosis of brainstem death—also known as 'death by neurological criteria'. The PICU consultant contacts the Specialist Nurse for Organ Donation (SNOD) to inform him of the test results so that he can come and speak to the family. She also informs the family that she has to make a referral to the lead consultant for child safeguarding owing to the nature of the injury, and that the coroner may need to be involved.

⊕ **Learning point** Organ donation in children

Organ donation should be a routine part of end-of-life care for children, as well as for adults; however, rates vary considerably internationally and between different units in the UK.[12] Donation may be following determination of death by neurological criteria—also known as donation after brain death—as in this case, or following determination of death by circulatory criteria—donation after circulatory death (DCD). In some rare cases, babies diagnosed with anencephaly and other life-limiting conditions have donated organs or tissues after death. Advances in transplantation techniques and in donor physiological optimization have allowed numbers of DCD donation in both adults and children to increase in recent years.

Intensivists must be aware that organ donation is a process that involves several stages: identification of a potential donor; referral to the specialist team; consent or authorization for donation; determination of death; donor management; and organ retrieval. Suboptimal management of any of these stages (along with unavoidable issues) may prevent or limit the possibility of donation. Family refusal is the greatest obstacle to organ donation in children, and rates of consent are higher where specialist nurses are involved in discussions with families[12]—(see Expert comment 'Role of the SNOD').

There is international and regional variation in policies and protocols for organ donation. In the UK, the Paediatric Intensive Care Society (PICS) has national standards for organ donation;[13] there is published National Institute for Health and Care Clinical Excellence guidance;[14] and the National Health Service Blood and Transplant Organ Donation and Transplantation website provides comprehensive and up-to-date data and resources on both adult and paediatric donation and transplantation.[15] In the USA, the American Academy of Pediatrics has published a policy statement on paediatric organ donation and transplantation,[16] and in addition to the ESPNIC Standards for End of Life Care,[11] an additional European resource is the European Society for Organ Transplant.[17]

⏱ Expert comment Role of the SNOD

The problem with the clinical team's approach here is the late involvement of the SNOD. Despite clear guidance, many PICU teams perform poorly in meeting organ donation standards: organ donation is a routine part of end-of-life care for children, as well as for adults.[10,12,16] Early referral, before performance of brain death tests, enables SNODs to attend and assess the child for potential donation. It also enables early consideration of organ optimization techniques once brain death tests have been completed.

The ideal point of referral was when the child returned to the PICU with fixed dilated pupils, if not earlier. In this situation presumably a conversation about brain death and death verification and post-death care, including postmortem and coronial issues, will have happened before the SNOD has even been called, let alone determined donor potential—which, of course, includes identifying potential recipients and planning retrieval teams to attend.

⏱ Expert comment End-of-life care in the PICU

Familiarity with excellent end-of-life care is a mandatory part of children's intensive care practice. This includes death verification processes, legal/coronial issues, palliative care, and, of course, organ donation. Brain death is a rare but crucial part of PICU practice and trainees need to become familiar with undertaking brainstem testing. Organ donation referral, donation after circulatory and brain death, and optimization of the donor are all in the domain of the PICU team working in collaboration with parents and organ donation teams. Failure to optimise donor potential from dying children may contribute to the unnecessary deaths of others.

Case history 3

You have just completed the PICU morning round and received a referral from a local emergency department: a 15-year-old boy found post-hanging. He had no cardiac output when the paramedics had arrived, but after commencement of cardiopulmonary resuscitation, there was return of spontaneous circulation after 25 minutes. His pupils are now fixed and dilated, although his acidosis is slowly improving. He has not made any spontaneous movements or breathing effort. His head CT showed a white cerebellum sign, with loss of grey–white matter differentiation—suggestive of irreversible, catastrophic hypoxic injury. The local team is requesting transfer to a PICU.

In the meantime, two other referrals are taken: a 3-week-old child who has bronchiolitis and is ventilated due to persistent apnoeas, and another for a 6-year-old child with cerebral palsy who presented with status epilepticus and was ventilated for respiratory depression. She has severe developmental delay, with hearing and visual impairment, and is on two antiepileptic drugs.

You only have one PICU bed: which patient should have it? There are no other paediatric intensive care beds in the region, with the nearest available bed 250 miles away.

You recognize the first child (child 1) has a very poor prognosis. He is likely to fulfil brainstem death criteria. However, he has the potential to be an organ donor.

This may benefit several other patients, including patients in your hospital. The child with bronchiolitis (child 2) has a much better prognosis and is very likely to be discharged without long-term sequelae. The child with status epilepticus (child 3) has had three previous PICU admissions, although her last admission was 18 months ago.

> ✪ **Learning point** Resource allocation
>
> Intensive care is resource-hungry and capacity limited. Even in the most resource-abundant setting, capacity can be overwhelmed by surges in activity, e.g. during pandemics, following natural disasters, or terrorist attacks.
>
> At such times, tragic choices may need to be made. In general terms, tragic choices are made based on one or a combination of four approaches:[18]
>
> - a pure market-based system—the highest bidder wins, or those who can afford the resource receive it;
> - an accountable political approach—a designated person/body make/s a decision;
> - a lottery—allocation is based on unbiased chance;
> - an evolutionary approach—allocations evolve naturally, not according to any explicit allocation process.
>
> In a universal healthcare service, such as the UK's National Health Service, a market-based approach is at odds with the universality of healthcare availability. Access to health care is based on clinical need rather than ability to pay. In all three cases, there is a clinical need: all three children need mechanical ventilation to stay alive.
>
> Intensive care services should have a prospectively agreed upon triage process, which is fair and transparent. This is recommended by most intensive care societies, including the UK PICS, the UK Faculty of Intensive Care Medicine (FICM), and the US Society of Critical Care Medicine (SCCM). Most allocation decisions in UK health care are based on John Rawls' 'Maximin' principle: that we maximize the minimum regret or loss.[19] We choose the alternative whose worst outcome is better than the worst outcome of all the other alternatives. This creates a shift of focus from the patient's need to the outcome.

> ✚ **Clinical tip** Evaluation of a child's resource requirements
>
> Although we earlier state that all three children have an equal need for intensive care, one could argue this is not strictly true: if all three children were disconnected from the ventilator, child 1 is likely to die instantaneously, the other two may recover over time. Therefore, child 1's need for ventilation is the greatest. However, he is highly likely to die even with intensive care. The other two are likely to survive: other outcome markers such as quality of life may need to be taken into account. From the information available, child 3 already has several disabilities that are likely to compromise her quality of life. Not providing an intensive care bed may diminish this further. Child 2, although very young, has no factors compromising her quality of life and the potential to recover fully. Not providing intensive care can lead to long-term disability and diminish future quality of life. Although it is difficult to quantify and therefore equate quality of life accurately in children, based on the likely possibilities, one could justify offering the intensive care bed to the child with bronchiolitis, based on the Maximin principle.
>
> If the first-come-first-serve rule should not be followed, and withholding and withdrawal of treatment are morally equivalent, then would it be justifiable to withdraw mechanical ventilation from an existing patient on the unit if they were deemed to have a poorer prognosis than the children referred? This is difficult to argue against (apart from the assumption that our prognostic tools are good enough to make this judgement). A patient already admitted to the Intensive Care Unit (ICU) has been deemed to have the potential to benefit from intensive care—while this remains the case, intensive care should be offered. With this, an element of the first-come-first-serve rule prevails.
>
> Finally, the argument of organ donation: although child 1 is likely not to benefit from intensive care, he has the potential to donate organs, which would benefit multiple patients. This is a utilitarian

argument for admitting this child to the intensive care bed: this will bring the greatest good to the greatest number of people. This is a common problem in many areas of health care, where decisions made for individuals may not benefit the population and vice versa. Yet, our decision has to be based on the individuals concerned: this is a fundamental duty of a doctor as stated by the UK General Medical Council (GMC).[20] To offer the last bed to the first child would not benefit him. We would therefore be treating him not as a means to an end: this is contrary to Kant's imperative to ' ... act in such a way that you treat humanity, whether in your own person or in the person of any other, never merely as a means to an end, but always at the same time as an end'.[21] However, is this not true of anyone donating organs? Organ donation is an altruistic act: the aim is to facilitate this opportunity for the donor. As a child, where individual wishes may not be known, parental wishes are taken into account. The possibility of organ donation by the first child therefore should not be abandoned. Given his age, organ harvesting may be managed in an adult centre: collaboration from the local team with the help of SNODs may still facilitate organ donation (see case 2).

⊕ Clinical tip Intensive care triage

Triage tools in intensive care have been considered widely, although there is no 'one-size-fits-all' tool. Most intensive care societies recommend adoption of local triage and admission policies as best suits the local service model. The SCCM has a framework to aid the formulation of local admission, discharge, and triage guidelines.[22] These are based on best available evidence; however, the latest iteration still acknowledges the paucity of evidence. Paediatric specific guidance is even scarcer.

Many efforts to create triage tools have focused on pandemics. Pandemics create a situation in which resources can be exhausted very quickly: triage becomes necessary, and triage rules need to be transparent and adhered to, in order to provide the best outcomes for patients. Triage protocols are designed to promote a system for allocating scare resources fairly, where, by definition, some groups are excluded.[23] Fortunately, triage tools have not been required to be used in critical care to date, yet the need for such triage protocols remains. Triage protocols need to be carefully designed, with the involvement of multidisciplinary teams to ensure engagement and transparency. Importantly, each protocol must have (a) a definition of when it should be activated; (b) inclusion and exclusion criteria; and (c) actions based on triage decisions. When used, triage criteria should be evaluated for effectiveness and fine-tuning.

★ Learning point Duty of doctors with respect to resource allocation

Managing resources effectively is part of the duty of a doctor, and should not be considered beyond the remit of medical practice, to be left to managers or administrators. As stated in the GMC's Good Medical Practice:[20]

> Whatever your role or level in your organization ... you should be willing to demonstrate leadership in managing and using resources effectively. This means that you should be prepared to contribute to decisions about allocating resources and setting priorities in any organization in which you work.

During the COVID-19 pandemic, the British Medical Association (BMA) issued a guidance note on ethical issues for doctors, including resource allocation and triage.[24]

❝ Expert comment Resource allocation in times of resource scarcity

Of course, while this example is an interesting theoretical construct, it misses several crucial elements of day-to-day PICU practice that readily resolve such not entirely infrequent scenarios, in the absence of a true pandemic or other cause of surge activity.

A 15-year-old, whatever the diagnosis, has very similar physiology to a young adult who would usually be cared for in the referring hospital. Referral to the local adult ICU services may resolve the issues, where organ donation discussions are arguably more prevalent. Child 2 had bronchiolitis causing single organ failure, and while transfer to PICU is recommended, management by paediatric services with support from adult ICU, paediatrics and neonatal services can be undertaken safely for a short time outside of the PICU. In the last case, the sedating anti-convulsants will eventually wear off and the child might be able to be successfully extubated after a few hours if the seizures do not recur.

Finally, intensivists have expertise in using their finite resources to accommodate patients: can children in the PICU be discharged, 'doubled up', or can any elective cases be deferred to accommodate these cases?

If there truly is such an emergency, escalation via regional PICU networks and local, regional, and national healthcare management is mandatory.

A final word from the expert

Decision-making in paediatric intensive care can be extremely challenging, particularly towards the end of life. Paediatric intensivists have a duty to act in the best interests of a child, but this can be very difficult in practice when it is at odds with the best interests of others—including the child's parents or carers—and when it may impact on the care (including potential/future care) of others. It is vital for all paediatric intensivists to be aware of the legal and ethical framework in which they work, understand their roles and responsibilities within that framework, and appreciate the importance of involving other members of the healthcare team at every stage.

References

1. Beauchamp TL, Childress J. *Principles of Biomedical Ethics*, 1st edition. New York: Oxford University Press; 1979.
2. Larcher V, Hutchinson A. How should paediatricians assess Gillick competence? *Arch. Dis. Child* 2010;95:307–11.
3. Larcher V, Craig F, Bhogal K, et al. Making decisions to limit treatment in life-limiting and life-threatening conditions in children: a framework for practice. *Arch. Dis. Child* 2015;100(Suppl 2): s1–s23.
4. In Re R (A Minor) (Wardship: Consent to Treatment): CA 1992.
5. Weise KL, Okun AL, Carter BS, et al. Guidance on forgoing life-sustaining medical treatment. *Pediatrics* 2017;140:e20171905.
6. Academy of Medical Royal Colleges (UK). A code of practice for the diagnosis and confirmation of death. Available at: https://www.aomrc.org.uk/reports-guidance/ukdec-reports-and-guidance/code-practice-diagnosis-confirmation-death/ (accessed 17 April 2020).
7. Wijdicks EFM. The diagnosis of brain death. *N. Engl. J. Med.* 2001;344:1215–21.
8. Nakagawa TA, Ashwal S, Mathur M, et al. Guidelines for the determination of brain death in infants and children: an update of the 1987 Task Force recommendations. *Crit. Care Med.* 2011;39:2139–55.
9. European Society of Paediatric and Neonatal Intensive Care. ESPNIC standards for end of life care. Available at: http://espnic-online.org/Media/Files/ESPNIC-Standards-for-End-of-Life-Care2 (accessed 17 April 2020).
10. Greer DM, Shemie SD, Lewis A, et al. Determination of brain death/death by neurological criteria. The World Brain Death Project. JAMA Published online August 3, 2020. doi:10.1001/jama.2020.11586.
11. Royal College of Paediatrics and Child Health (RCPCH). Diagnosis of death by neurological criteria (DNC) in infants less than two months old – clinical guideline. Available at: https://www.rcpch.ac.uk/resources/

diagnosis-death-neurological-criteria-dnc-infants-less-two-months-old-clinical-guideline (accessed 17 April 2020).

12. Hawkins KC, Scales A, Murphy P, Madden S, Brierley J. Current status of paediatric and neonatal organ donation in the UK. *Arch. Dis. Child* 2018;103:210–15.

13. Paediatric Intensive Care Society. National standards for organ donation 2014. Available at: https://nhsbtdbe.blob.core.windows.net/umbraco-assets-corp/1351/pics-standards-for-organ-donation-2.docx (accessed 22 April 2020).

14. National Institute for Health and Care Excellence. Organ donation for transplantation: improving donor identification and consent rates for deceased organ donation. Available at: https://www.nice.org.uk/guidance/cg135 (accessed 17 April 2020).

15. NHS Blood and Transplant. Organ donation and transplantation. Available at: http://www.odt.nhs.uk (accessed 17 April 2020).

16. Eichner JM, Chitkara MB, Lye PS, et al. Policy statement—pediatric organ donation and transplantation. *Pediatrics* 2010;125:822–8.

17. European Society for Organ Transplantation. Leading the way in organ transplantation. Available at: https://www.esot.org (accessed 17 April 2020).

18. Calabresi G, Bobbitt P. *Tragic Choices.* New York: Norton; 1978.

19. Rawls J. *A Theory of Justice.* Boston, MA: Harvard University Press; 1971.

20. General Medical Council. Good medical practice. Available at: https://www.gmc-uk.org/ethical-guidance/ethical-guidance-for-doctors/good-medical-practice (accessed 17 April 2020).

21. Kant I. *Grounding for the Metaphysics of Morals*, 3rd edition. Translated by Ellington JW. Indianapolis, IN: Hackett; 1993 [1785].

22. Nates JL, Nunnally N, Kleinpell P, et al. ICU Admission, discharge and triage guidelines: a framework to enhance clinical operations, development of institutional policies and further research. *Crit. Care Med.* 2016;44:1553–602.

23. Pagel C, Utley M, Ray S. Covid-19: How to triage effectively in a pandemic. *BMJ* 9 March 2020 https://blogs.bmj.com/bmj/2020/03/09/covid-19-triage-in-a-pandemic-is-even-thornier-than-you-might-think/.

24. Guidance. Available at: https://www.bma.org.uk/advice-and-support/covid-19/ethics/covid-19-ethical-issues (Accessed 5 August 2020).

13 Low cardiac output state in a postoperative cardiac patient

Arun Ghose

⊕ **Expert commentary** by Adrian Plunkett

Case history

A term baby presented at 4 hours of age with shock and central cyanosis. The antenatal/perinatal history was unremarkable. At the time of presentation, clinical observations revealed tachycardia, respiratory distress and poor peripheral perfusion. The pulse oximetry saturations were 72% in air. Venous blood gas demonstrated severe lactic acidosis.

He was transferred to the Neonatal Intensive Care Unit for resuscitation and stabilization. Initial interventions included intravascular volume expansion, antibiotics, mechanical ventilation, and maintenance intravenous fluids. The differential diagnosis at this stage included neonatal sepsis, persistent pulmonary hypertension of the newborn, and duct-dependent cyanotic heart disease. Oxygenation did not improve, despite 100% inspired oxygen with inhaled nitric oxide (iNO), so a prostaglandin infusion was commenced to maintain patency of the ductus arteriosus. Following this, the clinical condition partially improved. An echocardiogram (echo) demonstrated transposition of the great arteries (TGA) with intact ventricular septum; the ductus arteriosus was patent. There was restriction to flow at the atrial level via the patent foramen ovale. He was transferred to a Paediatric Intensive Care Unit (PICU).

The acidosis, cyanosis, and clinical signs of shock failed to improve. A balloon atrial septostomy procedure was carried out, following which the clinical condition stabilized. Corrective cardiac surgery—arterial switch operation—was carried out on day 4 of life.

The surgical team encountered an unanticipated technical complexity, resulting in a prolonged run of cardiopulmonary bypass (CPB) for a total of 230 minutes. On separation from CPB, left ventricular (LV) systolic function was impaired. The sternum was left partially open, and an adrenaline infusion at 0.1 µg/kg/min was required to maintain adequate cardiac output.

A postoperative echo was carried out shortly after arrival at the PICU. The echo showed significantly impaired LV systolic function and moderate mitral valve regurgitation. Electrocardiogram (ECG) did not show any evidence of coronary ischaemia, but the cardiac rhythm was slow and junctional (90–100 beats per minute (bpm)), requiring dual-chamber pacing to maintain adequate heart rate (HR) and atrioventricular (AV) synchrony. He was started on milrinone infusion at 0.3 µg/kg/min.

He was examined during the night ward round (~6 hours after return from surgery). Clinical signs demonstrated cool peripheries and weak peripheral pulses. Arterial blood gases showed severe lactic acidosis (lactate = 10 mmol/L), and the central venous saturations (from right internal jugular venous line) were low at 54%

⊙ Learning point Definition of low cardiac output state

Low cardiac output state (LCOS) may occur following CPB;[1] typically 6–18 hours postoperatively.[2] There is no consensus definition of this state.[3] LCOS is a clinical diagnosis. It is defined as a state resulting in inadequate organ perfusion and organ dysfunction.

(vs an arterial oxygen saturation of 98%). The initial central venous pressure (CVP) was 8 mmHg and mean arterial pressure (MAP) was 39 mmHg.

✓ Evidence base Low cardiac output syndrome in children

LCOS is defined by a cardiac index (CI) <2 L/min/m^2.

LCOS in paediatrics was first described in 1975 in a series of 139 children under 4 years of age following cardiac surgery. This cohort underwent a dye dilution technique to calculate cardiac output (CO) and CI (CI–CO adjusted for body surface area). The risk of mortality was higher in patients with a low mixed venous partial pressure of oxygen (pO$_2$) with a CI < 2 L/min/m^2.[4]

Wernovsky et al. described the incidence of low CI (<2 L/min/m^2) was 23.9% within the first 24 hours in paediatric patients post-arterial switch operation. In the majority of cases, the nadir of CI was reached between 9 and 12 hours after CPB.[2]

Mediastinal drain losses were improving. However, the haemoglobin concentration from the blood gas analyser was 89 g/L Packed red blood cells (10 mL/kg) were transfused following which the CVP and MAP increased to 12 mmHg and 45 mmHg, respectively. The clinical condition of cool peripheries and weak pulses did not improve. The lactic acidosis persisted, and the urine output was < 1 mL/kg/h. A clinical diagnosis of LCOS was made.

⊙ Learning point Risk factors for the development of low cardiac output state

Pre-operative

Ventricular hypertrophy/distension

- Chronically raised ventricular pressure leads to accelerated loss of high-energy nucleotides in the surrounding pool for adenosine triphosphate (ATP) production at a cellular level.
- Ventricular over-distension can lead to distension of the muscle beyond the inflexion point of the Starling curve, leading to inefficient relaxation and impaired contractility.[3]

Neonatal myocardium

Several intrinsic characteristics of the neonatal myocardium render it more susceptible to CPB-associated injury:[3]

- decreased sensitivity to insulin and increased dependence on glucose as the main substrate for cardiac myocyte activity;
- lower concentration of antioxidants;
- decreased coupling of β-adrenergic cells to adenylyl cyclase rendering inotropic medication less effective;
- decreased number of mitochondria;
- permeable sarcoplasmic reticulum leading to risk of intracellular calcium overload and reperfusion injury;
- transition from fetal to neonatal circulation.

Chronic cyanosis

Animal model data have shown an association between chronic cyanosis and accelerated loss of ATP; predisposing to myocardial injury.[3]

CPB itself stimulates an inflammatory response triggered by contact of blood with the bypass circuit and a period of ischaemia and reperfusion injury.

Intra-operative

Cardioplegia solutions

Cardioplegia solutions are used during surgery to cease cardiac activity, allowing for a clearer operative field. It is known that acidosis, free radical production, and myocardial injury are linked with LCOS.

① Expert comment Clinical assessment of low cardiac output state

Technical definitions of LCOS depend on measurement of CI and/or markers of oxygen delivery. While these definitions are arguably of use for research purposes, recognition of LCOS (and other shock states) depends on clinical judgement. The clinical markers of LCOS are detailed in the Examination and Investigation sections.

Therefore, the difference in the constituents of cardioplegia (free radical scavengers, acid buffers, and amino acid substrates) may affect how the myocardium recovers from CPB mitigating LCOS.[1]

Complexity of surgery: prolonged bypass or cross-clamp time

The duration of the ischaemic phase of CPB (and associated inflammatory stimulus) is directly related to the complexity of surgery.[1]

Protective factors for LCOS

Corticosteroids

Corticosteroids may dampen the CPB-associated inflammatory response. Survey data from paediatric cardiac centres show that corticosteroids are frequently used prior to CPB in paediatric cardiac surgery cases, although supportive evidence is inconclusive.[5]

Nitric oxide

Nitric oxide has multiple functions in the inflammatory response, including roles in apoptosis, platelet adhesion, white blood cell adhesion, and oxygen free radical production. It may attenuate the inflammatory response post-CPB.

Hypothermia

Period of hypothermia directly correlates with ischaemic time for the muscle. However, hypothermia reduces metabolic activity and might be protective.[1]

> **Evidence base** Nitric oxide during cardiopulmonary bypass
>
> Recent data from a single-centre randomized controlled trial (RCT) in 101 children undergoing bypass cardiac surgery showed a significant reduction in LCOS based on inotrope score (15% vs 31%; p = 0.007) in children randomized to receive iNO.[6] However, the results of this single-centre study are yet to be replicated, and routine use of iNO is not currently recommended practice.

Over the next 3 hours, the patient's skin developed a mottled appearance with poor perfusion, poor peripheral pulses, no urine output, tachycardia, narrow pulse pressure, a lactate increase, and blood gases demonstrating an arterial venous saturation gap of 54%. Initial renal panel results demonstrated early signs of acute kidney injury (AKI). His haemoglobin remained stable and he was not bleeding.

> **Learning point** Recognition of low cardiac output state: clinical signs, investigations, and monitoring
>
> **Examination**
>
> LCOS is a clinical diagnosis made in the context of a child post-CPB with some or all of the following features.
>
> **Tachycardia**
>
> An increased HR for age not related to pain, fever, or seizures.
>
> **Oliguria**
>
> Urine output <0.5 mL/kg/h, due to AKI related to decreased renal perfusion.
>
> **Poor peripheral perfusion**
>
> Assessed by prolonged capillary refill time, reduced peripheral palpable pulse volume, and an increased 'toe-core' temperature difference.
>
> **Hypotension**
>
> Hypotension is often a late sign of shock in children, but a rising requirement for inotropic support to maintain blood pressure in the normal range may be indicative of LCOS. LCOS may also be associated with normal or high arterial blood pressure in scenarios with elevated systemic afterload.
>
> **Altered pulse pressure**
>
> Pulse pressure may be reduced owing to low stroke volume, and/or increased systemic vascular resistance (SVR) following CPB. Conversely, a widened pulse pressure may occur in vasoplegia (also following CPB), resulting in low diastolic pressure and reduced mean arterial pressure.

Altered mental state

Rarely detected in postoperative cardiac patients, as the patients are usually deeply sedated in the immediate postoperative period. However, deterioration in mental state (including seizures, irritability, or new-onset drowsiness) is an important marker of low CO in children outside this period.

There was persistent hypotension with clinical signs of peripheral vasodilatation. A fluid challenge (5 mL/kg isotonic colloid) did not improve the clinical signs. A repeated echo demonstrated poor biventricular contractility with a small pericardial effusion. In view of refractory hypotension and worsening signs of LCOS, inotropic support was escalated (adrenaline was increased to 0.15 µg/kg/min, and noradrenaline was initiated at 0.1 µg/kg/min).

Learning point Investigations in a child with low cardiac output state

Laboratory blood tests

Important markers of end-organ dysfunction related to LCOS include renal and hepatic function tests and monocyte count. Abnormalities in these markers usually lag behind changes in the clinical condition.[1]

Lactic acidosis

Lactic acidosis may result from anaerobic metabolism due to inadequate oxygen delivery associated with LCOS. However, serum lactate concentration may also be raised owing to impaired clearance (e.g. hepatic dysfunction) or β-agonists such as adrenaline. A trend of rising serum lactate concentration following cardiac surgery is indicative of LCOS.[1]

Arterial:venous oxygen saturation difference

A decrease in central or mixed venous oxygen saturation can be indicative of LCOS, and, if sustained, is often followed by a rise in serum lactate and other features of LCOS. Venous measurements taken in the superior vena cava/inferior vena cava may differ, but trend analysis can be useful.[7]

Venous:arterial carbon dioxide difference (VACO$_2$)

An emerging concept in the diagnosis of LCOS is the elevated difference in the partial pressure of carbon dioxide (CO_2) between the venous and arterial blood gas samples.[8] Venous:arterial carbon dioxide difference (VACO$_2$) is hypothesized as a surrogate for impaired tissue perfusion. This is yet to be independently associated with LCOS.

Echocardiogram

This modality can be employed to assess the following scenarios:

- *Cardiac tamponade/effusion*—may be caused by haematoma, active bleeding, or iatrogenic causes (e.g. surgical gauze left postoperatively behind an open chest).
- *Residual lesions*—identification of residual or additional lesions amenable to surgery may lead to re-operation (see Evidence base 'Residual cardiac lesions').
- *Systolic function*—LV fractional shortening <30% is indicative of reduced systolic function. However, this can only be estimated in the absence of regional wall abnormalities.
- *Diastolic dysfunction*—can be estimated with a ratio taken between early and late peaks and troughs in ventricular filling. This can estimate relaxation of the ventricle and whether the ventricle is *restrictive*. Antegrade pulmonary artery flow coinciding with atrial systole is also characteristic with restrictive physiology.
- *Valvular abnormalities*—Doppler ultrasound measurement can provide estimates of pressure gradients across stenotic/regurgitant valves. The degree of valvular regurgitation at the AV level is dependent on the loading conditions, so may be affected by interventions which have an effect on afterload.
- *Regional ventricular wall abnormalities*—may signify coronary ischaemia.
- *Ventricular dilatation*—progressive ventricular dilatation in a failing circulation may herald cardiac arrest.

> **★ Learning point** Techniques for estimation of cardiac output
>
> Techniques for estimating CO should complement, but not replace, clinical assessments of adequacy of CO.[9] The following are some examples of techniques to estimate CO:
>
> - Pulmonary artery catheters allow estimation of CO and left atrial pressure (LAP); however, they are rarely utilized in paediatric practice, in part owing to increased risk of bleeding, arrhythmia, and vascular injury.
> - Oesophageal Doppler:[1,8] CO can be estimated by measuring velocity of ejection from the systemic ventricle across the outflow tract. There is more variability (10–40%) with this compared to pulmonary artery catheter measurements. In an anticoagulated child, oesophageal probes are associated with an increased risk of bleeding. Portable ultrasound Dopplers that utilize suprasternal aortic flow also exist.
> - Bioreactance haemodynamic monitoring is a non-invasive technique using electrical impedance to estimate CO. Electrodes on the chest wall emit a small current; pulsatile blood flow in the chest introduces a time delay in these currents. These are received and analysed giving CO monitoring data. The measurements can suffer from artefact and shunts in a congenital cardiac disease.
> - Arterial waveform analysis-based methods: several methods based on analysis of different aspects of arterial waveform using various algorithms with and without intermittent calibration using dilution methods exist. They are able to provide beat-to-beat monitoring capability.
>
> The usefulness of all of these techniques in a postoperative cardiac patient is limited by several problems, e.g. size of equipment, size of the child, anatomical shunts, abnormal rhythm, valvular incompetence, and accuracy of algorithms.

> **❝ Expert comment** Interpreting values and trends in low cardiac output state
>
> Be cautious interpreting absolute values of arteriovenous oxygen difference (AVO_2) or $VACO_2$ differences. Trend analysis, in conjunction with clinical signs, is more useful than analysis of single values to interpret 'direction of travel', i.e. deterioration or improvement.

> **❝ Expert comment** Monitoring modalities and clinical assessment
>
> No single monitoring modality is superior to regular clinical examination. Clinical judgement can be informed by looking carefully for changes in state over time and responses to changes in therapy. Regularly placing hands on the patient (e.g. palpation of pulse volume, peripheral perfusion, liver size, and other clinical signs) is essential to identify modifiable causes of LCOS and responses to treatments. See Table 13.1 for a systematic approach.

He was noted to be more tachycardic with a HR of 180 bpm. 'P' waves were not identifiable on the monitor and an atrial ECG demonstrated junctional ectopic tachycardia (JET). This was initially treated with correction of dyselectrolytaemia, along with sedation and muscle relaxation to reduce metabolic demand.

Table 13.1 Modifiable causes of low cardiac output state (LCOS) in postoperative cardiac surgery patients

Modifiable causes of LCOS	Clinical signs	Investigation	Management
Respiratory/ventilation failure (including airway size and position) Hypercarbia may promote vasodilation, or hypoxaemia may lead to impaired oxygen delivery	Auscultation—asymmetrical chest movement/leak from around the ETT	CXR Blood gas	May need ET movement or replacement/ventilation adjusting to optimize recruitment (and balance QP:QS in single-ventricle circulations)
Cardiac tamponade/bleeding Reduced ability for the myocardium to relax and fill in diastole impairing coronary perfusion and filling	Distended neck veins Muffled heart sounds Narrow pulse pressure Change in drain losses	Echo	May need drainage and surgical re-exploration Blood and coagulation factor replacement
Pulmonary hypertensive crisis Impaired ejection of RV against increased pulmonary arterial resistance	Systemic hypoxaemia (in the presence of shunt), and/or right-sided heart failure signs	Echo	Pulmonary vasodilators, i.e. iNO, and optimized sedation/analgesia
Arrhythmias (loss of AV synchrony/bradycardia/tachycardia) Loss of diastolic coronary filling time, leading to worsening myocardial acidosis and ischaemia	Loss of P-waves on ECG Discordance of P wave to QRS waves	ECG (three-lead monitoring, atrial wire study, or 12-lead)	Pacing Cardioversion, Electrolyte replacement Antiarrhythmic meds, Hypothermia (for rate control)
Residual lesions Depends on site of residual lesion	Nil improvement in spite of adequate medical management	Echo Cardiac catheterisation	May need further surgical intervention
Electrolyte abnormality (potassium/calcium/magnesium/phosphate) Impaired myocyte contractility	ECG changes Poor response to escalating inotropes	Blood gases/tests ECG abnormalities	Electrolyte correction

ETT, endotracheal tube; CXR, chest X-ray; ET, endotracheal; Echo, echocardiogram; RV, right ventricle; NO, nitric oxide; AV, atrioventricular; ECG, electrocardiogram.
Source: Reproduced from *Trends in Anaesthesia & Critical Care*, 16(6), Jones B, Hayden M, Fraser J, et al., Low cardiac output syndrome in children, pp. 347–358, Copyright (2005), with permission from Elsevier Ltd.

⊕ **Clinical tip** Rhythm, pacing, and importance of atrioventricular synchrony

Bradycardia

Bradycardia can be managed by atrial pacing provided there is adequate AV conduction. In the case of complete heart block, dual-chamber pacing is required. Patients receiving cardiac pacing via external pacing wires should undergo regular review of pacing thresholds and underlying cardiac rhythm.[10,11]

Tachycardia

The commonest tachyarrhythmia in the postoperative period is JET. It is due to abnormal automaticity produced from within or adjacent to the AV node.

Loss of AV synchrony

Loss of AV synchrony (e.g. nodal rhythm/JET) is common following paediatric cardiac surgery. This is of particular significance in cases of restrictive ventricular physiology, where the CO is reliant on the atrial contraction. CO may be improved by restoring AV synchrony through dual-chamber pacing via temporary pacing wires.

The principles of management of JET are:

1. Reduce oxygen and energy demand through adequate sedation, muscle relaxation, maintenance dextrose, and ventilation.
2. Rate control—interventions to reduce the HR, including induced hypothermia and antiarrhythmic medications, such as amiodarone.
3. Restore AV synchrony—after rate control is achieved, sequential AV pacing can temporarily restore AV synchrony.

Case history (continued)

Despite these measures, there was progressive hypotension and the arrhythmia (JET) persisted with a HR of 190 bpm. A bedside conference was held involving the bedside nursing staff, intensivists, cardiology, and cardiothoracic surgical teams. A systematic approach was taken to assess LCOS and options for further management.

⊕ **Learning point** Fluid and inotrope management: a systematic approach

Optimizing the CO through medical management requires a systematic approach (see Figure 13.1):

- assessing and optimizing ventricular preload;
- improving systolic and diastolic dysfunction;
- assessing and optimizing ventricular afterload;
- considering pulmonary and systemic circulations interdependently;
- considering cardiopulmonary interactions.

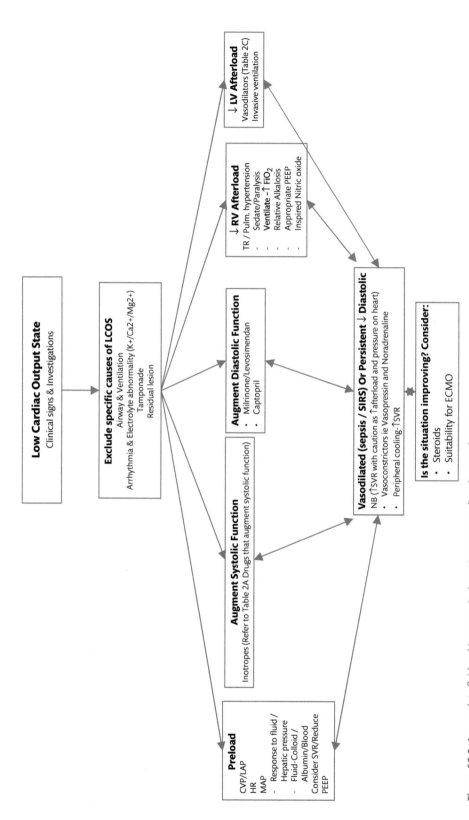

Figure 13.1 Approach to fluid and inotropes in the patient post-cardiopulmonary bypass.

LCOS, low cardiac output state; CVP, central venous pressure; LAP, left atrial pressure; MAP, mean arterial pressure; SVR, systemic vascular resistance; PEEP, positive end expiratory pressure; SIRS, systemic inflammatory response syndrome; ECMO, extracorporeal pulmonary bypass; RV, right ventricular; pulm., pulmonary; FiO₂, fraction of inspired oxygen; LV, left ventricular.

⚙ **Learning point** Ventricular preload

Ventricular preload is the end diastolic ventricular wall tension prior to cardiomyocyte contraction. In a child with suspected LCOS, the preload of the right and left side of the circulation should be considered separately.

Trends in CVP provide an estimate of changes in right ventricular preload. Trends in LAP—if available—correspond to the LV preload.

Signs suggestive of fluid responsiveness provide an indication of position on the Starling curve. Poor fluid responsiveness suggests that the plateau section of the Starling curve has been reached (see Figure 13.2). The left atrial (LA) pressure rising without filling can indicate a failing LV.[12]

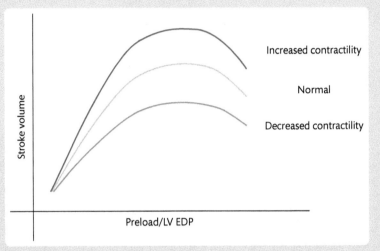

Figure 13.2 Starling's curve. Stroke volume versus left ventricular (LV) end diastolic pressure (EDP)

⚙ **Learning point** Systolic function

Systolic function can be augmented with the use of inotropic medications. However, the clinician needs to be mindful of the increase in metabolic demand (Table 13.2).[2,13,14]

Table 13.2 Drugs that augment systolic function

Drug	Dose (µg/kg/min)	Action	Comment
Adrenaline	0.01–0.1	α, β1, β2	Beta effect best in lower dose range; bronchodilation, inotropy, chronotropy, afterload reduction
	0.2–0.5	α1 and β1 >β2	Increases afterload—alpha and beta effects. Pupils can become dilated in higher doses especially in neonatal patients
Noradrenaline	0.1–0.5	α>β1	Vasoconstriction predominates, increases SVR, although some inotropy in higher doses
Dopamine	1–5	β1>α1	Inotropy, chronotropy
	5–20	α>β1	Vasoconstriction, inotropy, chronotropy
Dobutamine	5–15	β1>β2	Inotropy, chronotropy and vasodilatation, afterload reduction

SVR, systemic vascular resistance.

Calcium can also increase contractility post-CPB, and neonatal myocardium is particularly sensitive to calcium.

✪ **Learning point** Diastolic function

Diastolic dysfunction is defined by impaired relaxation of the ventricular myocardium, which results in reduced stroke volume under normal filling conditions.[1,13,14]

Augmentation of myocardial relaxation (lusitropy) with phosphodiesterase (PDE)-3 inhibitor medication could be considered. The PDE-3 inhibitors (i.e. milrinone) have two main effects (Table 13.3):

1. An inotropic function by reducing breakdown of cyclic adenosine monophosphate through inhibition of PDE.
2. Relaxation of the smooth muscles within the vasculature to cause afterload reduction.

Table 13.3 Phosphodiesterase 3 inhibitors

Drug	Dose (µg/kg/min)	Comment
Amrinone	5–20	Systemic and pulmonary vasodilator Lusitropy
Milrinone	0.25–1	Shorter half-life than amrinone. Inotropy, lusitropy, and vasodilatation

---

✪ **Learning point** Decreased right ventricular afterload and pulmonary hypertension

Right-sided afterload can be increased by increased resistance upstream (right ventricular outflow tract/pulmonary hypertension/LA/left AV valve incompetence/LV failure). Treatment for pulmonary hypertension crisis is to provide adequate sedation, analgesia (and neuromuscular relaxation if required), and promote pulmonary arterial vasodilatation with a high concentration of inspired fraction of inspired oxygen, iNO, and mild alkalosis.

An optimal ventilation strategy reduces pulmonary vascular resistance (PVR) through recruitment of alveoli when extra-alveolar vessels are at their least tortuous. This is around the point of functional residual capacity. If the lung volume is too high, there is compression of the alveolar vessels, and PVR increases; if too low then extra-alveolar vessels are compressed and tortuous increasing PVR. Adequate positive end expiratory pressure can help balance between the two (see Figure 13.3).[15]

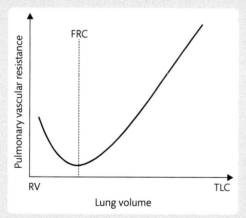

Figure 13.3 Image showing that the pulmonary vascular resistance (PVR) is lowest at functional residual capacity (FRC) of lungs. Both atelectasis and over-distension of lungs result in higher PVR. RV, Residual volume; TLC, total lung capacity.
Source: Reproduced from Cross M, Plunkett E, Physics, Pharmacology and Physiology for Anaesthetists: Key Concepts for the FRCA, Second Edition, Copyright (2014), with permission from Cambridge University Press.

⊗ **Learning point** Decreasing left ventricular afterload

Vasodilator medications may be used to reduce systemic afterload (see Table 13.4).

Table 13.4 Short acting vasodilators

Drug	Dose (µg/kg/min)	Comment
Sodium nitroprusside	0.5–5	Relaxation of smooth muscle and dilatation of pulmonary and systemic vessels
GTN (nitroglycerin)	5–10	Venodilator. Decreases preload and may decrease afterload
Calcium channel blockers (nicardipine)	1–5	Stops calcium from the sarcoplasmic reticulum to cytosol, causing arterial dilatation

GTN, glyceryl trinitrate.

Longer-acting vasodilator

Phenoxybenzamine is an α1 and α2 blocker that decreases peripheral resistance. It is used to maintain vasodilatation on CPB and post-CPB. Angiotensin-converting enzyme inhibitors are used for long-term afterload reduction in heart failure.

Positive pressure ventilation

Positive pressure ventilation (PPV) increases intrathoracic pressure and decreases afterload to the systemic ventricle. This is due to a decrease in transmural pressure gradient. Transmural pressure (~LV wall tension) is equal to systolic pressure minus the thoracic pressure. PPV also decreases the oxygen demand of the respiratory muscles.

⊕ **Clinical tip** Special considerations for ventricular preload in the postoperative child

- Post-tetralogy of Fallot repair: the right ventricle (RV) may be restrictive (poor compliance) necessitating a higher filling pressure (e.g. CVP = 12--18 mmHg).
- Post-arterial switch operation: the RV has been working as the systemic ventricle until the arterial switch operation and the LV will have to adapt to this new role. Clinicians must exercise caution with fluid administration and should watch changes in LAP.
- Post-Fontan operation: PPV reduces venous return and reduces preload, and therefore early extubation and spontaneous breathing is an optimal strategy.

Case history (continued)

It was decided to use therapeutic hypothermia (core temperature target of 35°C) to slow the JET, enable overdrive pacing, and re-establish AV synchrony. Amiodarone was considered, but the team was concerned about the degree of impaired ventricular function. Inotropic and vasopressor medications were continued but did not improve the persistent hypotension and LCOS. Therefore, steroids (hydrocortisone 2 mg/kg q6h) were initiated for catecholamine-resistant shock.

🕐 **Expert comment** Clinical assessment following fluid administration

Monitor liver size, venous pressure, peripheral perfusion, and pulse pressure when administering fluid. While not accurate proxies for fluid status, these clinical signs can give a guide and allow the intensivist to 'get a feel' for the circulatory status.

✓ **Evidence base** Other drugs considered in low cardiac output state

Corticosteroids

Corticosteroids may reduce the inflammatory response resulting from contact of blood with the CPB circuit, and during the ischaemic and reperfusion stages of CPB. Corticosteroids may work in a multimodal fashion; however, some studies have demonstrated immunosuppressive properties related to cumulative exposure to corticosteroids.[16,17]

A meta-analysis of prophylactic steroids in children undergoing cardiac surgery demonstrated no difference in the steroid-treated patient groups. However, the analysis included wide heterogeneity of steroid regimes.[18]

There is clinical equipoise on the use of steroids in LCOS. Low-dose corticosteroids are used in suspected catecholamine-resistant shock due to suppression of the hypothalamic–pituitary axis.[18]

Tri-iodothyronine

Tri-iodothyronine (T3) can increase cardiac contractility and lower SVR. T3 levels have been demonstrated to be reduced in some children following CPB. A multicentre, placebo-controlled, prospective RCT involving children aged <2 years undergoing CPB demonstrated no difference in the primary outcome of 'time to extubation'. T3 administration demonstrated reduction in inotropes used in the subgroup of children aged <5 months.[19,20]

Levosimendan

This is an inodilator (PDE-3 inhibitor similar to milrinone) and works as a calcium sensitizer (binds to troponin C and calcium complex, increasing stability of the compound).[21] These synergistic actions increase the efficiency of cardiac contractility. An observational study of 110 children demonstrated safety in a variety of postoperative children.[22]

> **⊕ Clinical tip** Steroids
>
> Consider low-dose steroid hydrocortisone 1–2 mg/kg q6h when LCOS is diagnosed with failure to respond to catecholamines and preload optimization, particularly if there is evidence of vasoplegia (e.g. wide pulse pressure).

Case history (continued)

After hypothermia, the child's HR had slowed down sufficiently to enable overdrive pacing at a HR of 160 bpm (DDD). However, the patient continued to deteriorate with rising requirements for inotropic support, and progressively increasing LA pressure. Echo demonstrated persistent impaired ventricular systolic function and pericardial clots.

Urgent surgical exploration was performed. During this procedure, the myocardium was noted to be dusky and there was loss of CO. Cardiac massage was commenced, resuscitation adrenaline administered, and the infant was placed on veno-arterial extracorporeal membrane oxygenation (ECMO; with a LA vent). Continuous veno-venous haemofiltration was incorporated into the ECMO circuit for fluid management, and heparin was used for anticoagulation. Antimicrobial spectrum was increased after repeat blood cultures, in case sepsis was driving the LCOS. The ventilation settings were reduced to 'rest settings'.

The patient remained on ECMO support for 4 days. Cardiac catheterization excluded any residual surgical lesions and revealed good coronary blood flow. After a reduction of ECMO circuit flow on day 4 and evidence of good myocardial contractility on stress echo, the patient was de-cannulated. Inotropic support was slowly weaned over the next 48 hours. Steroids were stopped on day 6, and full enteral feeding was recommenced on day 7.

He was eventually weaned from the ventilator after 10 days in the PICU. He spent another 4 days on non-invasive ventilation and was transferred to the ward on high-flow nasal cannula oxygen therapy.

He had a 4/52 stay in hospital establishing feeding and was discharged home with paediatric clinic follow-up owing to feeding concerns.

> **✔ Evidence base** Residual cardiac lesions
>
> Residual lesions are important to consider as a cause of LCOS and may be difficult to identify. There are few published data on the incidence of residual cardiac lesions in patients with postoperative LCOS.

Discussion

Role of ECMO

The decision to initiate ECMO is made between the intensivists, cardiac surgeons, and cardiology team. The primary question regarding suitability for ECMO concerns reversibility of the underlying organ failure. Post-cardiotomy LCOS often improves with supportive care and therefore would be an indication for ECMO.[25]

> **❝ Expert comment** Residual lesions
>
> It is essential to always consider residual lesions as a cause of persisting LCOS. Cardiac catheterisation may be indicated if echo is not diagnostic. This requires open communication between the intensivists, cardiologists and the cardiac surgeons.[23–25]

Common indications in a paediatric cardiac patient

1. Preoperative stabilization

   Rarely, ECMO is used preoperatively in infants with congenital cardiac conditions that lead to hypoxia (late presentation TGA, hypoplastic left heart (HLH) with inadequate shunting). ECMO may allow the PVR to fall, to improve surgical outcome.

2. Failure to wean post-cardiotomy or LCOS in the postoperative period

   This is the most common indication for the use of ECMO. Long periods on bypass, HLH, and pre-existing ventricular dysfunction are associated with severe postoperative myocardial dysfunction. These patients are more at risk of requiring ECMO. There is a high incidence of residual cardiac lesions in patients unable to wean off CPB following cardiac surgery (see Table 13.5), so these should always be ruled out.

3. Cardiac arrest (extracorporeal CPR)

   The International Liaison Committee on Resuscitation recommends ECMO CPR in 'paediatric patients with a cardiac diagnosis who experience an in-hospital cardiac arrest in an ECMO centre'. Timely cannulation and initiation of ECMO in these cases are associated with improved outcomes.

4. Arrhythmia

   ECMO may be used to mitigate shock due to life-threatening intractable arrhythmia while other therapeutic options are ongoing or planned.

Table 13.5 Key studies highlighting the prevalence of residual lesions on extracorporeal membrane oxygenation (ECMO)

Study	Aim and study design	Key results	Conclusion
Booth et al. (2002)[22]	Retrospective description of paediatric patients that underwent cardiac catheterization on ECMO (54/192 patients) at a single centre	Reasons for undergoing cardiac catheterization include 39% (n = 21/54) for consideration for surgical repair and 22% (n = 12/54) for consideration of left heart decompression	Cardiac catheterization can be performed safely in patients on ECMO to identify residual lesions
Agarwal et al. (2016)[23]	Retrospective analysis from a single centre; 119 paediatric patients on ECMO post-cardiac surgery	43/119 were evaluated for residual lesions and these were detected in 35 patients (29%). Detection within 3 days of ECMO improved de-cannulation rate (p = 0.004)	Residual lesions were present in 28% of postoperative patients requiring ECMO support
Howard et al. (2016)[24]	Retrospective analysis of a single centre of 84 neonates on veno-arterial ECMO post-cardiac surgery. (<28 days of age). Review of adequacy of surgical repair, timing of intervention, and ECMO time vs survival	83% on ECMO have residual lesions after cardiac surgery. Time to diagnosis/correction of residual lesions was significantly shorter in survivors (1 vs 2 days; p = 0.02)	Timely identification and repair of residual lesions may improve survival

Practical considerations for ECMO in LCOS

Cannulation for ECMO often uses the same sites as CPB for ease of access postoperatively. Post-cardiac surgery transthoracic cannulation with drainage through the right atrial appendage and flow provided through the ascending aorta is commonplace. This has the advantage over peripheral cannulation of rapid access to the surgical field, and the possibility of relatively large-bore cannula encouraging adequate drainage. The disadvantages of direct cannulation are of the risks of severe haemorrhage and infection, i.e. mediastinitis.[26]

A final word from the expert

LCOS following cardiac surgery is an archetypal problem faced by the intensivist. It typifies many other clinical states that occur as a final common pathway to multiple underlying processes (e.g. sepsis, AKI, and acute respiratory distress syndrome).

While definitions for this state (and others) exist in the literature, LCOS remains a clinical diagnosis. Therefore, recognition and management of this state are key skills for the cardiac intensivist.

Awareness of risk factors and careful monitoring with anticipation of clinical signs of deterioration are key components of the vigilant approach to respond appropriately to LCOS. Laboratory and monitoring data support, rather than confirm the diagnosis.

A systematic approach to identifying the underlying cause of LCOS will help identify potential treatments. The list in Table 13.1 is helpful, but it is important to keep an open mind and challenge assumptions while managing a patient with LCOS.

The value of putting hands on the patient and regularly assessing the impact of interventions cannot be emphasized enough. Along with this, it is essential to participate in early, open dialogue with other members of the multidisciplinary team, e.g. the nursing team, cardiologists, and cardiac surgeons. This is crucial not only to provide a deeper insight into possible underlying causes (e.g. residual lesions) but also to allow more timely intervention if and when required.

Finally, never forget the presence and role of parents and family. Be mindful of how they feel while they are watching their child in a critical condition. It is often useful to allocate a member of staff to liaise with the family during acute interventions and critical periods, in order to keep them updated without overloading them with information.

References

1. Jones B, Hayden M, Fraser J, Janes E. Low cardiac output syndrome in children. *Trends Anaesth.Crit. Care.* 2005;16:347–58.
2. Wernovsky G, Wypij D, Jonas R, et al. Postoperative course and hemodynamic profile after the arterial switch operation in neonates and infants. A comparison of low-flow cardiopulmonary bypass and circulatory arrest. *Circulation* 1995;92:2226–35.
3. Bautista-Hernandez V, Karamanlidis G, McCully J, Del Nido P. Cellular and molecular mechanisms of low cardiac output syndrome after pediatric cardiac surgery. *Curr. Vasc. Pharmacol.* 2016;14:5–13.
4. Parr G, Blackstone E, Kirklin J. Cardiac performance and mortality early after intracardiac surgery in infants and young children. *Circulation* 1975;51:867–74.
5. Checchia P, Bronicki R, Costello J, Nelson D. Steroid use before pediatric cardiac operations using cardiopulmonary bypass: an international survey of 36 centers. *Pediatr. Crit. Care Med.* 2005;6:441–4.
6. James C, Millar J, Horton S, et al. Nitric oxide administration during paediatric cardiopulmonary bypass: a randomised controlled trial. *Intensive Care Med.* 2016;42:1744–52.
7. Chandler H, Kirsch R. Management of the low cardiac output syndrome following surgery for congenital heart disease. *Curr. Cardiol. Rev.* 2016;12:107–11.
8. Rhodes L, Erwin C, Borasino S, Cleveland D, Alten J. Central venous to arterial CO_2 difference after cardiac surgery in infants and neonates. *Pediatr. Crit. Care Med.* 2017;18:228–33.

9. Schloss B, Tobias J. Cardiac output assessment in children: playing catch-up. *Pediatr. Anesth.* 2015;25:113–14.

10. Hoffman T, Wernovsky G, Wieand M, et al. The incidence of arrhythmias in a pediatric cardiac intensive care unit. *Pediatr. Cardiol.* 2002;23:598.

11. Hoffman T, Bush D, Wernovsky G, et al. Postoperative junctional ectopic tachycardia in children: incidence, risk factors, and treatment. *Ann. Thorac. Surg.* 2002;74:1607–11.

12. Starling EH. *The Linacre Lecture on the Law of the Heart.* London: Longmans, Green and Co.; 1918.

13. Wessell D. Managing low cardiac output syndrome after congenital heart surgery. *Crit. Care Med.* 2001;29(10 Suppl.):S220–30.

14. Barry P, Morris K, Ali T (eds). *Oxford Handbook of Paediatric Intensive Care.* Oxford: Oxford University Press; 2010.

15. Shekerdemian L, Bohn D. Cardiovascular effects of mechanical ventilation. *Arch. Dis. Child.* 1999;80:475–80.

16. Pasquali S, Hall M, Li J, et al. Corticosteroids and outcome in children undergoing congenital heart surgery: analysis of the Pediatric Health Information Systems database. *Circulation* 2010;122:2123–30.

17. Mastropietro C, Barrett R, Davalos M, et al. Cumulative corticosteroid exposure and infection risk after complex pediatric cardiac surgery. *Ann. Thorac. Surg.* 2013;95:2133–9.

18. Robertson-Malt S, Afrane B, El Barbary M. Prophylactic steroids for pediatric open heart surgery. *Cochrane Database Syst Rev.* 2007;(4):CD005550.

19. Mackie A, Booth K, Newburger J, et al. A randomized, double-blind, placebo-controlled pilot trial of triiodothyronine in neonatal heart surgery. *J. Thorac. Cardiovasc. Surg.* 2005;130:810–16

20. Portman M, Slee A, Olson A, et al.; TRICC Investigators. Triiodothyronine Supplementation in Infants and Children Undergoing Cardiopulmonary Bypass (TRICC): a multicenter placebo-controlled randomized trial: age analysis. *Circulation* 2010;122(11 Suppl.):S224–33

21. Braun J, Schneider M, Dohmen P, Döpfmer U. Successful treatment of dilative cardiomyopathy in a 12 year old girl using the calcium sensitizer levosimendan after weaning from mechanical bi-ventricular assist support. *J. Cardiothorac. Vasc. Anesth.* 2004;18:772–4.

22. Joshi R, Aggarwal N, Aggarwal M, Pandey R, Dinand V, Joshi R. Successful use of levosimendan as a primary inotrope in pediatric cardiac surgery: an observational study in 110 patients. *Ann. Pediatr. Cardiol.* 2016; 9:9–15.

23. Booth K, Roth S, Perry S, del Nido P, Wessel D, Laussen P. Cardiac catheterization of patients supported by extracorporeal membrane oxygenation. *J. Am. Coll Cardiol.* 2002;40:1681–6.

24. Agarwal H, Hardison D, Saville B, et al. Residual lesions in postoperative pediatric cardiac surgery patients receiving extracorporeal membrane oxygenation support. *J. Thorac. Cardiovasc. Surg.* 2014;147:434–41.

25. Howard TS, Kalish BT, Wigmore D, et al. Association of extracorporeal membrane oxygenation support adequacy and residual lesions with outcomes in neonates supported after cardiac surgery. *Pediatr. Crit. Care Med.* 2016;17:1045–54.

26. Di Nardo M, MacLaren G, Marano M, Cecchetti C, Bernaschi P, Amodeo A. ECLS in paediatric cardiac patients. *Front. Pediatr.* 2016;4:109.

14 Extracorporeal life support

Ryan P. Barbaro

ⓘ **Expert commentary** by Gail Annich and Roxanne Kirsch

Case history

A previously healthy 14-year-old male presented to emergency care with a 24-hour history of lethargy, fever, and myalgia. He arrived in extremis with severe acute respiratory failure and septic shock. Owing to impending cardiorespiratory failure, the patient was emergently intubated. The initial chest X-ray demonstrated bilateral infiltrates and the viral respiratory panel was positive for influenza, and tracheal aspirate had Gram-positive cocci in clusters (identified later to have both influenza A and methicillin-resistant *Staphylococcus aureus* (MRSA)). He immediately required rapid escalation of respiratory support to peak inspiratory pressure (PIP) of 45, positive end expiratory pressure (PEEP) of 20, and fractionated inspiratory oxygen level of 100%. He quickly demonstrated vasoactive refractory septic shock, despite rapid escalation of cardiovascular support, including vasoactive support with epinephrine and norepinephrine infusions escalated to 3 µg/kg/min, vasopressin infusion at 0.0003 U/kg/min, and the addition of stress dose steroids. He was treated with broad-spectrum antibiotics.

> ✪ **Learning point** Indications and relative contraindications for extracorporeal life support: evidence and expert consensus
>
> Extracorporeal life support (ECLS) is offered to critically ill children when we, the providing clinicians, believe the benefits of ECLS outweigh the complicating risk of ECLS.[1] ECLS is indicated when the medical team determines that conventional therapy is likely to cause harm or cannot achieve acceptable support. The exact point when the benefits of ECLS outweigh its risks is unknown, and likely vary from patient to patient. However, guideposts have been planted in the literature.
>
> More recently, other experts have suggested a ratio of PaO_2 to FiO_2 <80, despite a PEEP of 15–20 cm of water, for at least 6 hours; or uncompensated hypercapnia with a pH <7.15; or need for end inspiratory plateau pressure of >35–40 cm of water.[1] In each circumstance, markers of severe acute respiratory failure are used to identify patients with a trajectory of requiring unsustainable support.
>
> Relative contraindications to ECLS use generally fall into three categories: (1) patients who are unlikely to have a reversible condition; (2) patients who are at high risk of suffering an ECLS complication; and (3) patients for whom ECLS may provide suboptimal support. ECLS is supportive not curative. Consequently, patient selection requires that the underlying process can be reversed or treated. For this reason, the two aforementioned trials and expert recommendations also recommend the exclusion of patients with irreversible cardiopulmonary disease, irreversible brain injury, or untreatable metastatic cancer.[1,2] Along this same line of consideration, the CESAR trial also excluded patients who had received high pressure, >30 cm H_2O, or high FiO_2 >80% for more than 7 days because of concern that these patients might suffer unrecoverable lung injury from high ventilator support.[1,3] However, many centres elect to offer ECLS even beyond 14 days of mechanical ventilator support.

> ✔ **Evidence base** UK Collaborative ECMO and CESAR trials
>
> In the UK randomized control trial of neonatal extracorporeal membrane oxygenation (ECMO), neonates with an oxygenation index (OI) ≥40 or a partial pressure of carbon dioxide ($PaCO_2$) ≥90 mmHg for at least 3 hours were considered for ECLS (OI = mean airway pressure × fraction of inspired oxygen (FiO_2) × 100/partial pressure of oxygen (PaO_2) in mmHg).[2] In the Conventional ventilatory support versus Extracorporeal membrane oxygenation for Severe Adult Respiratory failure (CESAR) trial, adults with a Murray score ≥3 or pH <7.20 were considered candidates.[3]

Children placed on ECLS suffer a haemorrhage in 70% of cases and in certain instances that haemorrhage can be life threatening, with 16% of children having an intracranial haemorrhage (ICH). In contrast, only 12% of children supported with ECLS had a thrombosis and only 4% of children had an intracranial infarct. Given the high burden of haemorrhage suffered by children on ECLS, children with increased risk of life-threatening haemorrhage are often seen as poor candidates to receive ECLS. For example, children with known intraventricular haemorrhage or refractory thrombocytopenia are often precluded from ECLS.[2]

Expert comment Extracorporeal life support for septic shock

There are patients with potentially reversible conditions that are highly probable to have a difficult time on ECLS. Most notably in this group are patients with refractory septic shock and preserved left ventricular (LV) function.[4] In this case children should be placed on ECLS for respiratory failure not cardiovascular support. This is because these hyperdynamic children require more cardiac output (CO) than can be delivered via ECLS and, as a consequence, will continue to require exogenous vasoactive support and remain somewhat hypoxic, i.e. saturations not 100% on VA, more likely mid-80s.

Case history (continued)

The patient could only be handbag ventilated for transport and required intermittent bolus doses of epinephrine, to support intermittent drops in blood pressure. ECLS surgical and specialist teams were readied for ECLS cannulation via veno-arterial (VA) cannulation through the neck using the right carotid artery and right jugular vein. Within 6 hours of VA ECLS initiation the patient developed cardiac standstill and left atrial (LA) distension with significant pulmonary haemorrhage. Emergent LA vent was placed in the cardiac catheterization laboratory through the right femoral vein. The patient was then transferred to the Paediatric Intensive Care Unit for his management and care. Despite optimization of flow and oxygen carrying capacity, along with minimization of oxygen consumption by neuromuscular blockade and mild hypothermia, arterial oxygen saturations remained at 82%–85% on VA ECLS at flow of 5 L/min. Cardiovascular support required vasopressor infusions of epinephrine and norepinephrine despite full flow to maintain mean arterial pressures between 65 and 70 mmHg and central venous saturations between 60 and 65, with normal lactates. This intensive management was necessary for the first 7 days of ECLS support with minimal ability to wean any portion of it. Central cannulation for VA ECLS, although discussed, was not performed owing to lack of experience with such support for sepsis aetiology. By the end of week 2 of VA ECLS support the patient was finally fully supported without the need for other interventions to reduce oxygenation consumption or exogenous vasopressors. Antibiotics were switched based on sensitivities.

Clinical tip Drug dosing on extracorporeal life support

There are significant uncertainties about pharmacokinetics and appropriate drug dosing while on ECLS. Therapeutic drug level monitoring is recommended, where possible. Consideration should be given to a higher initial loading dose for some drugs such as antibiotics and sedatives, to minimize the possibility of sub-therapeutic drug levels.

Learning point Choice of veno-arterial, veno-venous, or veno-arterio-venous cannulation and need for left atrial vent

When purely respiratory support is required most clinicians prefer veno-venous (VV) cannulation over VA cannulation, in order to avoid the theoretical complications of VA cannulation. VA cannulations are generally performed through the neck using the jugular vein and carotid artery, or centrally in the right atrium and aorta, and occasionally in the femoral artery and vein. However, groin cannulations are generally reserved for children weighing >20–25 kg because prior to this the vessels are too small. In children who receive VA cannulations there is a higher risk of neurological complications in children cannulated through the carotid artery.[5] Children who receive VA cannulations through the groin also have a moderate risk of limb ischaemia, limb amputation, and north-south syndrome (see Clinical tip 'North-south syndrome or Harlequin syndrome'). For these reasons, VV cannulation is generally preferred when possible, for pure respiratory support, either through dual-lumen single cannulae placed in the right jugular vein or via two single-lumen cannulae placed in the femoral vein (drain) and jugular vein (re-infusion).

However, many times patients have acute respiratory failure in the setting of catecholamine-resistant shock. This combination of cardiorespiratory failure comes in two mechanisms of shock: (1) depressed ventricular function with reduced CO; and (2) preserved LV function and hyperdynamic CO that is failing to meet extreme cardiac demand. Both cases require careful clinical assessment. In case 1, simply improving oxygenation may reduce the pulmonary vascular resistance that was impeding right ventricular function, and improve myocardial oxygenation and therefore LV output. However, some cases will continue to exhibit severe ventricular dysfunction even with improved oxygenation, and these children will require VA cannulation. Those extreme cases that progress to complete absence of LV ejection may require a LA decompression. This is because even on ECLS, blood will continue to drain into the LA through the pulmonary veins both via uncaptured blood that is ejected from the right ventricle and through the bronchial veins. This blood can accumulate, generating increased LA pressure, which can eventually lead to pulmonary haemorrhage. There are several approaches to decompression of the LA. This is usually accomplished in the cardiac catheterization suite by a femoral venous approach, through which a radiofrequency perforation is made to allow passage of a wire to perform a balloon atrial septostomy. When this intervention does not provide enough decompression then a cannula can be placed across the atrial membrane and incorporated into the venous drainage system of the ECLS circuit. This is often called a LA vent.[6,7]

In case 2, where there is preservation of LV function and hyperdynamic CO that is failing to meet extreme cardiac demand, VA through the neck or groin generally cannot meet this extreme demand. Consequently, the patient will continue to need vasoactive support, and ventilator support on top of ECLS, unless central cannulation is considered to meet the CO demands.

In some instances a combination of VA and VV ECLS can be considered. Veno-arterio-venous (VAV) ECLS is rarely used, but is most useful when a patient has cardiac and respiratory failure where cardiac recovery is anticipated prior to respiratory recovery. It is usually used in larger patients (adolescent age) where groin cannulation can be performed for arterial support.

⊕ **Clinical tip** North-south syndrome or Harlequin syndrome

In patients who are supported with VA ECLS with femoral arterial cannulation, if lungs remain completely opacified when cardiac function has returned, then the native CO competes with the ECLS CO and creates a north-south syndrome. This is where the upper part of the body (north) is blue, whereas the lower part of the body (south) remains pink. Addition of a venous re-infusion cannula in the right internal jugular vein to provide ECLS oxygenated blood to the LV outflow tract, and therefore upper body, may be required (VAV support). Alternatively, once cardiac function has returned, the ECLS support can be narrowed to VV ECLS and the arterial cannula can be removed. The venous cannulation can be accomplished with either a double-lumen VV cannula in the right internal jugular vein or single venous cannulation of an internal jugular and femoral vein.

🄰 **Expert comment** Cannulation options

VV support for patients with sepsis and acute respiratory distress syndrome is the first line of support to be considered in a patient failing conventional therapies. However, anticipation of further decompensation must be considered at the initiation of ECLS and escalation to VA must

⊕ **Clinical tip** Left atrial decompression

In patients without a LA vent, in addition to routine serial echocardiograms, a low threshold for ad-hoc urgent scans, to look at LA decompression in response to change in clinical condition, such as cardiac standstill, is recommended.

be anticipated and quickly performed if necessary. Additionally, as in this case, once VA support is initiated the myocardium may stun and the resultant loss of contractility will cause LA distension and the need for emergent LA decompression. As such, the surgical and interventional teams involved with ECLS cannulation must remain on standby for these potential procedures after initial cannulation has been performed.

Central cannulation for sepsis is not performed in all ECLS centres and therefore, as in this case, is not an option when peripheral cannulation/support is not enough. Escalation of support to central cannulation must be done in a centre where protocols are in place and a well-established team of cardiothoracic surgery and ECLS practitioners is prepared to perform the procedure. This must be in place before attempting this escalation.

VAV ECLS is a reasonable option in larger patients who can be cardiac supported through groin cannulation. Therefore, this is usually used in the adolescent population, requires careful decision-making, and preservation of distal limb perfusion is imperative.

⚙ **Learning point** When gas exchange is not required: mechanical circulatory support maybe an option

While a full review of paediatric cardiac mechanical circulatory support (MCS) lies outside the scope of this chapter, it is important to understand the increasing use of ventricular assist devices (VADs) as options for MCS use when gas exchange is not required but rather in isolated cardiac dysfunction/disease. The numbers of children with advanced cardiac disease continues to grow and with it a commensurate rise in the utilization of mechanical support devices.[8] ECLS for cardiac support is most commonly used in the peri-operative setting, either initiated for pre-operative stabilization or, more often, in the postoperative period. Non-operative conditions also require ECLS for cardiac support, such as acute myocarditis, arrhythmias, and cardiomyopathies. Largely, MCS encompasses the realm of device utilization for bridge to recovery, bridge to a bridge (ECLS or temporary VAD to bridge to durable VAD), or bridge to transplant, although VADs are also utilized in adult and some adolescents as destination therapy. The transition from temporary support with ECLS to chronic support with VAD or total artificial heart is influenced by acuity of illness, comorbidities, potential for recovery, and anticipated duration of support.[9]

Limitations remain in paediatrics, with most devices too large for paediatric use. Additionally, there is greater anatomical complexity, with many having congenital heart disease, potential for somatic growth of the patient, and a tendency towards higher complications with anticoagulation given their immature coagulation systems. The development of paediatric VADs was initiated and continues to be largely driven by the utilization of adult devices in children, although recent US Food and Drugs Administration (FDA) approval of the paediatric-specific Berlin Heart EXCOR (Berlin Heart GMBh, Berlin, Germany) in Canada and the USA has expanded utilization. Additionally, there has been a recent focus of efforts and resources into paediatric VAD development.[10] By and large, the majority of patients will have VADs placed (either right, left, or both ventricles) to support CO while awaiting transplant. However, for older patients who have a wider availability of VADs available, including those approved by the FDA for outpatient use, may utilize VAD as a destination therapy. This use of VAD is to provide symptomatic relief of heart failure and allow adequate CO for outpatient continuous 'lifetime' use, with a recent case report of >5 years of use.[8,10,11]

❝ **Expert comment** Ventricular assist devices

The utilization of paediatric MCS is growing and paediatric VAD teams are building an extensive literature to support and inform use. Additionally, current recommendations are to put into place a preparedness plan that includes key stakeholders (cardiology, surgery, transplant, physician, VAD nurse, palliative care team, social work, nursing) and the patient and family to make clear both the purpose of the VAD and to initiate discussions, including possible management of complications and advanced care planning for potential need for device discontinuation.[8]

The recent publication of the International Society of Heart and Lung Transplantation monograph series 'Pediatric Ventricular Assist Devices', provides a thorough review of the medical, surgical, practical, and ethical implications of paediatric VAD use.[8]

Case history (continued)

One of the major issues with the case was related to the pulmonary haemorrhage and subsequent clot formation within the bronchi secondary to the MRSA pneumonia/sepsis. At the time of intubation active haemorrhage was identified with the need for high PEEPs to tamponade the pulmonary haemorrhage allowing for oxygenation and ventilation. Once ECLS was initiated owing to failure of conventional respiratory therapies, lung rest settings were implemented on the ventilator. At this time there continued to be pulmonary haemorrhage, as evidenced by blood coming up the endo-tracheal tube and draining into the ventilator circuit. Protocols for management of haemorrhage on ECLS were employed. Platelets were maintained at $> 100,000 \times 10^9$/L and the heparin infusion was adjusted to maintain activated clotting times (ACTs) at the lowest range according to the institutional protocol for bleeding during ECLS. If bleeding continued, the heparin infusion was held and re-evaluated every 4 hours to determine timing for re-initiation of anticoagulation. As bleeding subsided, heparin management reverted back to standard protocol.

Once bleeding had stopped, flexible bronchoscopy was performed and revealed a large occlusive thrombus straddling the carina and causing mechanical blockage of the distal trachea. The clearance of this was challenging but was carried out with two methods. Mechanical removal via flexible bronchoscopy was utilized, as rigid bronchoscopy was considered too aggressive, and performed every second day. In addition, chemical dissolution with a combination of nebulized tissue plasminogen activator (TPA) and 3% normal saline treatments were used. Over the course of a week these methods were applied and the occlusive blood clots in the large airways were removed, clearing them for lung recruitment once the lungs recovered.

⊕ Learning point Anticoagulation strategy in the face of diffuse pulmonary haemorrhage during extracorporeal life support

Haemorrhage during ECLS is one of the leading complications. This includes complications within both the circuit and patient. The most devastating of these haemorrhagic complications are those associated with ICH and usually lead to withdrawal of life-sustaining therapies. Other haemorrhagic complications are challenging to manage on ECLS, the most common being surgical site bleeding (mostly at the cannulation site), or bleeding at other access sites, including intravenous, arterial line, central venous access, and chest tube sites. When the source of bleeding cannot be locally or surgically controlled, such as in postoperative heart surgery where a source cannot be identified, or in this case with necrotizing pneumonia and pulmonary haemorrhage, then each ECLS centre must rely upon their centre-specific anticoagulation/bleeding protocols. There are anticoagulation guidelines available on the Extracorporeal Life Support Organization (ELSO) website and also in the ELSO Red Book.[12,13] However, these are guidelines, and therefore each programme requires more specific and detailed protocols for bedside management to appropriately approach both bleeding and thrombosis during ECLS. For the earlier-described diffuse bleeding within the pulmonary bed where neither a specific surgical nor technical intervention is an option, optimization of haemostasis within the patient with prevention of thrombus formation within the circuit must be achieved. There are similarities from centre to centre as to how to approach this, and these include ranges of ACTs to be followed if they are used to monitor ECLS anticoagulation as in this case. The application of low, moderately low, and normal anticoagulation ranges can be applied to other monitoring tests as well, such as activated partial thromboplastin time, antifactor Xa levels, or heparin levels, and this again is centre specific. In addition to these strategies, ensuring platelet counts are ≥100,000 × 10^9/L is important so that there is a continual source of functional platelets to provide initial response at the site of bleeding.[14] Antifibrinolytics are utilized during ECLS to prevent breakdown of the haemostatic clots at the site of bleeding, but this is more frequently added if a patient on ECLS undergoes a surgical intervention in anticipation of bleeding.[15] Tranexamic acid or Σ-aminocaproic acid are the main agents used. Once fibrinolysis is activated during ECLS it is difficult to reverse the process with these agents; nonetheless, they are often used as part of haemorrhage control protocols during ECLS.[15] If haemorrhage is not controlled by these interventions then holding anticoagulation may also be indicated. With technological advancements to the ECLS circuit itself, circuit longevity and anticoagulant use have changed. In fact, in some instances entire ECLS runs have occurred without the use of anticoagulation owing to bleeding risks in the patient.[16,17]

🕐 Expert comment Anticoagulation on extracorporeal life support

Anticoagulation during ECLS can be extremely challenging in patients who suffer haemorrhage from their underlying disease. Anticoagulation/bleeding protocols are necessary and standard practice for ECLS programmes. Guidelines provided by ELSO should be the basis upon which each centre constructs protocols for their programme.[13,15] Involvement of haematology experts with an understanding of extracorporeal circuitries is important in the development of these protocols and the maintenance of this part of the ECLS programme; this is most especially important as technology and anticoagulants continue to evolve. It is important to note that despite protocols not every patient will behave the same with anticoagulation and therefore there must always be customization capability for the patient, depending upon their individual response to the ECLS circuit and anticoagulation.

Holding the anticoagulant used to be something that was not done in the early history of ECLS; however, with the advancement of technology and development of circuit coatings this has changed such that holding anticoagulation can be done with very specific guidelines about length of time off anticoagulation and length of time between re-assessments to resume anticoagulation. This interval varies but is generally about 4–6 hours, which coincides with the half-life of heparin.

🕐 Expert comment Pulmonary haemorrhage on extracorporeal life support

As for the formation of an occlusive thrombus after management of the pulmonary haemorrhage, there are few scientific data to support how to manage this. Nebulized TPA has been used successfully in the management of plastic bronchitis.[18] Its use in this case was carefully reviewed and with no sign of airway haemorrhage on flexible bronchoscopy, despite manipulation of the airway during bronchoscopy, nebulized TPA was administered every 6 hours. In between these times nebulized treatments of 3% saline were administered. This allowed for softening of the thrombus straddling the carina and mechanical removal of it with routine gentle suctioning of the endotracheal tube (ETT) and flexible bronchoscopy. In times such as this it is important to have group discussion, opinion, and consensus. One thought in a retrospective review of this case was that leaving the airway completely without manipulation during the acute pulmonary haemorrhage likely caused the maturation of the thrombus. Therefore, maintaining routine airway care, including ETT suctioning with regular nebulized and lavage saline should be part of regular pulmonary hygiene provided to patients on ECLS, even in the face of pulmonary haemorrhage. Again, this should be customized to the patient's presentation.

Case history (continued)

After 2 months of ECLS support the lungs had still not recovered to support oxygenation or ventilation owing to persistent bronchopulmonary fistulae related to areas of pulmonary necrosis caused by the MRSA. During this period, all other organ fail-ures/dysfunctions had recovered and the patient was neurologically intact, undergoing daily mobilization and reconditioning while on ECLS. Uncertainty regarding lung re-covery was at the forefront of concerns as this patient was now the longest paediatric patient that had been supported for respiratory failure at our institution. This forced new clinical and ethical dilemmas about how best to proceed.

The first clinical dilemma was prognostication about lung recovery and the length of time it would take for this recovery to occur. At 60 days of support, the previous longest paediatric ECLS run for respiratory failure at our institution, this patient's lungs were only partially open, despite some success in weaning ECLS support. The patient had converted from two oxygenators for support to one oxygenator. Blood flow rates were less and sweep gas flows were also reduced. There was some success with patient self-recruitment by spontaneous breathing, but this also resulted in the expansion of several pneumatoceles and the opening of multiple bronchopleural fis-tulae (BPFs) bilaterally. Bilateral chest tubes were in place to deal with the BPFs, but the expanding pneumatoceles would often impinge upon the adjacent functional lung tissue and cause it to collapse, limiting or even preventing recruitment. It was at this time that prognosis was unclear and discussion regarding the patient's candidacy for lung transplantation was entertained, despite him being an unconventional candidate who in previous years would not have been considered.

As the patient was the size of a small adult, the initial lung transplant consultation was requested from our institution's adult lung transplant team. The patient was not deemed suitable and there were great concerns regarding the aetiology of the lung failure—MRSA sepsis/pneumonia. The consult was then expanded outside the insti-tution to several paediatric lung transplant centres. Several provided considerations for review. As potential transport to these centres was being organized, the parents decided that lung transplant was not desired and they would remain hopeful for lung recovery. Thus, began the journey into uncharted territory of when or if lung recovery would occur.

Simultaneous to these consultations, the patient continued his course on ECLS. Owing to continual volume loss with initiation of lung recruitment because of the mul-tiple BPFs, the patient underwent several bedside bronchoscopies where lung segments with the BPFs were identified and Spiration® endobronchial valves, 6 and 7 mm in size, were placed. After this placement, lung recruitment improved and the patient converted completely from hypoxic respiratory failure to hypercarbic respiratory failure. The course continued to be challenging with a sepsis episode on day 69 requiring 12 hours off ECLS to replace all lines. With resumption of ECLS, the patient was converted to VV ECLS with continued support to maintain the health of all organ systems. He also was placed on a daily schedule, which included wake/sleep times, physiotherapy, occupational therapy, school, television, and recreational times. During these scheduled events, some caregivers were concerned that he was suffering and that daily routines were 'cruel'. His parents and his core team of caregivers, however, advocated for con-tinuing these rehabilitation routines, recognizing them as necessary to maximize any chance for recovery. In addition, as a team, we saw slow but steady daily improve-ments, and the potential to survive an otherwise fatal illness. We heard and addressed concerns by implementing more active mental health support for the patient.

Sweep gas flows were weaned in a stepwise fashion, slowly allowing the patient to accommodate a potential rise in $PaCO_2$ with each wean. This approach allowed the patient to separate successfully from ECLS on day 87 of support. Thereafter, the patient remained in hospital for 6 months. He was discharged home with a tracheostomy and ventilator on minimal oxygen support. Six months after discharge he no longer required any mechanical ventilatory support and by 12 months after discharge he was decannulated from his tracheostomy tube. He is presently device free and oxygen free. He suffers no ill effects of chronic pulmonary failure and leads an active life similar to his pre-illness baseline.

> ✪ **Learning point** Long-term extracorporeal life support for respiratory failure: when to consider lung transplant, who is a candidate, and who will recover without transplant
>
> There is no clear timing for when to consider a patient for lung transplant in such a case. Prolonged ECLS is becoming more common across ECLS centres worldwide and experiences of 60 or more days, with one >500 days, is pushing providers to alter prognosis.[19] What was once thought to be non-recoverable lung injury at 4 weeks of ECLS support is now an indeterminate time and with that a wavering confidence in prognosticating quality of life (QoL) and expectation for recovery. Therefore, while we hoped for lung recovery, we explored consideration for lung transplant, asking ourselves what needed to be accomplished to enable lung transplant candidacy. Paediatric lung transplant is an uncommon and morbid procedure but with relatively good long-term outcomes for those children who survive to 5 years. Only approximately 15 US centres per year perform paediatric lung transplants. In 2015, 21 children aged 12–17 years and 78 children aged 0–11 years received a lung transplant. For both age groups the 5-year survival was approximately 55%. Despite the high mortality, 93% of survivors reported functional status as fully active at 5 years post-transplant.
>
> When ECLS is used as a bridge to lung transplant, it is recommended for young adults, without multiorgan dysfunction and good rehabilitation potential. It should be avoided in septic shock, multiorgan dysfunction, and prior prolonged mechanical ventilation. With this in mind our patient did present with septic shock and multiorgan failure, but 2 months later on ECLS support, he was a young, near-adult-aged male with single-organ failure.[20] In addition, he was awake and although significantly deconditioned was able to participate in daily rehabilitation. ECLS has been used to support maintenance of physical conditioning and to enable regaining physical condition in children and adults.[21,22] Thus, consideration for lung transplantation was explored as the management plan evolved. As noted previously, the parents declined this option, and the decision to continue support for single-order failure was made with no set end point unless the clinical condition of the patient deteriorated.

> ⓺ **Expert comment** Longer-term extracorporeal life support
>
> ECLS for acute respiratory failure can easily become a 'chronic' ECLS run depending upon the aetiology. Such single organ failure can be well supported on ECLS. During such support, the patient's condition must be optimized to support all organ systems, prevent organ failures, ensure adequate nutrition, and prevent and reduce deconditioning. Regardless of whether the patient is on ECLS for bridge to lung transplant or for a bridge to recovery, the care plan should not differ. The timing for deciding when to consult and list for transplant if a candidate, versus waiting for recovery is not set in advance, nor static. This timing must be dynamic; the potential for lung transplant must be part of the future discussions when long-term ECLS is inevitable. In this case, the patient may have undergone lung transplantation prior to day 87 (time of separation form ECLS) at other centres. There is yet to be a perfect algorithm to go by as to when to transplant versus waiting longer. Preservation of good organ function and prevention of deconditioning all increase the time one can wait, but this requires the entire team, including family and the patient themselves, being on board.

Discussion

Ethical decision-making dilemma around timing of decision to lung transplant versus continuing long-term ECLS

Although a rare case, with the lengthening course of ECLS support beyond our longest previous run for paediatric respiratory support, the timing of review or consideration for lung transplant candidacy became a major point of challenge. Retrospectively, as a team we all feel justified in not pursuing lung transplant and even more relieved that we did not stop at a time where in previous years we might have, owing to no signs of recovery. As successful cases of recovery are described with long-term ECLS, so are successful cases of bridging to lung transplant, after severe respiratory failure from acute infection.

Regardless of the path, the broad purpose of the ECLS support should inform the goals of the multidisciplinary team as the course of therapy evolves. If the goal was support until achieving organ replacement, then a point at which transplant (or long-term mechanical support device) is no longer an option is an important moment to review and reflect on whether a change in broad purpose is warranted.[8] If the patient is not a candidate for transplant the reasons for lack of candidacy, or loss of previous candidacy, may significantly affect their overall morbidities and current QoL. For example, a large stroke or renal failure may significantly affect a patient's QoL, even within that Intensive Care Unit (ICU) stay. If the patient or family refuse transplant, the reasons for their refusal may also underlie concerns for current or future QoL and should be explored. Herein, the discussions with family that framed the purpose of the ECLS support and the values, beliefs, and preferences for what constitutes an acceptable QoL, and what burdens are acceptable to achieve a likelihood of acceptable QoL, are very important in framing solutions. Palliative care teams can be valuable in exploring, understanding, and helping to articulate family goals.[23] The team, with an understanding of what constitutes acceptable patient and family burdens, must then decide if there is reasonable potential (now or in future) for organ recovery to allow successful decannulation of ECLS. This may also constitute a more thorough discussion of the long-term implications of late organ recovery. For example, discussing the potential for tracheostomy and chronic ventilation, or life limitation due to late progressive lung disease. Often, potentials cannot be informed by evidence-based data, but it is worth sharing some sense of the possibilities as the team and family undertake a journey laden with uncertainty.

Preparation of the team for a long-term course of mechanical support is important. The VAD literature for both adults and paediatrics has many recommendations for preparedness plans surrounding VAD implantation.[24-26] With an intent to continue ECLS for lung support across months, it is sensible to choose a similar approach. This would entail that the team that will primarily manage the device and care for the patient assembles to work through processes for both success and failure over the longer term.

A final word from the expert

Deciding to stop or continue when the purpose of the ECLS has changed requires multidisciplinary and patient or family input. Finding a stopping point when a team has already traversed a lengthy ECLS course can be difficult. Agreeing on set time points (calendar or clinical) to review the course, agreeing on what constitutes acceptable progress to continue ECLS, and agreeing on what constitutes potential burdens that would prompt discussions for stopping ECLS will provide a 'roadmap' for the longer duration. Institutional readiness can be enhanced by making known that a process exists for assessing, reviewing, and stopping long-duration ECLS support. This can provide clarity for others on the ethical, legal permissions, and the medical decision-making process. Assembling a core group from ICU physician(s), critical care nurses, ECLS specialists, surgeon(s), transplant teams (where relevant), the pulmonary team (or alternate subspecialist), social work, physiotherapy, child life, bioethics, and palliative care can offer a robust process for designing and implementing a preparedness plan. As a patient's disease progresses, or with changes in their clinical status, the plan should be revisited and reviewed. Maintaining a core team of clinical providers can help with consistency in communication, care, and sustaining knowledge of the preparedness plan. Ideally, preparedness planning is started prior to answering questions of organ replacement, as soon as a 'short' or 'usual' course for recovery is recognized.

References

1. Brodie D, Bacchetta M. Extracorporeal membrane oxygenation for ARDS in adults. *N. Engl. J. Med.* 2011;365:1905–14.
2. UK Collaborative ECMO Trial Group. UK collaborative randomised trial of neonatal extracorporeal membrane oxygenation. *Lancet.* 1996;348:75–82.
3. Peek GJ, Mugford M, Tiruvoipati R, et al. Efficacy and economic assessment of conventional ventilatory support versus extracorporeal membrane oxygenation for severe adult respiratory failure (CESAR): a multicentre randomised controlled trial. *Lancet* 2009;374:1351–63.
4. Schmidt M, Brechot N, Combes A. Ten situations in which ECMO is unlikely to be successful. *Intensive Care Med.* 2016;42:750–2.
5. Teele SA, Salvin JW, Barrett CS, et al. The association of carotid artery cannulation and neurologic injury in pediatric patients supported with venoarterial extracorporeal membrane oxygenation. *Pediatr. Crit. Care Med.* 2014;15:355–61.
6. Kirsch R, Schwartz SM. Medical managment of neonates and children with cardiovascular disease. In: Brogan TV, Lequier L, Lorusso R, MacLaren G, Peek GJ (eds) *Extracorporeal Life Support: The ELSO Red Book*, 5th ed. Ann Arbor, MI: Extracorporeal Life Support Organization; 2017, pp. 367–78.
7. Peek GJ, Hammond I. Neonatal and pediatric cardiac cannulation. In: Brogan TV, Lequier L, Lorusso R, MacLaren G, Peek GJ (eds) *Extracorporeal Life Support: The ELSO Red Book*, 5th ed. Ann Arbor, MI: Extracorporeal Life Support Organization; 2017, pp. 347–55.
8. Lorts A, Schweiger M, Conway J (eds). *Pediatric Ventricular Assist Devices. ISHLT Monograph Series*, Vol. 11. Birmingham, AB: UAB Printing; 2017.
9. Jaquiss RD, Bronicki RA. An overview of mechanical circulatory support in children. *Pediatr. Crit. Care Med.* 2013;14(5 Suppl. 1):S3–6.
10. Stiller B, Adachi I, Fraser CD, Jr. Pediatric ventricular assist devices. *Pediatr. Crit. Care Med.* 2013;14(5 Suppl. 1):S20–6.

11. Purkey NJ, Lin A, Murray JM, et al. Long-term pediatric ventricular assist device therapy: a case report of 2100 + days of support. *ASAIO J.* 2018;64:e1–e2.

12. Bridges BC, Ranucci M, Lequier L. Anticoagulation and disorders of hemostasis. In: Brogan TV, Lequier L, Lorusso R, MacLaren G, Peek GJ (eds) *Extracorporeal Life Support: The ELSO Red Book*, 5th ed. Ann Arbor, MI; 2017, pp. 93–103.

13. Lequier L, Annich GM, Al-Ibrahim O, et al. (eds) ELSO anticoagulation guidelines. Available at: https://www.elso.org/Resources/Guidelines.aspx (accessed 20 April 2020).

14. Annich GM. Extracorporeal life support: the precarious balance of hemostasis. *J. Thromb. Haemost.* 2015;13(Suppl. 1):S336–342.

15. Winkler AM. Transfusion management during extracorporeal life support. In: Brogan TV, Lequier L, Lorusso R, MacLaren G, Peek GJ (eds) *Extracorporeal Life Support: The ELSO Red Book*, 5th ed. Ann Arbor, MI; 2017, pp. 105–16.

16. Muellenbach RM, Kredel M, Kunze E, et al. Prolonged heparin-free extracorporeal membrane oxygenation in multiple injured acute respiratory distress syndrome patients with traumatic brain injury. *J. Trauma Acute Care Surg.* 2012;72:1444–7.

17. Robba C, Ortu A, Bilotta F, et al. Extracorporeal membrane oxygenation for adult respiratory distress syndrome in trauma patients: a case series and systematic literature review. *J. Trauma Acute Care Surg.* 2017;82:165–73.

18. Gibb E, Blount R, Lewis N, et al. Management of plastic bronchitis with topical tissue-type plasminogen activator. *Pediatrics* 2012;130:e446–50.

19. Courtwright AM, Robinson EM, Feins K, et al. ethics committee consultation and extracorporeal membrane oxygenation. *Ann. Am. Thorac. Soc.* 2016;13:1553–8.

20. Abrams D, Brodie D, Arcasoy SM. Extracorporeal life support in lung transplantation. *Clin. Chest Med.* 2017;38:655–66.

21. Turner DA, Rehder KJ, Bonadonna D, et al. Ambulatory ECMO as a bridge to lung transplant in a previously well pediatric patient with ARDS. *Pediatrics* 2014;134:e583–5.

22. Fuehner T, Kuehn C, Hadem J, et al. Extracorporeal membrane oxygenation in awake patients as bridge to lung transplantation. *Am J. Respir. Crit. Care Med.* 2012;185:763–8.

23. Feudtner C. Collaborative communication in pediatric palliative care: a foundation for problem-solving and decision-making. *Pediatr. Clin. North Am.* 2007;54:583–607.

24. Whellan DJ, Goodlin SJ, Dickinson MG, et al. End-of-life care in patients with heart failure. *J. Card. Fail.* 2014;20:121–34.

25. MacIver J, Ross HJ. Withdrawal of ventricular assist device support. *J. Palliat. Care.* 2005;21:151–6.

26. Scheel J, Ploutz M, Blume E, Kirsch R. Paediatric ventricular assist devices. In: Lorts A, Schweiger M, Conway J (eds) *ISHLT Monograph Series*. Birmingham, AB: UAB Printing; 2017, pp. 172–7.

Status epilepticus in the Paediatric Intensive Care Unit

Justin Q.Y. Wang

ⓘ **Expert commentary** by Hari Krishnan

Case history

A 5-year-old boy was brought by paramedics to the Emergency Department of a district general hospital with ongoing generalized tonic-clonic seizures. The paramedics had administered one dose of rectal diazepam en route 5 minutes earlier. There was no significant past medical history other than fever and cough a few days previously. As the seizures continued, he was diagnosed to have status epilepticus (SE). He was managed according to the UK Advanced Paediatric Life Support algorithm for management of SE. Initial management included care of the airway; breathing; circulation, including administration of supplemental oxygen; obtaining intravenous access; blood culture; and venous blood gas analysis. Blood glucose and electrolytes were normal. He had a dose of intravenous (IV) lorazepam followed by a loading dose of phenytoin 10 minutes later owing to unresponsive tonic-clonic seizures. These were also unsuccessful in terminating the seizures. He was commenced on empirical broad-spectrum antibiotic (cefotaxime) and antiviral (aciclovir) at meningitic doses. Senior paediatric and anaesthetic help was requested, and with their assistance, the child was intubated after rapid sequence induction of anaesthesia.

✪ Learning point Definition and initial management

Seizures often become more refractory with time. Hence, despite the debates about the duration-based definition of SE, it is widely accepted that any seizure lasting longer than 5 minutes could be considered SE and merits treatment. Guideline-based standardized management of SE is recommended in many parts of the world. This usually starts with clinical assessment and support of airway, breathing, and circulation, and correction of glucose and electrolyte levels (see Clinical tip ABC-DEFG-HI). At most, two doses of benzodiazepine are administered, ideally at least 10 minutes apart, with at least one of them being an IV or intraosseous dose. Be mindful of the prehospital dose(s) of benzodiazepines, as more than two doses may result in significant respiratory depression. If seizures persist, the next step is to administer an antiepileptic. In the UK, standard guidelines suggest phenytoin as the first choice antiepileptic. However, in other parts of the world, other antiepileptics, such as fosphenytoin, valproate, or levetiracetam are also used.[1] Phenobarbitone is the commonly used alternative in young infants. Clinical trials such as EcLiPSE, ConSEPT, and ESETT have shown that levetiracetam may be as effective as phenytoin. It is anticipated that the results of these trials may inform future versions of SE management algorithms. If seizures continue despite antiepileptics, induction of general anaesthesia with thiopentone or pentobarbital, along with intubation and ventilatory support, is performed. This is usually successful in controlling SE.

> **⊕ Clinical tip** Don't forget the viral infections
>
> Consider administering aciclovir in cases of prolonged seizure with fever, particularly if the seizures are focal and/or liver function test results are abnormal, to treat for herpes simplex encephalitis.

> **⊕ Clinical tip** Nasopharyngeal airway
>
> Nasopharyngeal airway insertion (in the absence of contraindications such as trauma or coagulopathy) is useful in airway management of a convulsing or postictal child. It is easier to insert and much better tolerated than the oropharyngeal airway in this situation, and allows for improved oxygenation and ventilation either until spontaneous recovery or during assisted mask ventilation. An appropriately sized lubricated endotracheal tube (ETT) may be used as the nasopharyngeal airway. This is usually inserted to a depth equivalent to the distance from the nostril to the tragus of the ear.

> **⊕ Clinical tip** ABC-DEFG-HI
>
> Hypoglycaemia is a common cause of seizure, especially in neonates, and can be easily corrected. A bedside glucose test should be performed as soon as possible. As the famous adage goes, 'don't ever forget glucose' (DEFG). Similarly, hyponatraemia and hypocalcaemia are also known to cause seizures. Blood gas analysis is helpful in obtaining an immediate diagnosis. Infection is probably the most important and commonest treatable cause and therefore prompt antibiotic therapy should be initiated when this is suspected. Therefore, in this instance, the mnemonic to remember might be 'ABC-DEFG-HI'.

Case history (continued)

The child was intubated uneventfully with a size 5 uncuffed oral ETT. Accurate tube placement was confirmed with capnography followed by a chest X-ray. He was started on morphine and midazolam infusions after intubation. His pupils were noted to be dilated and sluggishly reactive, with associated episodic unexplained tachycardia and desaturations. Abnormal tonic posturing was noted after recovery from neuromuscular blockade. Continuing electrical seizure activity was suspected. He was therefore re-sedated and a referral was made to the regional paediatric intensive care (PIC) retrieval team for transfer to a Paediatric Intensive Care Unit (PICU). An urgent brain computed tomography (CT) was performed, which was reported as normal. He had further boluses of midazolam followed by an increased infusion rate to 4 µg/kg/min. Rocuronium infusion was continued to facilitate safe retrieval. He was then transferred to the PICU by the retrieval team.

> **✪ Learning point** Neuroimaging
>
> The purpose of neuroimaging in SE is to exclude neurosurgical causes (intracranial bleed), find a structural explanation for the seizures (space-occupying lesions), or presence of complications (such as midline shift and cerebral oedema). Neuroimaging is often performed in children with a history of prolonged seizures with unclear aetiology, especially in young infants; seizures of an unusual pattern in those known to have seizure disorders; with the presence of focal neurology; a history of trauma; and those with a high-risk past medical background, including brain tumour, stroke, ventricular shunt in situ, coagulopathy, sickle cell disease, and cardiac defects. The Neurocritical Care Society recommends neuroimaging within an hour of onset of SE.[2]
>
> CT brain is the most commonly used neuroimaging modality during and after SE as it is readily available in most places and quick to perform. In paediatric SE, up to 20% of brain CTs and 58% of brain magnetic resonance imagings (MRIs) were abnormal. Neuroimaging was relevant in altering acute management in 24% of patients.[3] More detailed parenchymal abnormalities can be detected with MRI of the brain, particularly in infants and those with prolonged or focal seizures. MRI is often not available, especially out of hours; is more expensive; requires a significantly longer imaging time; and is perhaps more difficult to interpret without expertise. While CT is the first-choice neuroimaging modality, MRI should still be considered subsequently. In one series, MRI brain detected abnormalities not identified by CT in 47% of cases.[3]

> **⊄ Expert comment** Don't forget the underlying aetiology
>
> Although termination of seizures/SE remains the first priority, identification of the trigger should remain a key focus. Early identification of the underlying aetiology would mean prompt specific therapy.

> **ⓘ Expert comment** Decision-making regarding transfer to the PICU
>
> In countries with healthcare systems with centralized PIC services, such as in the UK, children with continuing requirement for mechanical ventilation, antiepileptic infusions, or other intensive care interventions may need transfer from the local hospital that provided the initial management of SE. However, there are several situations when children with SE may be safely managed locally without PIC transfer. Most children who do not require induction of anaesthesia and intubation are managed by paediatricians in local hospitals. Children who are intubated owing to respiratory depression from antiepileptic medications rather than ongoing seizures are good candidates for discontinuation of sedation and for extubation locally. Patients with SE from aetiologies such as atypical febrile seizures, hypoglycaemia, hyponatraemia, recurrence of seizures in patients with known epilepsy, or those with similar transient episodes in the past are candidates for consideration of extubation rather than continued intensive care. Easy intubation, ease of oxygenation and ventilation during mechanical ventilation, stable haemodynamics, control of seizures, normal neuroimaging (if performed), and ability to perform continuous monitoring for a short period of time are all pre-requisites for successful extubation in the local hospital.

Case history (continued)

On admission to the PICU, cerebral function monitoring (CFM) was initiated and he was noted to remain in SE. The dose of midazolam infusion was escalated in a stepwise manner. However, frequent breakthrough seizures were noted on CFM. He had arterial and central venous lines inserted for better haemodynamic monitoring. He remained easy to ventilate. Upon reaching the maximum dose (24 µg/kg/min of midazolam infusion) without termination of seizures, he was commenced on thiopentone infusion, aiming for burst suppression on CFM. Midazolam infusion was discontinued. Blood results, including full blood count, renal and liver function, electrolytes, bone profile, coagulation profile, and C-reactive protein were unremarkable. Metabolic screen, urine toxicology, and repeat blood cultures were sent. Lumbar puncture was deferred. A neurology consult was requested and anti-N-methyl-D-aspartate (NMDA) and glutamic acid decarboxylase antibodies were also sent.

> **⊕ Clinical tip** Escalation in supportive therapy
>
> Patients on high-dose midazolam and thiopentone are at increased risk of hypotension and cardiovascular collapse. Central venous line insertion, arterial line monitoring, and inotropes/vasopressors are often required.

> **⊕ Clinical tip** Cerebrospinal fluid analysis
>
> Cerebrospinal fluid (CSF) analysis is often required to establish the diagnosis in SE, especially if an infective aetiology is likely. However, the optimal timing for lumbar puncture is uncertain. Many paediatric intensivists defer lumbar puncture, despite normal CT brain during the acute stages in the presence of uncontrolled SE, owing to the possibility of transient SE-associated cerebral oedema. CT is not sensitive enough to rule out any increase in intracranial tension. Even if lumbar puncture is deferred, antibiotics should be administered immediately, without any delay, as they may be life-saving. Lumbar puncture should then be performed at the earliest possible opportunity after termination of seizures unless other contraindications exist. CSF culture after antibiotics may result in a false-negative result; however, polymerase chain reaction (PCR)-based techniques can offset this issue. Moreover, CSF pleocytosis may persist for several days and useful information may still be obtained after antibiotic therapy.

> **✪ Learning point** Refractory status epilepticus
>
> Refractory status epilepticus (RSE) has been defined as seizures observed clinically or detected on electroencephalogram (EEG) after adequate doses of initial benzodiazepines and loading dose of an antiepileptic medication. In practice, this often refers to seizures that are ongoing for longer than an hour or two, despite appropriate antiepileptic therapy. Studies have revealed that SE lasts >1 hour in 26%–45% of children with SE >2 hours in 17%–25%, and >4 hours in 10%.[4] Rapid sequential treatment rather than reliance of time-based definitions is the key. RSE accounts for 25%–50% of children with SE, and makes up 4% of all PICU admissions, according to some studies.[5,6]

> **✪ Learning point** Management of refractory status epilepticus
>
> Midazolam infusion is the most frequently used first-line treatment option, in up to 80% of patients.[6] The aim remains to terminate seizures as rapidly as possible with the use of an escalation pathway. This would provide time for conventional antiepileptics to work. One suggested pathway can be seen in Figure 15.1. Midazolam infusion is successful in terminating RSE in 40%–70% of patients.[6]

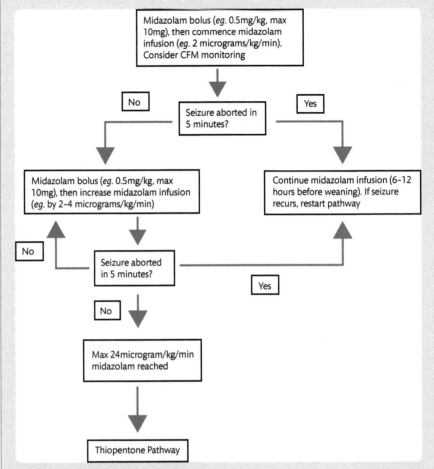

Figure 15.1 Midazolam pathway.
CFM, cerebral function monitor.

Midazolam is a fast-acting, water-soluble benzodiazepine with a half-life of approximately 1–12 hours. It binds to type A γ-aminobutyric acid (GABA$_A$) receptors and enhances GABAergic transmission.[7] Tachyphylaxis commonly develops within 24–48 hours; hence, dose adjustments will be required if on prolonged infusion.[8]

If SE continues despite the maximum recommended dose of midazolam infusion, then a barbiturate infusion (e.g. thiopentone) is often chosen as the second-line treatment of choice. In those requiring a barbiturate infusion, seizure termination occurred in a median of 30 hours versus <6 hours if first-line treatment was successful. The need for a second agent significantly increases the children's length of stay in the PICU.[6] One suggested barbiturate pathway can be seen in Figure 15.2, with burst suppression as the treatment target.

Barbiturates such as thiopentone and pentobarbital have multiple actions; this may explain their effectiveness, even in patients resistant to benzodiazepines. They activate GABA receptors and inhibit NMDA receptors, with changes to the conductance of calcium and potassium channels.[5] However, barbiturates have a relatively poor safety profile compared to midazolam. Barbiturates are thought to uncouple oxidative phosphorylation, which leads to decreased adenosine triphosphate production and subsequently cardiac complications. A large majority of children requiring pentobarbital or thiopentone infusions for RSE will need inotropic and/or vasopressor support. Other complications include ileus, immune dysfunction with resultant increased likelihood of hospital-acquired infection, respiratory depression, myocardial depression, hypotension, and pulmonary oedema. Once burst

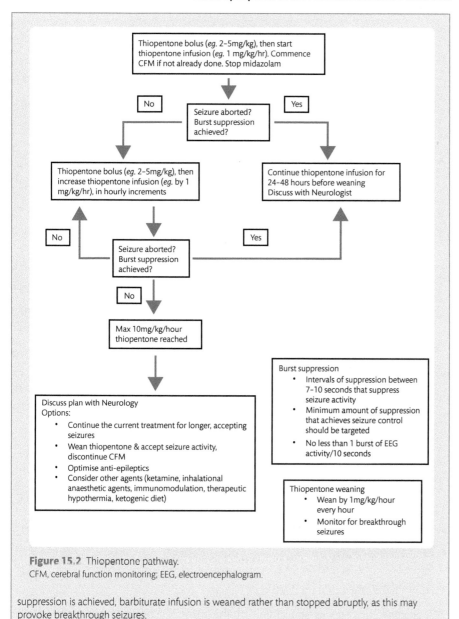

Figure 15.2 Thiopentone pathway.
CFM, cerebral function monitoring; EEG, electroencephalogram.

suppression is achieved, barbiturate infusion is weaned rather than stopped abruptly, as this may provoke breakthrough seizures.

❝ Expert comment Electroencephalogram monitoring

Continuous multi-channel EEG (cEEG) monitoring is considered the 'gold standard' of monitoring in patients with suspected non-convulsive SE and in those who need titration of antiepileptics to achieve seizure termination or burst suppression. cEEG has high sensitivity and specificity (~100%) with regard to the aforementioned indications. When cEEG monitoring was used to identify seizures needing treatment, considerably higher doses of midazolam were used (2.8 vs 10.7 μg/kg/min) and time to seizure control was longer, compared to studies where cEEG was not used. These observations suggest that non-convulsive seizures and SE may be undertreated when cEEG monitoring was not used as a treatment target.[9] However, conclusive evidence of benefit in outcomes associated with cEEG is lacking. Moreover, cEEG is often not available around the clock in many PICUs. Even when available, the frequency of expert bedside interpretation of the cEEG is limited, with half of such monitoring episodes being reviewed only once or twice a day.[10]

Quantitative EEG (qEEG) techniques aim to overcome some of these disadvantages of cEEG (i.e. availability and interpretation) by using fewer channels of EEG and quantitative processing techniques that aid ease of bedside interpretation by the intensive care team. This facilitates prompt delivery of therapeutic interventions and bedside guidance for titration of medications. The commonly used and most well-known of qEEG is amplitude integrated EEG (aEEG). However, other techniques, such as colour density spectral array (cDSA) and envelope trends, are also available. The author's institution uses an eight-electrode montage (four scalp electrodes—two for each hemisphere, earth, reference, and two electrocardiogram electrodes) to generate a combination of two-channel aEEG, cDSA, and display of raw EEG waveforms as the CFM method of choice. Owing to the limited number of channels and the processed nature of EEG, the sensitivity and specificity of this technique may be lower than that of cEEG. However, there is some evidence for comparable accuracy when a combination of qEEG methods are used, as suggested earlier and when CFM interpretation is backed up by robust education and training.

⊕ Expert comment Indications of quantitative electroencephalogram monitoring

1. Diagnosis of non-convulsive seizures or SE, and other paroxysmal events. This also applies to detection of seizures that might be rendered non-convulsive because of neuromuscular blockade.
2. Assessment of treatment efficacy for SE.
3. Identification of cerebral ischaemia.
4. Assessment of severity of encephalopathy and prognostication.

Common clinical situations where CFM is used are:

- traumatic brain injury;
- post-cardiac arrest;
- admission diagnosis of seizures or SE;
- post-neurosurgery;
- stroke;
- acute liver failure;
- metabolic disorders (hyperammonaemia, diabetic ketoacidosis, etc.);
- other mechanically ventilated patients who require neuromuscular blockade and might be at risk of cerebral ischaemia or seizures.

It has to be noted that despite the benefits of CFM, there is still uncertainty about whether the treatment goal should actually be termination of seizure or induction of burst suppression.[11] It also remains unclear how long the patients should remain in pharmacological coma.[4]

Case history (continued)

Thiopentone infusion was titrated up with the intent of achieving burst suppression on CFM. Four hours later, burst suppression was achieved on an infusion rate of 5 mg/kg/h. However, he became hypotensive and required inotropic, vasopressor support. He developed feed intolerance, which was initially managed with nasojejunal feeds. However, he developed ileus and was supported with parenteral nutrition. Figure 15.3 demonstrates CFM images with their corresponding interpretations. Burst suppression was maintained for 24 hours. Levetiracetam was added to maintenance phenytoin to facilitate better seizure control and barbiturate weaning. Thiopentone infusion was gradually weaned,

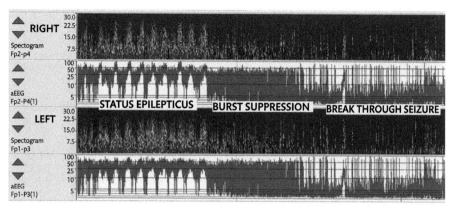

Figure 15.3 Screenshots from cerebral function monitoring showing evolution of electroencephalogram patterns over a four-hour time period. Status epilepticus evolves to adequate burst suppression after thiopentone infusion, then to excessive burst suppression with a break through seizure despite excessive suppression. Changes in the colour density spectral array imaging appear less prominent than amplitude integrated electroencephalogram here because of the grayscale image.

> **☼ Learning point**
> Investigations
>
> In addition to routine investigations, Table 15.1 demonstrates other investigations that may be useful in RSE.

with only a few infrequent, brief breakthrough seizures on CFM. MRI of his brain was performed, which was reported as normal; in particular, there was no evidence of demyelination. CSF analysis showed neither white nor red cells; normal protein, glucose, and lactate; and no abnormal oligoclonal bands. CSF herpes simplex and enteroviral PCRs were negative. Cefotaxime and aciclovir were subsequently discontinued.

Table 15.1 Investigations to consider in refractory status epilepticus

Investigations	Comments
Plasma amino acid, urine organic acid	Variety of metabolic conditions
Blood/urine for α-AASA	Pyridoxine-dependent epilepsy, particularly in infants
CSF lactate	Mitochondrial disease
CSF oligoclonal bands	Multiple sclerosis; may be transiently present in ADEM
Urine toxicology	Substance abuse, poisoning (safeguarding implications)
NMDA receptor antibody	Anti-NMDA receptor encephalitis
Anti-GAD antibody	Epilepsy syndromes associated with several conditions, including Miller Fisher syndrome, stiff person syndrome, limbic encephalitis, paraneoplastic syndromes, etc.
POLG mutation	Epilepsy associated with mitochondrial DNA depletion syndromes

AASA, aminoadipic semialdehyde; CSF, cerebrospinal fluid; ADEM, acute disseminated encephalomyelitis; NMDA: *N*-methyl-d-aspartate; GAD, glutamic acid decarboxylase.

☼ Learning point Super-refractory status epilepticus

SRSE pertains to SE that continues for 24 hours or more after the onset of general anaesthesia, including recurrent seizures on weaning or withdrawal of anaesthesia.[12] SRSE has been associated with various new unexplained SE manifesting in people without pre-existing comorbidities or identifiable aetiological factors, coined new-onset RSE, which include febrile infection-related epilepsy syndrome (FIRES), devastating epilepsy in school-age children, and acute encephalitis with refractory repetitive partial seizures.[4] SRSE is also associated with high morbidity and mortality.

☼ Learning point Management strategies for super-refractory status epilepticus

Owing to the relatively infrequent incidence of SRSE, evidence for management strategies is scarce, consisting mainly of case reports, case series, and retrospective reviews. While SRSE treatment is ongoing, a combination of two or three antiepileptic medications ought to be retained at high doses, without frequent alterations.[13] A variety of management strategies have been suggested, which include:

- **Ketamine**—as down-regulation in GABA receptors may occur in SRSE, the alternative NMDA receptor-blocking effect of ketamine has been successfully exploited.[14] Several reports of successful resolution of SRSE using ketamine exist.[15]
- **Propofol** has been successfully used in SRSE in adults. However, concerns relating to development of propofol infusion syndrome limit the usefulness of this medication in children.[16]
- **Inhalational anaesthetic agents** like isoflurane probably work on multiple receptors to provide good control of seizure activity in SRSE, but the logistics of delivering, monitoring, and scavenging mean that their use is usually confined to operating theatres and exceptional circumstances.[5] The use of an anaesthetic conservation device such as 'AnaConDa' may facilitate the use of inhalational anaesthetics for SRSE in the PICU environment.[8] While this strategy may be effective, significant morbidity associated with prolonged inhalational anaesthetics include hypotension, ileus, and prolonged mechanical ventilation, etc. Abrupt discontinuation after prolonged use of isoflurane may lead to extreme agitation and psychomotor disturbances.[5]
- **Immunomodulation** using steroids, immunoglobulins, plasma exchange, cyclophosphamide, and rituximab—on their own or in combination—may be effective in treating SRSE where paraneoplastic syndromes or autoimmune encephalitis are suspected.[17]
- **Therapeutic hypothermia**—the role of therapeutic hypothermia in SRSE is unclear. This method reduces cerebral metabolism and oxidative stress. A temperature target of 32–35°C for 24–48 hours has been suggested for seizure control and neuroprotection in the Intensive Care Unit for refractory epilepsy. However, clinical trials have not confirmed the effectiveness of therapeutic hypothermia in SE.[18]
- **A ketogenic diet** promotes the formation of ketone bodies, leading to an increase in fatty acid levels that open adenosine triphosphate-sensitive potassium channels, thereby enhancing membrane hyperpolarization to reduce seizure activity.[17] This has been shown to be effective in cases of FIRES, immune-mediated encephalitis, non-ketotic hyperglycinaemia, and genetic epilepsy.[19,20] This strategy is only suitable for those able to feed enterally, and input from an experienced dietician is required, with regular monitoring for severe hypoglycaemia and hypertriglyceridaemia.

Case history (continued)

A diagnosis of FIRES was made based on the consistent clinical syndrome and absence of alternative diagnoses. Inotropic support was weaned off after discontinuation of thiopentone. Over the next 48 hours, his neurology improved gradually and he was extubated. His Glasgow Coma Scale score was 12 (E3, M5, V4). His pupils were equal and reactive. No focal neurological deficit was immediately apparent. Nasogastric feeding was established after ileus improved. He was subsequently discharged from the PICU, 10 days after the initial admission with SE, under the care of neurologists. He had a prolonged in-hospital stay with persistent encephalopathy and infrequent break-through seizures. Some further improvement was noted after ketogenic diet. He was discharged with ongoing neurology and community paediatric follow-up on pheny-toin, levetiracetam, and a ketogenic diet.

✪ Expert comment
Neurologists are partners

Expert neurology help should always be sought to help with investigation and management of any child with refractory or super-refractory status epilepticus (SRSE).

Discussion

Febrile infection-related epileptic syndrome and other differential diagnoses

FIRES is thought to be a postinfectious neurological disorder with refractory epilepsy, causing profound and often persistent encephalopathy. The exact aetiology of FIRES is unknown. It typically occurs in school-age children, who within 2 weeks of a mild febrile illness, develop extremely frequent seizures that are difficult to manage with conventional therapy.[21] Ketogenic diet and immunoglobulins may be beneficial.[22] Prognosis is poor, and children have marked cognitive impairment with refractory epilepsy. Differential diagnoses include acute bacterial meningitis or an alternative infective meningoencephalitis, acute disseminated encephalomyelitis (ADEM), or anti-NMDA receptor encephalitis. Children with ADEM may present with multifocal symptoms, meningoencephalitis, optic neuritis, and encephalopathy. Anti-NMDA receptor encephalitis is another progressive autoimmune condition often seen in females. Non-specific upper respiratory tract illness is followed, typically after 2 weeks, with seizures and altered behaviour with occasional psychiatric manifestations.

A final word from the expert

Mortality due to or related to SE is significantly lower in children than adults, with common estimates suggesting a mortality rate of around 2%–7%.[23] Protocol-based management of SE is usually successful in terminating seizures and prevents the need for intensive care. Even when intensive care is required, the vast majority of children with SE admitted to the PICU only require a brief stay in the PICU. Paediatric index of mortality score categorizes SE or seizure-related admissions to the PICU to the low-risk diagnosis group. However, there could be significant morbidity and mortality associated with ICU admissions due to RSE and SRSE. Predictors of poor prognosis include afebrile seizures, history of perinatal problems, preceding developmental delay, abnormal neurological examination, abnormal neuroimaging, and infant age group.[24] The morbidity incurred is associated with aetiology, duration of SE, and age of the patient. It may also be related to the interventions required in PICU such as mechanical ventilation, vasopressor therapy, and adverse effects of prolonged sedative or suppressive medications. Short-term morbidity includes secondary bacterial infections, atelectasis, paralytic ileus, and persistent encephalopathy, and so on. Longer-term problems include cognitive decline, behavioural problems, and developmental delay. Up to one-third of children developed epilepsy with some developing refractory epilepsy, and up to half of children with a history of SE have recurrence of these episodes.[24] There is some concern that the risk of sudden unexpected death in epilepsy increases following SE; however, this is rare in children.[25] Mortality may be a result of multiorgan failure (e.g. Dravet syndrome), underlying brain damage (such as in fulminant bacterial meningitis), adverse effects of antiepileptic therapy (cardiovascular collapse associated with thiopentone), or due to direct neurotoxicity related to the underlying diagnosis.

While SE remains a medical emergency in children, rapid sequential antiepileptic treatment (see Figure 15.4—stepwise approach) with good supportive care, along with specific therapies relevant to the possible differential diagnoses, is often successful in preventing significant health impairment.

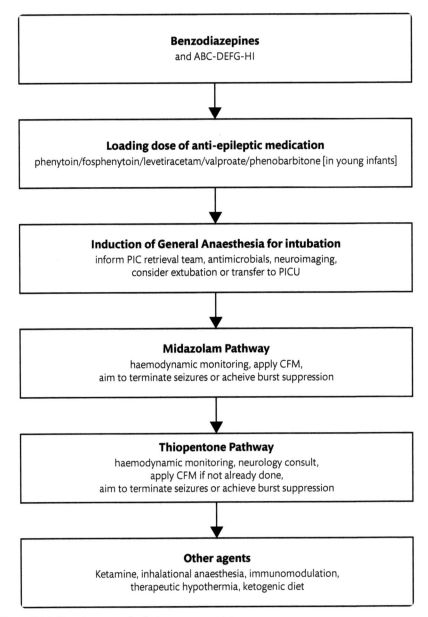

Figure 15.4 Stepwise approach of seizure management.
ABC-DEFG-HI, airway, breathing, circulation–don't ever forget glucose–hyponatraemia, hypocalcaemia, and infection; PIC, Paediatric Intensive Care; PICU, Paediatric Intensive Care Unit; CFM, cerebral function monitoring.

References

1. Glauser T, Shinnar S, Gloss D, et al. Evidence-based guideline: treatment of convulsive status epilepticus in children and adults: report of the Guideline Committee of the American Epilepsy Society. *Epilepsy Curr.* 2016;16:48–61.
2. Brophy GM, Bell R, Claassen J, et al. Guidelines for the evaluation and management of status epilepticus. *Neurocrit. Care* 2012;17:3–23.
3. Singh RK, Stephens S, Berl MM, et al. Prospective study of new-onset seizures presenting as status epilepticus in childhood. *Neurology* 2010;74:636–42.
4. Smith DM, McGinnis EL, Walleigh DJ, et al. Management of status epilepticus in children. *J. Clin. Med.* 2016;5:47.
5. Wilkes R, Tasker RC. Pediatric intensive care treatment of uncontrolled status epilepticus. *Crit. Care Clin.* 2013;29:239–57.
6. Tasker RC, Goodkin HP, Sanchez Fernandez I, et al. Refractory status epilepticus in children: intention to treat with continuous infusions of midazolam and pentobarbital. *Pediatr. Crit. Care Med.* 2016;17:968–75.
7. Claassen J, Hirsch LJ, Emerson RG, et al. Continuous EEG monitoring and midazolam infusion for refractory nonconvulsive status epilepticus. *Neurology* 2001;57:1036–42.
8. Lionel KR, Hrishi AP. Seizures—just the tip of the iceberg: critical care management of super-refractory status epilepticus. *Indian J. Crit. Care Med.* 2016;20:587–92.
9. Wilkes R, Tasker RC. Intensive care treatment of uncontrolled status epilepticus in children: systematic literature search of midazolam and anesthetic therapies. *Pediatr. Crit. Care Med.* 2014;15:632–9.
10. Abend NS, Arndt DH, Carpenter JL, et al. Electrographic seizures in pediatric ICU patients: cohort study of risk factors and mortality. *Neurology* 2013;81:383–91.
11. Claassen J, Hirsch LJ, Emerson RG, et al. Treatment of refractory status epilepticus with pentobarbital, propofol, or midazolam: a systematic review. *Epilepsia* 2002;43:146–53.
12. Hocker S, Tatum WO, LaRoche S, et al. Refractory and super-refractory status epilepticus--an update. *Curr. Neurol. Neurosci. Rep.* 2014;14:452.
13. Shorvon S. Super-refractory status epilepticus: an approach to therapy in this difficult clinical situation. *Epilepsia* 2011;52(Suppl. 8):53–6.
14. Zeiler FA. Early use of the NMDA receptor antagonist ketamine in refractory and superrefractory status epilepticus. *Crit. Care Res. Pract.* 2015;2015:831260.
15. Rosati A, L'Erario M, Ilvento L, et al. Efficacy and safety of ketamine in refractory status epilepticus in children. *Neurology* 2012;79:2355–8.
16. Iyer VN, Hoel R, Rabinstein AA. Propofol infusion syndrome in patients with refractory status epilepticus: an 11-year clinical experience. *Crit. Care Med.* 2009;37:3024–30.
17. Bayrlee A, Ganeshalingam N, Kurczewski L, et al. Treatment of super-refractory status epilepticus. *Curr. Neurol. Neurosci. Rep.* 2015;15:66.
18. Legriel S, Lemiale V, Schenck M, et al. Hypothermia for neuroprotection in convulsive status epilepticus. *N. Engl. J. Med.* 2016;375:2457–67.
19. Nabbout R, Mazzuca M, Hubert P, et al. Efficacy of ketogenic diet in severe refractory status epilepticus initiating fever induced refractory epileptic encephalopathy in school age children (FIRES). *Epilepsia* 2010;51:2033–7.
20. Appavu B, Vanatta L, Condie J, et al. Ketogenic diet treatment for pediatric super-refractory status epilepticus. *Seizure* 2016;41:62–65.
21. van Baalen A, Hausler M, Boor R, et al. Febrile infection-related epilepsy syndrome (FIRES): a nonencephalitic encephalopathy in childhood. *Epilepsia* 2010;51:1323–8.
22. Caraballo RH, Reyes G, Avaria MF, et al. Febrile infection-related epilepsy syndrome: a study of 12 patients. *Seizure* 2013;22:553–9.

23. Chin RF, Neville BG, Peckham C, et al. Incidence, cause, and short-term outcome of convulsive status epilepticus in childhood: prospective population-based study. *Lancet* 2006;368:222–9.
24. Barnard C, Wirrell E. Does status epilepticus in children cause developmental deterioration and exacerbation of epilepsy? *J. Child Neurol.* 1999;14:787–94.
25. Sperling MR. Sudden unexplained death in epilepsy. *Epilepsy Curr.* 2001;1:21–23.

16 Safeguarding children in the Paediatric Intensive Care Unit

Thomas D. Jerrom

Expert commentary by Padmanabhan Ramnarayan

Case history

A tertiary paediatric intensive care (PIC) retrieval service received a referral regarding a 3-year-old boy who had 'fallen down the stairs' at home. He was unconscious when the paramedics arrived and was transferred to the Emergency Department (ED), intubated, and ventilated. The referring doctor said that the boy's parents had been acting strangely in the ED and that the boy was unkempt and very thin. They were concerned about the possibility of non-accidental injury (NAI) being the mechanism for the boy's injuries. The PIC retrieval service suggested that the boy should have an urgent computed tomography (CT) scan of his brain and arranged for transport to the nearest neurosurgical Paediatric Intensive Care Unit (PICU).

> **⭐ Learning point** Introduction to child abuse
>
> Brandon et al.[1] estimated that 85 children (0.77/100,000 children) die each year in England as a result of violence or maltreatment. In the USA it is estimated that in 2014, 1580 children died of abuse or neglect, at a rate of 2.13/100,000 children.
>
> Overall, children <1 year of age are more likely to be killed by another person (most commonly a parent) than any other age group, and are seven times more likely to be killed than older children. Abused children have poorer long-term outcomes across a range of measures, including educational, mental health problems, and difficulties functioning in society.

> **Ⓒ Expert comment** Duties of medical professionals
>
> Trying to protect children from suffering harm is a key duty of all health professionals and is a concept supported by the World Health Organization, the United Nations Children's Fund (UNICEF) and medical regulatory bodies throughout the world.
>
> In the UK, the General Medical Council (GMC)[2] clearly describes how 'All children and young people have a right to be protected from abuse and neglect—all doctors have a duty to act on any concerns they have about the safety or welfare of a child or young person ... [and that] this includes doctors who treat adult patients'.
>
> In the USA the American Medical Association (AMA) describes similar responsibilities for doctors. Despite the AMA requiring physicians to report suspected cases of child abuse, several retrospective studies indicate that this is not universal practice.[3]

Clinical tip Risk factors for child abuse

The presence of risk factors for child abuse obviously does not in itself mean that the child is being abused and the inverse is also true. Some affluent, well-educated parents with no risk factors abuse children. It is in these cases where keeping an open mind about how an injury has been sustained is most important.

Learning point Types of child abuse

Child abuse is often divided into four different types:

- neglect;
- emotional abuse;
- physical abuse;
- sexual abuse.

Child abuse severe enough to be the primary reason for admission to PICU is most often physical and involves severe head injury.[4] An increase in the number of severely disabled children who are being admitted to PICU necessitates a good understanding of child protection issues for PICU doctors. Disabled children are three times more likely to be victims of abuse (primarily neglect) than children without disabilities, and many are unable to express what is happening to them. Table 16.1 lists known risk factors for child abuse, which should be considered and documented in every case.

Table 16.1 Risk factors for child abuse

Risk factors for perpetration	Parent/individual's risk factors: • a lack of understanding of the child's needs • a history of abuse in the perpetrator's childhood • substance abuse and other mental health issues • non-biological caregivers • specific parental characteristics: young age, low education achievement, single parenthood, large number of dependent children, low income Family risk factors: • social isolation • domestic violence
Child risk factors	• Children <4 years of age • Increased dependency: disabilities, developmental delay, mental health issues, and chronic physical illnesses

Source: Adapted from Risk and Protective Factors. Centers for Disease Control and Prevention. Available at https://www.cdc.gov/violenceprevention/childabuseandneglect/riskprotectivefactors.html

Case history (continued)

The referring doctor spoke in more detail to the parents and Children's Social Care (CSC) team. CSC said that the child had missed a series of his mandatory health checks but had not previously been referred for child protection concerns. The only contact that they had was to organize accommodation for the mother. The mother apparently said that her partner (the boy's father), who was recently been released from prison, had been staying with them for the last 3 months. She went out to see a friend earlier in the evening but received a call from her partner, who said that their son had fallen down the stairs. The mother called the ambulance when she got home, having found her son unresponsive on the floor.

Learning point Features in the history of an injury that raise the suspicion of physical abuse

The Royal College of Paediatrics and Child Health (RCPCH)[5] describes the following features in the history of an injured child that should raise suspicion of physical abuse:

- significant injury where there is no explanation, or the explanation does not fit with the pattern of injury/seem plausible (i.e. does not fit with the motor developmental stage of the child);
- multiple injuries;

- inconsistent explanation for the injury;
- inappropriate delay in seeking medical care;
- inappropriate parent/carer response, e.g. unconcerned or aggressive;
- a history of inappropriate child response (e.g. didn't cry, felt no pain);
- child or family known to CSC or subject to a child protection plan;
- repeated attendance with injuries;
- previous history of unusual injury/illness, e.g. unexplained apnoea.

⊕ **Expert comment**
Recognition of physical abuse

The RCPCH emphasizes how paediatricians need to 'adopt a forensic approach to the assessment of a child with suspected physical abuse, matching the history to the clinical findings to determine the likelihood of intentional injury. Ask yourself the question: "Does the explanation match the clinical findings?"'.5

✪ **Learning point**   Initial assessment of the child

The principles of history taking in cases of NAI are fundamentally the same as that of any child admitted to the PICU. What you are trying to achieve is a full understanding of the events leading up to the child's illness or injury.

A child protection history should include child development; history of domestic violence; parental mental health issues; addiction; previous contact with social care; who had access to the child (supervised/unsupervised including childcare settings); and if there are other children who may be at risk. Meticulous documentation of exactly what was said by whom is particularly important as the medical notes may form part of the evidence presented in court to secure a conviction. Details about the proposed mechanism of injury (the height of the fall, type of surface impacted, who was where, etc.) and timings are vital. Asking the parent/carer to draw a diagram of how an injury was sustained can be particularly insightful. Children admitted to the PICU have often had their history documented on a number of occasions before they arrive in the unit (paramedics, ED, retrieval team, etc.). Looking for inconsistencies in these histories can provide clues that the child has been abused. It is good practice to take the history with a chaperone present.

Although expert review in cases of potential child abuse is invaluable, the ability to carry out and clearly document the examination findings on admission is also important. However, it may not be possible to perform a full child protection examination on admission owing to ongoing resuscitation. The safeguarding examination should include inspection of the child's entire skin surface, with documentation of any bruises or marks. The inside of the mouth (checking for a torn frenulum), nose, and ears (checking for haemotympanum) should be thoroughly examined. The perineum and external anus should be examined, but it is not appropriate to perform an internal examination if you are not an expert. Fundoscopy should be performed and then repeated by an experienced ophthalmologist. The child's clothes should be stored and given to the police if requested. All positive and important negative findings should be documented on a body map with annotation to describe any lesion's shape, colour, measurements, site relative to bony landmarks, and any explanation given for them by the parents/carer. Medical photographic documentation of any marks should be performed swiftly following admission and the parents should be informed of this.

Clear handover of child protection information between members of the same team and communication with other agencies is crucial. The RCPCH provides further child protection guidance and useful documents on their website (www.rcpch.ac.uk).

⊕ **Clinical tip**   Interactions with families in cases of potential non-accidental injury

It is important to remember that as medical professionals our job is to safeguard the child, but not to decide whether or who, if anyone, is guilty of inflicting the injury. We provide information to CSC and the police, who will decide if they are going to pursue child protection proceedings. Sometimes explanations that seem highly improbable when described by parents/carers prove to be plausible when CSC or the police perform a home visit. Because of this, unless there are concerns that a parent poses a risk to their child or others, they should be allowed into the PICU (while chaperoned) and their child's care discussed with them, as we would with any other parent.

> **✪ Learning point** Parental responsibility and consent
>
> The exact legal definitions of parental responsibility and consent differ around the world, but certain key concepts are universally accepted. UNICEF's Convention on the Rights of the Child describes how both parents share rights and responsibility to direct and guide their children's life. This parental autonomy in how they wish to bring up their child is balanced against the best interests of the child, with the latter superseding any other parental rights if the child is at risk of harm. For this reason when there are concerns that a child is being abused, parents cannot refuse to consent for their child to be investigated, but this may need to be discussed with CSC, the police, or the courts.
>
> It is accepted good practice that information should be shared with parents/carer when there are child protection concerns, and that parents/carers should be informed that a referral is being made to CSC. The only exception to this practice is the rare case where doing so might compromise an investigation (e.g. fabricated or induced illness), or when you are concerned that disclosure might put the child or other children at immediate risk.

Case history (continued)

His CT head showed multiple skull fractures and significant parenchymal brain injury. He was safely transported to the PICU, where he was met and reviewed by the neurosurgical team. He was found to have unilateral dilated and unreactive pupil. He was hypotensive and needed fluid resuscitation. He also received a dose of 3% saline as a hyperosmolar agent to reduce cerebral oedema.

> **✔ Evidence base** Non-accidental brain injury
>
> Non-accidental brain injury (NABI) is defined as damage to the brain caused by an external abusive physical force and is a significant cause of acquired brain injury in children. The terms inflicted brain injury and abusive head trauma describe the same diagnosis. NABI is predominantly inflicted on young infants (median age 2.2 months). In some studies 40%–50% of all significant abusive injuries are head injuries and around 80% of deaths due to isolated head injuries are due to abuse.[6] Other research has suggested that when compared to other forms of traumatic brain injury, NABI is more commonly associated with apnoea and seizures.[7] A significant proportion of survivors suffer permanent cognitive or neurological disability.[6]
>
> Perpetrators of NABI are most commonly family members and studies have shown are most commonly (in descending order) the father, mother's boyfriend, female babysitter, and then the mother.
>
> Infants are particularly vulnerable to head trauma for a number of reasons:[8]
>
> - they are unable to defend themselves;
> - their subarachnoid space is relatively large;
> - they have large heads relative to body size;
> - myelination is incomplete and their brain has a high water content;
> - their neck musculature is weak leading to poor head control;
> - they have soft non-ossified skull bones with unfused sutures and open fontanelles;
> - their cerebral blood vessels are very fragile.

> **✪ Learning point** Specific types of non-accidental injury
>
> **Shaken baby syndrome**
>
> Shaken baby syndrome (SBS) is a subtype of NABI described in young infants in which the victim is held by the torso or the extremities and violently shaken, causing abrupt uncontrolled head movements with a marked rotatory component leading to an acceleration/deceleration injury. Infants with SBS present with encephalopathy, thin subdural haemorrhages (SDHs; demonstrated in >90%

of cases), and retinal haemorrhages (RHs) due to traumatic shearing of the subdural veins and retinal vessels. They also often have associated rib fractures and suffer apnoeas, leading to further hypoxic damage.

SBS has as an annual incidence of 24.6/100,000 children[9] and occurs in all social strata. Risk factors include a baby that 'cries all the time' with young, overstressed parents with a low frustration threshold and poor control of impulses. The defence in court of those accused of causing SBS often concentrates on the medical team failing to exclude the rare differential diagnoses described in Table 16.2.

Table 16.2 Differential diagnoses of shaken baby syndrome

Alternative diagnoses	Features
Accidental head trauma	Serious accidents normally cause SDH associated with skull fractures without RH and are rare in infancy
Perinatal birth trauma	SDH are found in 8% of newborns RH are found in 34% of newborns but generally resolve within 4 weeks
Increased intrathoracic pressure	RH have been described after resuscitation or seizures There is no evidence that vomiting or coughing causes SDH or RH in normal children
Arachnoid cyst/benign enlargement of the subarachnoid spaces	SDHs are possible in these children following trivial trauma. Associated RHs are rare but described. Diagnosed by imaging over a prolonged time frame
Meningoencephalitis	Can lead to postinfectious hygroma Associated RH are rare but described
Coagulopathies	SDH and RH possible. Need to be excluded on blood tests at admission as coagulopathies can be transient
Menkes syndrome	SDH described in rare cases Characteristic clinical picture featuring microcephaly and typical trichopathy
Glutaric aciduria type 1	SDH and RH are described in this condition Children suffer characteristic crises and it is now screened for on UK blood spot neonatal testing
Galactosaemia	RH are rare but described Characteristic clinical picture, including hepatosplenomegaly, jaundice, sepsis, and cataracts
Osteogenesis imperfecta type 1/type 4	Atypical skull fractures are possible. Characteristic clinical picture with positive family history, blue sclera and Wormian bones. Molecular genetic diagnosis

SDH, subdural haemorrhage; RH, retinal haemorrhage.
Source: Reproduced from *Dtsch Arztebl Int.*, 106(13), Matschke J, Herrmann B, Sperhake J, et al., Shaken baby syndrome, pp. 211–7, Copyright (2009), with permission from *Deutsches Ärzteblatt International.*

In SBS, the Royal College of Radiologists suggest performing a CT scan first (if acute MRI is not available) and then an MRI on day 3–5 (if the patient still has an encephalopathy or if the CT was abnormal), with a follow-up MRI at 3–6 months if the previous MRI was abnormal. Cerebral ultrasonography is not sensitive enough to be used in isolation. Their full guidance on imaging in suspected NAI can be found at www.rcr.ac.uk.

Retinal haemorrhages

SBS is associated with RH in 85% of cases.[10] The pathogenesis of the RH is thought to be due to vitreoretinal traction and bleeding can be pre-retinal (flame/splinter haemorrhages), intraretinal, subretinal (dot/blot haemorrhages), and potentially associated with vitreous haemorrhages. Traumatic retinoschisis describes the splitting of the layers of the neurosensory retina causing an intraretinal cavity where a haematoma can form and is highly indicative of NABI. It is well accepted that ophthalmological haemorrhages seen in NABI may be unilateral.[10]

The examination for and documentation of RH (both pre- and postmortem) is a vital part of the clinical assessment of children who are suspected to have suffered NAI. The presence of RH is likely to be a key piece of evidence in a potential future court case. For this reason it is accepted practice for the ophthalmological examination to be performed and documented by a consultant ophthalmologist with extensive paediatric experience. In a study of 123 children admitted with SDH caused by abuse, non-ophthalmologists failed to detect RH in 29% of affected children.[11]

✚ Clinical tip Fundoscopy in the PICU

Unless the child already has very dilated pupils, the ophthalmologists will normally need the child to be given mydriatic eye drops. In a PICU setting where it is important to be able to carefully monitor a ventilated patient's pupillary response following a head injury, it is far safer to use tropicamide 0.5% (length of action of 4–8 hours), rather than cyclopentolate 1% (length of action up to 24 hours). Missing a new unilaterally dilated pupil (sign of significantly raised intracranial pressure with impending herniation) because the child's pupils are still dilated from mydriatic drops could clearly have devastating consequences.

✪ Learning point Specific types of non-accidental injury

Spinal trauma

There is an increasing awareness that physical abuse can cause spinal injuries in two patterns, involving the chest and lower back, or the cervical spine. Cervical injuries are most commonly seen in children with a co-existing NABI and/or RH in infants <4 months of age. Thoracic or lumbar injuries are seen more commonly in toddlers aged >9 months and are often accompanied by a neurological deficit or an obvious bony deformity. Children with NABI may also have a spinal SDH. Spinal injuries are difficult to detect, especially if the child is obtunded as a result of a co-existing NABI. Infants who are awake may be distressed when their neck is moved.

Spinal views are part of a standard skeletal survey. But if there are any concerns about a spinal injury, an MRI should be performed to rule out spinal cord injury without radiographic abnormality.

Other bony injuries

Examining for fractures in a patient on PICU is often difficult as the child may be sedated or unresponsive due to an encephalopathy. For this reason, careful examination looking for bruising, swelling, signs of crepitus, and high-quality imaging are essential. Rib fractures in the absence of major chest trauma strongly suggests physical abuse but can also be seen following chest compressions. Spiral fractures of the humeral shaft are significantly more common in abused children, as are femur fractures in babies who are not yet walking. Multiple fractures at various stages of healing are always concerning.

✪ Learning point Specific types of non-accidental injury

Abdominal injuries

Although abusive abdominal injuries are rare they carry a high mortality and morbidity. They are predominantly seen in children aged <5 years. Bruising over the abdomen is often absent. High levels of suspicion and blood/radiological investigations are needed to diagnose these injuries.

---

❻ Expert comment
Anal gaping

Trauma or dilation of the anus is an important sign of sexual abuse, but another condition called 'anal gaping' is sometimes seen in patients in the PICU. Anal gaping describes atraumatic dilatation of the anus and can be seen in patients receiving anaesthetic agents, regional anaesthetic techniques, or postmortem. If you are concerned about abnormal findings on examination of the anus, it is vital to seek an expert opinion.[14]

Examination of the skin

As described before, the size, location, shape (could a specific implement have been used?), and pattern (finger/bite marks or immersion burns) of bruises or burns should be accurately recorded on a body map and photographed. Recent studies have shown that the age of bruises cannot be accurately assessed visually.[12] There are several conditions that may be confused with abusive bruises, such as Mongolian spots, haemangiomas, idiopathic thrombocytopenic purpura, clotting deficiencies, and leukaemia.

Any human bite could be abusive and should be fully assessed by a forensic dentist (see www.bafo. org.uk) who can take serial photographs and casts of the bite, and possibly retrieve DNA to identify the perpetrator.

Two to thirty-five per cent of burns in childhood are due to abuse (45% for genital and perineal burns).[13] Cigarette burns should always raise concern of abuse, as should any delay in seeking medical treatment.

⊗ **Learning point** Specific types of non-accidental injury

Sexual abuse

Sexual abuse is rarely a primary cause of admission to PICU, but it is an important potential comorbidity that needs to be considered. Sexual abuse in children can be discovered in a variety of ways, depending on the child's ability to describe what has happened to them and the type of sexual abuse that they are suffering. Children may demonstrate an emotional change with anxiety/depression, deliberate self-harm/attempted suicide (potentially leading to PICU admission), drug use, combative behaviour, sleep disturbance, sexualized behaviour, or new encopresis. Children may also present with physical symptoms, including signs of a sexually transmitted infection, urinary tract infections, constipation, or genital trauma. However, a significant number of children have no physical signs of sexual abuse, even if they have been recently assaulted.

Genital examination is an important part of the initial assessment of the child with child protection concerns, but internal examination should only be performed by specialists who are able to formally document the findings and take forensic samples.

Female genital mutilation (FGM, also known as 'cutting' or 'female circumcision') describes a range of cultural practices involving the removal of certain parts of the female genitals. Although FGM is common in many parts of the world, it is illegal in Western Europe, the USA, and many other countries. Children with FGM should be referred to urology, the local child protection team, and the police, who will consider the safety of the individual child, as well as female siblings who may also be at risk.

⊗ **Learning point** Specific types of non-accidental injury

Poisoning

Most developed healthcare systems have some form of national poisons advice service. In the USA the Poison Help Line (1-800-222-1222, www.poisonhelp.hrsa.gov) provides poisoning information and advice for healthcare professionals, and in the UK the National Poisons Information Service (telephone 0344 892 0111, www.toxbase.org) undertakes a similar task. A poisoning expert should always be contacted regarding the management of any critically unwell poisoned child.

It is important to have a systematic approach to managing the critically unwell poisoned child. Using the 'RRSIDEAD' mnemonic is a useful way to remember the key steps in the assessment and management of these complex patients:

R (resuscitation)
R (risk assessment)
S (supportive care)
I (investigations)
D (decontamination)

E (enhanced elimination)

A (antidotes)

D (disposition, *where to manage them*)

Specific investigations and treatments will depend on the child's presentation and if the type of poison is known. Basic investigations that should be performed on every patient include:

- full set of observations;
- electrocardiogram;
- blood gas, glucose, anion gap, carbon monoxide;
- paracetamol and salicylate level.

Hypoxaemia and hypoglycaemia are two common causes of altered mental status in the poisoned child that should be excluded.

⚙ Expert comment Diagnosing poisoning and the 'chain of custody'

A high level of suspicion is needed to correctly diagnose poisoning where there is no clear history. It should always be part of the potential differential diagnosis in the collapsed patient with metabolic derangement.

Many of the samples taken in child protection cases may potentially be used as evidence in court. The 'chain of custody' (also known as the 'chain of evidence') is the chronological documentation of the collection, transfer, receipt, analysis, storage, and disposal of samples, which helps to ensure that their results are admissible in court. This documentation provides evidence that the sample have not been tampered with and definitely came from the correct person. Most hospitals in the UK have specific documentation that can be completed when taking such samples.

The key aspects are:

- Complete documentation on the sample and in the patient's notes of patient demographic information (name, date of birth, hospital number, and address) and your own details (full name, signature, grade, bleep, and GMC number).
- Clear documentation of which samples have been taken and when, with a witness co-signing that all of this has been done correctly.

✪ Learning point Specific types of non-accidental injury

Fabricated or induced illness

Fabricated or induced illness (FII; previously known as Munchausen syndrome by proxy) describes two subtly different situations where a parent/carer deliberately makes the child sick (induced illness), or convinces others (most commonly medical professionals) that the child is sick (fabricated illness), for their own emotional or psychological benefit. The perpetrators of FII often seem like very caring parents/carers who simply want to find the cause for the often complex and concerning range of symptoms their child is suffering. As a result, well-meaning medical professionals often start a range of medications, hospitalize the child to perform multiple investigations, and there have been cases where children have received surgery for purely fictional ailments.

It is the high mortality rate of fabricated illness that makes it an important diagnosis for doctors working in the PICU to know about. Children with FII can be admitted to the PICU following smothering, poisoning (with drugs or by putting salt into a baby's milk, etc.), or when a parent has convinced a medical team to escalate seizure management to the point that the child needs intubation. The key to gaining the diagnosis is to keep an open mind and good interdisciplinary working. As described before, this is one of the few situations where it may be appropriate not to discuss child protection concerns with the family or carers before making a formal referral to CSC. Despite the increased understanding of the condition, less than one case of FII is escalated to a level of a Child Protection Conference per week in the UK.

> **✔ Evidence base** Fabricated or induced illness
>
> Many children suffering FII will have a past or co-existing genuine medical disorder, making diagnosis more complex. Perpetrators of FII are usually caregiving mothers who, in research studies, report high rates of early childhood deprivation and abuse. Over 50% of perpetrators have a somatoform or factitious disorder, and more than 75% have a co-existing personality disorder.[15]
>
> A review of 451 cases of FII showed the time elapsed from onset to diagnosis averaged 21.8 months. Of these 451 cases:[15]
>
> - 6% had died (the majority of these children suffered induced illness);
> - 7% were judged to have suffered long-term or permanent injury;
> - 25% of victims' known siblings were dead;
> - 61% of siblings had illnesses similar to those of the victim or which raised suspicions of FII.

Case history (continued)

The child had an external ventricular drain inserted and was transferred to the PICU for ongoing neuroprotective management. His chest X-ray showed multiple healing rib fractures. He was cachectic, with multiple small round burns on his torso. All teams involved were very suspicious that the child was being abused. The CSC and the police were contacted. The PICU consultant requested a child protection panel of investigations.

> **★ Learning point** Panel of investigations in suspected non-accidental injury
>
> The purpose of investigations in NAI are twofold (Table 16.3). Firstly, one needs to delineate the known illness/injury and search for any associated injuries, both to aid treatment and, if the findings are consistent with abuse, provide evidence for future legal proceedings. The second indication is to identify alternative (non-abusive) explanations for the physical findings. This aim is equally important as missing a non-abusive cause may result in children being unnecessarily removed from the parents and their condition not being treated appropriately. Failure to exclude diagnoses can also introduce 'reasonable doubt' to court proceedings and lead to children being returned to abusive parents.

Case history (continued)

The baby's skeletal survey showed multiple healing fractures and all investigations looking for an underlying medical explanation were negative. Sadly, in this case, the injury that the boy had suffered was fatal. After a period of neuroprotection he was assessed and confirmed dead by neurological criteria and he was extubated on the unit. The police arrested the father and pursued a conviction for murder. The medical professionals involved were required to provide statements to the court. The subsequent serious case review highlighted failings in communication between agencies, an unacceptably common finding in such cases. The father had a previous conviction for domestic violence, and health and social care teams were criticized for losing track of the child.

> **❻ Expert comment** Organ donation
>
> Child protection concerns in themselves do not preclude organ donation. So, if the child is certified as dead by neurological criteria, early discussion with the Coroner (or an equivalent authority elsewhere) can sometimes allow organ donation if the history and investigation findings are sufficient. However, there may be issues with gaining consent. Significant variation in legal and medical practices might exist worldwide, and practitioners should familiarize themselves with those requirements.

Table 16.3 Investigations in potential non-accidental injury

Patient type	Investigation	Purpose of investigation
Physical abuse with bruising or fractures	**22-film skeletal survey**	Exclude other fractures potentially of different ages
	Consideration of CT/MRI head if other fractures are found in an infant	Exclude NABI
	FBC, basic clotting profile, platelet function activity, and extended factor screen if needed	To be taken on admission to identify or avoid the defence of 'transient coagulopathy'
	Urinalysis, LFTs, and serum amylase. Consider need for USS/CT abdomen	Exclude occult abdominal injury
	Bone metabolism investigations to include serum calcium, phosphorus, alkaline phosphatase, parathyroid hormone, and 25-hydroxyvitamin D	Exclude bone fragility
	Photographic documentation of injuries	Documentation and forensic information
	Documentation of fundoscopy by an expert	Documentation of retinal haemorrhages
	Consideration of skin biopsy for fibroblast culture and/or venous blood for DNA	Osteogenesis imperfecta
	Consideration of radionuclide bone scan	Exclude and age fractures
Head injury	Urgent CT, MRI day 3–5 and 3–6 months if concerns	Exclude cerebral pathology
	If there are subdural haemorrhages, send urine organic acids	Exclude glutaric aciduria type 1
	Consider spinal CT/MRI on top of skeletal survey	Exclude spinal injuries
Sexual abuse	Expert forensic examination, documentation, and sampling	Exclude signs of sexual abuse
Bite marks	Expert forensic examination, by a forensic odontologist for documentation and sampling	Documentation of injury and sampling
Poisoning	Urine and blood for basic toxicology (compliant with chain of evidence practice) and a save sample	Exclude poisoning. Should be taken as early as possible before started on IV sedation

Bold indicates tests that should be carried out in all cases. CT, computed tomography; MRI, magnetic resonance imaging; NABI, non-accidental brain injury; FBC, full blood count; LFT, liver function test; USS, ultrasound scan; IV, intravenous.

Discussion

Writing reports and attending court

Attending court and writing medical reports are now a relatively routine part of working in the PICU. The RCPCH provides guidance and templates for writing medical reports and police statements on their website (www.rcpch.ac.uk). The report should start with professional information about yourself and when/where you saw the child. You should then describe the history (noting exactly what was said by whom) and your clinical findings. It is important to only state facts and where you are required to provide a medical opinion try to support it with evidence if discussing a particular type of fracture or injury. The resource, formerly known as the 'Cardiff Child Protection Systematic Reviews project (CORE info)', which produced systematic literature reviews of physical abuse and neglect in children, is now run as 'Child Protection Evidence' reviews by the RCPCH (https://www.rcpch.ac.uk/key-topics/child-protection/evidence-reviews). This is a good resource of supporting evidence when writing reports. You should write in plain language (explaining any medical terms used) and ask an experienced colleague to read your report before submission.

In the UK, doctors may be called to court as three different types of witness:

- *ordinary witnesses*, provide evidence unrelated to their professional work;
- *professional witnesses*, or a 'witness to fact', provide evidence of what they personally witnessed happen during the medical care they provided the patient;
- *expert witnesses*, provide an expert opinion relevant to the case but did not provide care for the individual patient.

Most legal systems around the world have a similar approach, although the nomenclature may differ. As a junior doctor or new PICU consultant you are most likely to be called to attend court as a 'professional witness' to provide first-hand information about a case you were involved in. You will be asked to write a report detailing your involvement with the patient and can be compelled via a summons to attend court in person. As a professional witness you should describe your personal observations and understanding of the case but avoid providing opinions beyond your level of experience (it is the job of the expert witness to provide this information). Try to keep your answers concise and do not be afraid to say that you 'don't know' if you are asked a very specific question. The various medical indemnity societies provide further information on their websites about attending court and will provide individual legal advice to their members if needed.

A final word from the expert

Safeguarding children is everyone's business and is a key skill in the PICU. Sadly, child abuse is endemic in all societies and social strata, and is an important differential to consider in every patient. The children that we care for are often the most vulnerable and may have suffered the most terrible forms of abuse. Following good child protection practices can help protect our patients and their siblings from further abuse, and save lives. It is our job as clinicians to raise concerns and provide evidence for the police and social care to act upon. Caring for children who have suffered severe abuse is emotionally distressing for all members of the team involved. Supporting your colleagues and having a forum to discuss the emotional impact that these cases have on staff is important.

Although child protection procedures differ between countries the key aspects are the same around the world. Maintaining an open mind about the aetiology of injuries or illnesses, always putting the safety and best interests of the child first, good documentation, and effective liaison with other agencies is vital in these challenging cases.

References

1. Brandon M, Sidebotham P, Bailey S, et al. New learning from serious case reviews: a two year report for 2009–2011. Available at: https://www.gov.uk/government/publications/new-learning-from-serious-case-reviews-a-2-year-report-for-2009-to-2011 (accessed 21 April 2020).
2. General Medical Council. *Protecting Children and Young People: The Responsibilities of all Doctors*. London: General Medical Council; 2012.

3. American Medical Association. Report 2 of the Council on Science and Public Health (I-09) Identifying and Reporting Suspected Child Abuse (Resolution 426, A-08) (Reference Committee K). Available at: https://www.ama-assn.org/sites/ama-assn.org/files/corp/media-browser/public/about-ama/councils/Council%20Reports/council-on-science-public-health/i09-csaph-suspected-child-abuse.pdf (accessed 21 April 2020).

4. Zenel J, Goldstein B. Child abuse in the pediatric intensive care unit. *Crit. Care Med.* 2002;30:S515–23.

5. Royal College of Paediatrics and Child Health. *Child Protection Companion* London. Paediatric Care Online and Royal College of Paediatrics and Child Health; 2013.

6. Case ME. Abusive head injuries in infants and young children. *Legal Med.* 2007;9:83–7.

7. Ferguson NM, Sarnaik A, Miles D, et al. Abusive head trauma and mortality—an analysis from an international comparative effectiveness study of children with severe traumatic brain injury. *Crit. Care Med.* 2017;45:1398–407.

8. Matschke J, Herrmann B, Sperhake J, Korber T, Glatzel M. Shaken baby syndrome. *Dtsch. Arztebl. Int.* 2009;106:211–17.

9. Barlow KM, Minns RA. Annual incidence of shaken impact syndrome in young children. *Lancet* 2000;356:1571–2.

10. Wygnanski-Jaffe T, Morad Y, Levin AV. Pathology of retinal hemorrhage in abusive head trauma. *Forensic Sci. Med. Pathol.* 2009;5:291–7.

11. Morad Y, Kim YM, Mian M, Huyer D, Capra L, Levin AV. Nonophthalmologist accuracy in diagnosing retinal hemorrhages in the shaken baby syndrome. *J. Pediatr.* 2003;142:431–4.

12. Maguire S, Mann M. Systematic reviews of bruising in relation to child abuse—what have we learnt: an overview of review updates. *Evid. Based Child Health* 2013;8:255–63.

13. Paul AR, Adamo MA. Non-accidental trauma in pediatric patients: a review of epidemiology, pathophysiology, diagnosis and treatment. *Transl. Pediatr.* 2014;3:195.

14. Royal College of Paediatrics and Child Health and The Royal College of Physicians of London and its Faculty of Forensic and Legal Medicine UK. *The Physical Signs of Child Sexual Abuse: An Evidence-based Review and Guidance for Best Practice.* Sudbury: Lavenham Press; 2015

15. Bass C, Glaser D. Early recognition and management of fabricated or induced illness in children. *Lancet* 2014;383:1412–21.

17 Inherited metabolic disorders in the Paediatric Intensive Care Unit

Dilanee Sangaran

ⓘ **Expert commentary** by Mike Champion

Case history

A female term infant was born by ventouse delivery. She was the first baby born to consanguineous parents. The pregnancy was uneventful, with no concerns on antenatal scans. She required no resuscitation and there were no known risk factors for intrapartum sepsis. She began to breast feed, passed urine and meconium appropriately, and had a normal neonatal check by the paediatrician. She was discharged home at 24 hours of age breastfeeding well. However, over the following 24 hours she became progressively less responsive, was feeding less frequently, and was vomiting. This was associated with a decreased urine output.

By 72 hours of life, with ongoing deterioration, her parents presented to their local Emergency Department. After history and examination, she was diagnosed with neonatal sepsis and had a full septic screen performed. This included full blood count, C-reactive protein, blood, urine, and cerebrospinal fluid cultures, and was commenced on benzyl penicillin and gentamicin for broad-spectrum empirical antibiotic cover.

She was admitted to the paediatric ward and was later noted to have some abnormal movements of her upper and lower limbs, as well as abnormal eye movements. At the point of reassessment there were concerns of reduced responsiveness associated with possible seizures. She was given a loading dose of phenobarbitone, which terminated the apparent seizure and magnetic resonance imaging (MRI) of her brain was performed. This showed symmetrical diffusion restriction in the ventrolateral thalami, putamina, and peri-rolandic cortices—a pattern usually associated with acute hypoxic–ischaemic encephalopathy but which can be seen in some metabolic disorders.

> ⊗ **Learning point** Neonatal presentation of inherited metabolic disorder
>
> Neonatal presentation of IMDs can be varied and difficult to identify. They are often non-specific, with lethargy and poor feeding, and it is easy to overlook IMDs from the list of differential diagnoses. The other challenge is that these infants often present collapsed and in need of acute resuscitation. Therefore, the rapid management of shock and often treatment of multiorgan dysfunction needs to occur in parallel with investigation of the underlying diagnosis (see Case 2).

> ⓘ **Expert comment** Considering the diagnosis of inherited metabolic disorder
>
> Inherited metabolic diseases (IMDs) pose a particular challenge to diagnosis. There is a combination of non-specific symptoms and signs, with their rarity leading to limited exposure of medical staff outside the main metabolic centres, and the need for specific investigations to make the diagnosis. Individual disorders are rare but, collectively, are common with an incidence of <1 in 750. Clinicians, therefore, need to consider IMDs within the differential in undiagnosed patients and liaise early with the local IMD team to target investigations and expedite results. Earlier diagnosis significantly improves outcome in a number of acute disorders of intermediary metabolism.

⊕ **Clinical tip** History-taking in inherited metabolic disorder

The key to identifying the underlying disease process in a collapsed neonate is to take a careful and detailed history from the family. This will include asking about:

- parental consanguinity—increases the risk of a genetic disorder;
- family history of sudden unexpected infant death, especially in males—consider X-linked inheritance such as ornithine transcarbamylase (OTC) deficiency (the commonest of the urea cycle defects (UCD))—potential for previously affected siblings;
- family history of specific conditions within the extended family;
- pregnancy history, including early fetal losses, growth scans, and fetal movements—potential for previously affected pregnancies;
- maternal health in pregnancy—liver dysfunction associated with some IMDs;
- a symptom-free period of variable duration post-delivery;
- symptoms triggered by a period of illness, change in diet, or poor feeding;
- seizures;
- unusual odour, e.g. isovaleric acidaemia (IVA; pungent sweaty-feet smell), maple syrup urine disease (MSUD; slightly sweet smell to nappies; descriptions other than maple syrup have included curry, cappuccino, and marmite!).

⊕ **Expert comment** Maternal symptoms in pregnancy suggestive of inherited metabolic disorder in the fetus

Maternal acute fatty liver of pregnancy, and haemolysis, elevated liver enzymes, and low platelets (HELLP) syndrome are associated with carrying an affected fetus with a fat oxidation defect in a minority of cases. However, there is specific management for these conditions so acylcarnitines should always be checked in the infants of these mothers to avoid missing the potential therapeutic window to avoid decompensation or the development of cardiomyopathy. Maternal hepatic symptoms develop as the mother, being an obligate carrier, has reduced capacity to metabolize the metabolite that the affected fetus is producing in greater quantities, combined with the metabolic stress of pregnancy.

It is important to ask about increased fetal movements, especially rhythmic, as this may be a clue to in utero seizures in conditions such as non-ketotic hyperglycinaemia where early diagnosis allows timely counselling regarding prognosis and management options.

⊕ **Learning point** Neonatal presentations

IMDs can be considered in four broad groups in the neonatal period and those listed in Table 17.1 will more likely require input from intensive care, either at presentation or during a crisis, for supportive management and potential treatment.

Intoxication disorders

The intoxication arises from a block in intermediary metabolism, leading to an accumulation of a toxic metabolite. The key feature is the symptom-free period during which time the toxic metabolite accumulates, followed by the intoxication episode in which the baby can develop lethargy, poor feeding, vomiting, encephalopathy, and coma.

Energy deficiency disorders

These patients are unable to either produce energy or utilize it appropriately. Symptoms may be present at birth (no symptom-free period) or may appear more slowly. Interruption of feeding may provoke symptoms such as failing to establish feeds in medium-chain acyl-CoA dehydrogenase deficiency (MCADD), or poor feeding during illness in an hepatic glycogen storage disorder. They present with hyperlactataemia and/or severe hypoglycaemia, generalized hypotonia, myopathy, cardiomyopathy, and sudden infant death. Fat oxidation defects, and glycogenosis and gluconeogenesis defects respond well to treatment, but congenital lactic acidoses have a poor prognosis.

Complex molecule disorders

This group of patients is unable to either synthesize or catabolize complex molecules. Complex molecules play key roles in embryogenesis and so problems with synthesis may present with dysmorphic features at birth, whereas failure to breakdown complex molecules results in storage. With the exception of I-cell disease, dysmorphic features tend to develop with time as storage material accumulates and presentation in the neonatal period is uncommon.

Seizures

These patients are rarer in their presentation to intensive care. However, there are certain diagnoses that are key to identification, as they are a potentially treatable group of patients. Treatable conditions include pyrixodine-dependent seizures, folinic acid-responsive seizures, biotin-responsive multicarboxylase deficiency, and congenital malabsorption of magnesium. Treatment includes supplemental B6, folinic acid, biotin, or intramuscular magnesium sulfate, respectively. In practice, the IMD specialist may recommend empirical treatment with all of these therapies whilst the correct diagnosis is sought.

Table 17.1 Main subgroups of inherited metabolic diseases presenting in the neonatal period

Intoxication	Energy deficiency	Making and breaking complex molecules	Seizures
Aminoacidopathies MSUD Tyrosinaemia type 1	**Mitochondrial disorders** Pyruvate disorders Pyruvate dehydrogenase deficiency	**Lysosomal disorders** I-cell disease	**Vitamin disorders** Pyridoxine-dependent seizures Pyridoxal phosphate dependent seizures PROSC deficiency Biotinidase deficiency
Organic acidaemias Methylmalonic acidaemia Propionic acidaemia Isovaleric acidaemia	**Fatty oxidation disorders** MCADD VLCADD LCHADD MADD	**Peroxisomal disorders** Biogenesis disorders, e.g. Zellweger Rhizomelic chondrodysplasia punctata	**Aminoacidopathies** 3-Phosphoglycerate dehydrogenase deficiency Non-ketotic hyperglycinaemia
Urea cycle defects OTC deficiency Carbamoyl phosphate synthetase deficiency Citrullinaemia	**Glycogenoses and gluconeogenesis defects** Glycogen storage disorders Fructose 1,6-bisphosphate deficiency	**Inborn errors of cholesterol synthesis**	**Creatine synthesis defects** Creatine transporter defect GAMT deficiency
Sugar intolerances Galactosaemia		**Congenital disorders of glycosylation**	**Molybdenum cofactor deficiency** Sulfite oxidase deficiency **Glucose transporter defect (GLUT1)**

MSUD, maple syrup urine disease; PROSC, pyridoxal phosphate-binding protein; MCADD, medium-chain acyl-CoA dehydrogenase deficiency; VLCAD, very-long-chain acyl-CoA dehydrogenase deficiency; LCHAD, long-chain hydroxyl acyl-CoA dehydrogenase deficiency; MADD, multiple acyl-CoA dehydrogenase deficiency; OTC, ornithine transcarbamylase; GAMT, guanidinoacetate methyltransferase deficiency; GLUT1, glucose transporter 1.

⊕ **Clinical tip** Differential diagnoses of acute encephalopathy

- Sepsis: bacterial, viral, fungal
- Neurological: infective, vascular, traumatic
- Metabolic disorders
- Endocrine disorders: congenital adrenal hyperplasia
- Poisoning
- Drug withdrawal

Other conditions, including non-ketotic hyperglycinaemia, sulfite oxidase deficiency, and peroxisomal disorders present with an excess of seizures in the context of severe neurological insult. Electroencephalography (EEG) or cerebral function analysing monitoring (CFAM) with quantitative EEG is useful in the paediatric intensive care setting and will show periodic patterns of intense activity alternating with almost flat segments.

It is important to note that infants with UCD, MSUD, and organic acidaemia (OA) may also experience seizures, but this is a result of other pathological changes, including coma, encephalopathy, and hypoglycaemia.

⦅ ❝ **Expert comment** Metabolic encephalopathies

Metabolic encephalopathies may go undiagnosed owing to the requirement for specific assays to be undertaken. Notoriously, MSUD causes minimal acidosis, ketosis, and hypoglycaemia until decompensation is advanced. The diagnosis will not be made unless leucine is specifically requested in a plasma amino acid sample. Similarly, the early associated encephalopathy frequently goes unnoticed. Some IMD centres provide rapid tandem mass spectrometry (TMS) analysis on liquid or dried blood spot samples to confirm or rule out the diagnosis. On the same sample, fatty acid oxidation disorders, UCD, creatine disorders, tyrosinaemia type 1, and the common OAs can all be diagnosed/excluded.

The scan result prompted the team to seek advice from the local tertiary metabolic service, who suggested a baseline screen for IMDs and encephalopathy, including assessment of ammonia. The ammonia was 1165 µmol/L and, immediately, the local team requested transfer to the tertiary hospital for paediatric intensive care and specialist metabolic input.

⊕ **Clinical tip** Investigation of a suspected inborn error of metabolism

- Blood:
  - blood gas (arterial or venous);
  - glucose;
  - lactate (free flowing sample);
  - ammonia (free flowing sample);
  - acylcarnitines;
  - amino acids.
- Urine:
  - ketones (dipstick);
  - organic acids, including orotic acid;
  - reducing substances—if galactosaemia suspected (NB: these disappear once feeds are stopped and therefore unreliable in the acute PICU patient who will be nil by mouth on intravenous (IV) fluids).
- Newborn screening blood sample (if not yet sent). (NB: IVA and MSUD often present prior to the screening result being available. MCADD can present as early as the first 48 hours if feeding fails to be established.)

Depending upon the clinical condition of patient and acuity of situation consider:

- brain imaging (CT or MRI);
- EEG/CFAM.

If the child is deteriorating significantly and withdrawal of intensive care support and palliation need to be offered, then consideration must be given to obtaining samples for diagnosis perimortem. Conditions more likely to present like this are mitochondrial disorders and advanced decompensation in UCDs and OAs. The parents should be counselled about this and the following should be taken, with advice from a metabolic specialist:

- heparinized blood samples (10 mL)—sample separated in the laboratory (red cells stored at 4°C, plasma stored at –20°C);
- ethylenediaminetetraacetic acid (EDTA) samples for DNA analysis;
- four blood spots on Guthrie card- can be used for TMS and DNA;
- urine 10-20 mL stored at –20°C;
- skin biopsy—culture medium or sterile saline stored at 4°C (refrigerator; *do not freeze*);
- muscle and liver biopsies (if indicated—discuss with local IMD team) need to be snap frozen in liquid nitrogen or rapidly transported to a –80°C freezer;
- postmortem examination may be requested for medical, legal purposes to establish a cause of death.

ⓖ Expert comment Perimortem tissue sampling

Previously, muscle and liver biopsies were taken perimortem, with the family's prior consent, within 30 minutes of death to reduce the risk of the degrading of samples due to autolysis. Beyond this, samples are unhelpful/impossible to interpret. The timing was to spare the families the distress of such invasive samples when their child was so sick and to avoid increasing the child's pain and discomfort taking samples that ultimately could hasten their death. Coroners (in England) increasingly will not allow such biopsies after death and so this critical opportunity to make a diagnosis may be lost. Discussion with the coroner's office or similar medico-legal entities elsewhere is essential to clarify local requirements and whether such samples are permitted within their jurisdiction, as this will inform the timing and discussions with families.

✪ Learning point Hyperammonaemia

- Ammonia is a powerful central respiratory stimulant that drives hypocarbia and so infants can present with a respiratory alkalosis (uncommon in sick neonates and infants). Ammonia is also unusual in that it promotes its own toxicity. At physiological pH, 95% is in the ammonium form, but as levels and pH rises this drives the equilibrium towards ammonia, which more readily diffuses into cells.
- Blood ammonia levels should be taken as a free-flowing sample (venous or arterial) and collected, ideally, into a prechilled sample container (or on ice) with either EDTA or lithium heparin (but must have been confirmed to be free of ammonia contamination). The sample should be separated in the laboratory within 15 minutes of collection and analysed immediately. Non-free-flowing samples and non-urgent samples will lead to spuriously elevated results, as the ammonia level of standing blood increases spontaneously due to generation and release of ammonia from red blood cells.
- In the case of intensive care retrieval, a repeat sample should always be requested of the local team before the retrieval team leaves base. This ensures that the repeat sample will be available on arrival and will give a sense of the trend and the subsequent urgency of treatment. Note: if the original sample has an ammonia >200 µmol/L do not delay initiation of treatment.

On arrival of the retrieval team she was intubated and ventilated with fentanyl, ketamine, and rocuronium. She remained haemodynamically stable. Her feeds were stopped and she was started on maintenance fluids of 10% dextrose with 0.9% sodium chloride via a peripheral IV cannula. Specialist scavenging medications were not available immediately during retrieval.

➕ Clinical tip Testing for hyperammonaemia

Respiratory alkalosis in a sick neonate/or infant should prompt clinicians to assess the blood ammonia level, if this has not already been done. In any child of any age with unexplained cerebral oedema, encephalopathy, seizures, or coma, ammonia level *must* be checked.

Ammonia levels in the newborn and treatment thresholds

- Normal <100 µmol/L.
- Severe illness (including IMDs) >180 µmol/L.
- Hepatic failure, UCD, OA, transient hyperammonaemia of the newborn (THAN) >400 µmol/L.
- UCD, OA, THAN >1000 µmol/L.
- Ammonia >100 µmol/L will cause encephalopathy.
- Ammonia >150 µmol/L *must* be investigated thoroughly for IMD.
- Ammonia >350 µmol/L will require haemofiltration if ammonia levels are rising in spite of medical management
- 1 month of age <50 µmol/L.

Expert comment Transient hyperammonaemia of the newborn

THAN is a rare, but treatable, cause of high ammonia levels, which may be significantly greater than 1000 µmol/L. Prognosis is excellent if the hyperammonaemia is recognized early and ammonia controlled rapidly, owing to its transient and reversible nature. Onset is earlier than classical UCDs—usually within the first 24–36 hours—and is thought to result from temporary shunting of blood, bypassing hepatocytes, so although urea cycle function in the liver is normal, ammonia is not cleared. Biochemically, THAN is characterized by a low plasma glutamine:ammonia ratio of <1.6.

In the PICU, she had a repeat ammonia sample sent. A metabolic screen was taken (including blood and urine samples). She had a vascath and central line placed in order to facilitate continuous veno-venous haemofiltration (CVVH) and the administration of alternative pathway medications—arginine hydrochloride, sodium benzoate, and sodium phenylbutyrate. The ammonia level, obtained prior to initiation of CVVH, had fallen to 732 µmol/L.

Learning point Emergency treatment of acute crisis or presentation

The plan should always be to resuscitate first, identify key elements of the diagnosis, and then treat symptomatically in the first instance before specialist intensive care or metabolic help can be sought. If the child already has a diagnosis of IMD then the parents may present with an emergency management plan.

- Manage airway, breathing, circulation, and neurological disability as per life support guidelines.
- Manage cause of decompensation, e.g. identify and treat sepsis. Consider antibiotics—bacterial sepsis can be fatal in these patients.
- Stop all feeds and promote anabolism by starting IV 10% dextrose (at a rate of >8 mg/kg/min) with added electrolytes as required.
- Check glucose, ammonia, and lactate urgently, and initiate appropriate treatment.
- Manage hyperglycaemia of >12 mmol/L with a low-dose insulin infusion at 0.05 units/kg/h.
- Start relevant alternative pathway treatments.
- Engage help from specialist team.

Priority must be given to elimination of toxic metabolites that accumulate and cause symptoms, as well as managing the potentially significant metabolic acidosis.

The choice of drugs will depend upon the biochemical toxicity of the patient. In patients with high ammonia, treatment should begin with an IV infusion of L-arginine, which will allow conversion of ammonia to urea in arginine-deficient states. Arginine is made in the body within the urea cycle and therefore becomes an essential amino acid when the cycle is impaired (with the exception of arginase deficiency) and so can be depleted.

Start IV infusions of sodium benzoate, which will conjugate with glycine, and sodium phenylbutyrate, which conjugates with glutamine, forming water-soluble metabolites that can be excreted in the urine, bypassing the urea cycle. Always start these drugs together in severe decompensation situations and monitor closely for hypokalaemia while these infusions are running. The conjugation process creates an increase in phenylacetylglutamine and hippurate, both of which enhance renal potassium loss.

Loading doses are indicated where the patient is not regularly on these medications. They can be given in 5% or 10% dextrose. The former is preferred in small infants as hyperglycaemia may ensue following loading over the prescribed 90 minutes if 10% dextrose is used. These alternate pathway medications include a significant sodium load and so sodium is often omitted from maintenance fluids and sodium levels monitored carefully.

Often the diagnosis is unknown at the outset and therefore all treatments are started concurrently, and scaled back once the diagnosis is apparent. Therefore, start carnitine if there is a high anion gap acidosis, as it allows the elimination of organic acids as carnitine esters. A warning, however: carnitine can cause fatal arrhythmias if used in some fatty acid oxidation defects. Specialist advice *must* be sought.

Carglumic acid (Carbaglu; Orphan Europe, Paris, France) is indicated in hyperammonaemia if there is a deficiency of the hepatic enzyme *N*-acetylglutamate synthase and should be started under specialist metabolic advice. While awaiting a diagnosis, consideration can be given to augmenting residual enzyme activity by starting cofactors, for example biotin (carboxylase deficiency), thiamine (MSUD), and vitamin B12 (methylmalonic acidaemia).

The acidosis can be managed initially with IV sodium bicarbonate; however, owing to the ongoing catabolic state of the patient, this may not be sufficient to correct it. Use of potassium bicarbonate or acetate may help alleviate the hypokalaemia. It is common to have to these as continuous infusions throughout the acute period of decompensation.

Throughout this process, adequate amounts of glucose should be delivered to encourage anabolism— at least 8 mg/kg/min but may well be higher. Insulin will not only manage the hyperglycaemia, but also helps to promote anabolism.

Her ammonia cleared within 24 hours and CVVH was discontinued. Metabolic screen showed a markedly raised plasma citrulline along with urinary orotic acid, indicating a deficiency in arginosuccinate synthetase (a urea cycle enzyme that converts citrulline to arginosuccinate). A diagnosis of citrullinaemia was made (see Figure 17.1).

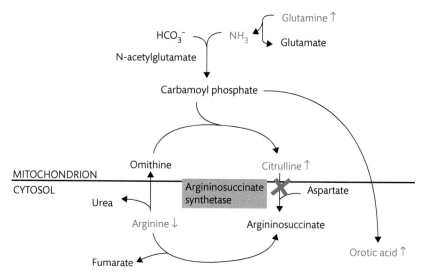

Figure 17.1 Urea cycle with the enzyme defect causing citrullinaemia shown.
Source: Adapted from Mew NA, Simpson KL, Gropman AL, et al., Urea Cycle Disorders Overview. In: Adam MP, Ardinger HH, Pagon RA, et al. [Eds.], GeneReviews, Copyright (1993–2020), with permission from University of Washington, Seattle.

While on the ICU, an anabolic state was promoted aggressively by restricting protein completely and starting Intralipid (Baxter, Deerfield, IL, USA) at 1 g/kg/day. While on alternative pathway medications, enteral feeds of expressed breast milk were reintroduced, initially with a protein load of 0.5 g/kg/day, increasing to 2 g/kg/day as tolerated with minimal change to her ammonia levels. She was moved to the paediatric ward and arginine supplementation was continued.

➕ **Clinical tip** Calculating the glucose infusion rate

Glucose infusion rate (mg/kg/min) = (infusion rate (mL/h) × dextrose %)/ (6 × weight (kg))

🕮 **Expert comment** Feeding children with inherited metabolic disorders in the PICU

Nutrition must be delivered in a form that is appropriate for the patient's clinical condition; either tailored total parenteral nutrition or formula for an enteral diet. Specialist dietetic and pharmacy advice should be sought. Energy will need to come from a carbohydrate and/or fat source, to avoid exogenous nitrogen intake (for the first 48 hours). If there is clinical improvement with good ammonia clearance, then protein can be reintroduced at 0.5 mg/kg/day and increased as tolerated. The challenge lies in finding the ideal balance between switching off catabolism—and the volume of nutrition required to allow this—and managing the expected fluid restriction in a sick, ventilated patient in intensive care. Promoting anabolism, thereby utilizing exogenous protein, rather than sending it down the impaired pathway to be broken down, is the key to successful management—switching off the increased production of ammonia. Adequate nutritional support is central to successful management and therefore greater daily fluid volumes are often required versus other non-IMD PICU patients. As the patient improves the aim is for early extubation and the promotion of enteral specialist feed.

Deciding whether to feed or what fluids to use in the undiagnosed patient can be a challenge. The standard fluid used in these patients is 10% dextrose with 0.9% sodium chloride, with added potassium. However, carbohydrate loads in mitochondrial patients can drive lactate levels much higher. Five per cent dextrose-based fluids are preferred in these patients. It is important to supply adequate dextrose to meet the glucose requirements for age to avoid iatrogenic hypoglycaemia due to fluid restriction in the PICU without compensatory increase in dextrose provision. A newborn's hepatic glucose production rate is 7–8 mg/kg/min. Breast milk and most formulas approximate to 7% glucose concentration, which can be used when enteral feeding is allowed.

Further anabolism can be promoted by the early introduction of Intralipid as a fat source in suspected IMDs, for example UCD and OAs, once a fatty oxidation defect has been excluded on acylcarnitine profile.

Protein cessation, in the initial management stage should be for a maximum of 48 hours, which should also take into account from the history the time that regular feeds stopped prior to retrieval. This may have already stretched to several days in the presentation.

Discussion

Haemofiltration in hyperammonaemia

Hyperammonaemia is a medical emergency. The decision to use CVVH is critical in preventing or minimizing irreversible central nervous system damage. When in doubt in the face of a markedly elevated ammonia levels failing to respond to stopping protein and IV medications, the decision should be to haemofilter as soon as possible.

Prior to starting haemofiltration it is imperative to ensure that blood is taken for DNA storage, in order to maximize the chances of securing the diagnosis. Allogenic blood exposure is high in critically ill children and haemofiltration circuits will often be blood primed in patients < 10 kg.

Hyperammonaemia causes a metabolic encephalopathy due to the conversion of large amounts of glutamate to glutamine, mostly within the astrocytes. In response to the osmotic effect of the glutamine, the astrocytes swell, resulting in cerebral oedema, intracranial hypertension, and cerebral hypoperfusion. Both the peak ammonia level and the duration of hyperammonaemia will have a direct effect on neurocognitive function. The mortality rates of neonates presenting with hyperammonaemia is much higher than in older children who have repeated episodes or present later in life. This shows the non-linear relationship between ammonia levels and encephalopathic damage.

In the majority of children with UCD who survive, there are varying degrees of cognitive impairment. The degree of developmental disability and brain abnormalities relates to the severity, duration, and age of onset of hyperammonaemia. The speed at which hyperammonaemia is recognized and reduced is the key to good outcomes.

If the ammonia level is > 350 µmol/L or is rising rapidly despite maximal scavenging treatment (within the first 4 hours), then the only other way of removing ammonia is by haemofiltration. Peritoneal dialysis is less effective in these patients and haemodialysis alone can cause significant fluid shifts in the already compromised patient; therefore, the safest management strategy is CVVH or continuous veno-venous haemodiafiltration. In all patients in the PICU, it is advisable to intubate and ventilate and ensure adequate levels of sedation and neuromuscular blockade (as required) prior to inserting vascath and central venous lines. Vascaths are generally placed into the right internal jugular; the tip placement should be confirmed by both plain chest radiograph and echocardiogram. The line should lie almost parallel to the spine and not cross the midline; if it does it is much more likely to be in the right atrium and will need manipulating. On echocardiogram, the tip should be at the right atrium–inferior vena cava junction (see Case 9 for more information on renal replacement therapy RRT).

The largest double-lumen catheter for the size of the patient is ideal. For effective use of CVVH for the clearance of ammonia, the removal has to occur at a higher rate than production. The patient will remain on all scavenging infusions while on CVVH to maximize the excretion of ammonia, as well as continuing to achieve an anabolic state. There may be a period of instability when the patient is started on CVVH initially, especially in those weighing < 10 kg. This will need to be managed judiciously with fluid boluses and inotropes as indicated.

The clearance of any substance during filtration is dependent upon many factors— its volume of distribution in the plasma, the sieving coefficient of the membrane, and the rate of ultrafiltration. The passage of solutes is dependent upon their molecular weight and the design of the membrane in the haemofilter. Most membranes will allow the passage of molecules between 20,000 and 30,000 Da. This includes ions and small chemicals such as sodium, potassium, magnesium, calcium, phosphate, bicarbonate, glucose, and ammonia. The patient must have strict biochemical monitoring throughout the duration of CVVH and the use of appropriate replacement haemofiltration fluid.

Although ammonia will be freely filtered, in order to ensure maximum clearance, the ultrafiltration rate on the CVVH will need to be higher than in other circumstances, i.e. > 100 mL/kg/h. The blood flow rate will also need to be high to support the increased ultrafiltration rate. However, with this higher rate there may be more evidence of recirculation, noted by the decrease in rate of ammonia clearance. In neonates this is usually around 10% but can be as high as 50%.

CVVH can be utilized in other IMD conditions, where the rate of lactate (pyruvate disorders) or leucine (MSUD) production is also too high and unsuitable for other methods of clearance. Both these molecules are small enough to be freely filtered freely across the standard membranes and a more conservative ultrafiltration rate will suffice as the consequences on the developing brain of these molecules is far less devastating.

In general, CVVH will be effective at rapidly clearing toxic metabolites, including ammonia. The duration of therapy will be patient and disease specific and is guided by tracking serial ammonia measurements. Once the level remains < 100 µmol/L, then challenging the patient off haemofiltration may be appropriate. There will always be a rebound rise in ammonia, but this should be managed with the continuation of alternative pathway medications and the ongoing promotion of anabolism via adequate nutrition. It may become clear that the patient will need to have a further period of time of filtration and this may be the prompt to re-evaluate prognosis and the continuation/discontinuation of treatment.

The technical limit for CVVH and patient size is typically around 2.5 kg. For smaller infants cross-flow peritoneal dialysis may be considered using two indwelling catheters, which ensures that the dialysate enters the abdomen and clears the catheter internal volume.

> ⓕ **Expert comment** Liver and hepatocyte transplantation
>
> In some patients with UCDs who have recurrent hyperammonaemic episodes, the only remaining option may be liver transplantation. This is dependent upon many factors, including the availability of a suitable donor and the degree of overall neurological insult sustained. Transplant offers excellent survival, metabolic correction, and overall improved quality of life with a normal protein diet. It has also been shown to improve, although not completely reverse, some neurological deficits
>
> In acutely unwell neonates with minimal encephalopathic damage, it may be appropriate to recommend an hepatocyte transplant as a suitable treatment option, commonly known as a 'bridge to transplantation'. The technique has been used internationally in children with UCDs and is improving, but the availability is dependent upon suitable donor cells. Once this treatment strategy has been embarked upon, the clinical trajectory would require a full liver transplant.

A final word from the expert

The advent of next-generation sequencing, facilitating whole-exome and whole-genome sequencing, is fundamentally changing our ability to diagnose IMDs, both previously described and novel. In recent years a number of new conditions have been recognized using this strategy in conjunction with detailed phenotyping. Examples include TANGO2 (encephalopathy, hypoglycemia, hyperammonaemia, episodic rhabdomyolysis, cardiac tachyarrhythmias, developmental delay) and carbonic anhydrase VA deficiency (CAVA; encephalopathy, hyperammonaemia, acid–base disturbance, ketosis, hypoglycaemia) to add to the hyperammonaemia differential. DNA samples should be taken for storage at the time of referral, prior to transfusion, to allow further molecular studies as the clinical picture develops.

Good links with the local IMD and genetics teams are important for an effective PICU to keep up with developments and evolution of management strategies. Newborn screening is likely to continue to expand as therapeutic options increase, including genetic therapies that are now beginning to come to clinical trial. IMDs are an increasingly significant part of modern intensive care and a working knowledge of investigation and first-line management is an essential skill for the intensivist.

Further reading

British Inherited Metabolic Disease Group. Emergency guidelines. Available at: www.bimdg.org.uk/guidelines.asp (last accessed 21 April 2020).

Saudubray J-M, Baumgartner MR, Walter JH. *Inborn Metabolic Diseases: Diagnosis and Treatment*, 6th edition. New York: Springer; 2016.

Auron A, Brophy PD. Hyperammonemia in review: pathophysiology, diagnosis, and treatment. *Paediatr. Nephrol.* 2012;27:207–22.

Leonard JV, Morris AAM. Diagnosis and early management of inborn errors of metabolism presenting around the time of birth. *Acta Paedictr.* 2006;95:6–14.

Champion MP. An approach to the diagnosis of inherited metabolic disease. *Arch. Dis. Child Educ. Pract. Ed* 2010;95:40–6.

Dhawan A. Clinical human hepatocyte transplantation: current status and challenges. *Liver Transplant.* 2015;21:S39–44.

18 Nutritional considerations in the Paediatric Intensive Care Unit

Ben D. Albert and Katelyn Ariagno

ⓘ Expert commentary by Nilesh M. Mehta

Case history

Lilly, an 8-year-old female, is admitted to the Paediatric Intensive Care Unit (PICU) after developing acute respiratory insufficiency in the oncology unit. She has been hospitalized for the past several weeks after being diagnosed with acute lymphoblastic leukaemia (ALL), being treated with an intensive chemotherapy regimen. The oncology staff became concerned 2 days ago when she developed a fever in the setting of neutropenia. Her illness began with a cough and nasal congestion 3 days prior to her fever. Lilly's mother reports that her daughter has been losing significant weight over the past several months. She is concerned about Lilly's low energy and limited food intake, which she attributes to severe mouth pain, dysphagia, decreased appetite, and nausea in the past weeks.

> **✪ Learning point** Nutritional challenges in children with cancer
>
> Children undergoing treatment for an oncological diagnosis are at high risk for poor nutrient intake and malnutrition. Decreased intake and increased gastrointestinal (GI) losses may be a consequence of the disease process and/or side effects of treatment. Children may experience significant nausea and vomiting because of chemotherapy and/or radiation. They may develop complications such as mucositis, pancreatitis, colitis, and pneumatosis intestinalis.[1] Mucositis is particularly common in children undergoing stem cell transplantation, leading to decreased oral intake until it resolves after engraftment. Graft-versus-host disease, which can affect multiple organs including the GI tract can lead to intolerance of enteral nutrition (EN) secondary to pain, abdominal discomfort, and diarrhoea. Inadequate intake in addition to the increase metabolic demand from disease or infections may result in the conversion from a state of anabolism to catabolism, which can result in loss of muscle mass.[1]

This morning, in the oncology unit, the medical team noticed that Lilly's work of breathing had increased, with an elevated respiratory rate and evidence of accessory muscle use. She was requiring 2 litres of oxygen delivered via nasal cannula to maintain her oxygen saturation above 95%. On physical examination, she was febrile, flushed, and warm to the touch. She was promptly initiated on broad-spectrum antibiotics. A normal saline bolus was administered for hypotension and the Intensive Care Unit (ICU) team was consulted with a request to transfer to an escalated level of care. Upon arrival in the ICU, Lilly was started on bilevel positive airway ventilation to alleviate work of breathing. A second peripheral intravenous (IV) catheter was placed for additional access. A chest X-ray (CXR) was performed, which revealed right lower and middle lobe infiltrates. Initial diagnosis included a respiratory infection with early acute lung injury in the setting of febrile neutropenia (immunocompromised host).

A more detailed medical history was obtained from her mother. Lilly was born full term at 39 weeks' gestation. She had never been hospitalized before she was diagnosed with ALL 4 weeks ago. She has no other medical problems and did not take any medications before starting chemotherapy. Her treatment course has been significant for alopecia, intermittent headaches, severe nausea, emesis, and mucositis. Nausea has been a consistent issue since she began chemotherapy. Certain foods, especially those with a strong odour, tend to trigger nausea. During chemotherapy, Lilly would have 2–3 episodes of emesis per day, requiring ondansetron for relief. Lately, her mucositis has worsened and has resulted in an even greater decline in her ability to tolerate food. She has one older brother at home who has not been sick. She is in the third grade and doing well in school.

Once the patient was stabilized, other members of the multidisciplinary team began to introduce themselves to the family. The social worker provided an orientation of the ICU, as well as an overview of support services available to Lilly and her family during her admission. The dietitian introduced herself and explained she would obtain a more detailed history and nutritional assessment.

Clinical tip A detailed nutrition history

Nutrition-related interview questions should be focused to obtain information related to the patient's historical and current nutritional status. These questions include dietary intake (parenteral or enteral), including any vitamin and dietary supplements. Recent intended or unintended weight changes. Oral and GI symptoms should be questions to assess barriers to appropriate nutrient intake. Brief questions about swallowing and oral coordination can be signs of aspiration risk. Lastly, a family and social history should be obtained to understand the environmental and socio-economic factors to appropriate nutrition.[2]

Learning point Assessment of nutritional status

All children should have initial nutritional screening within 24 hours of admission to the PICU.[3] Screening allows for identifying patients admitted with malnutrition or at risk of nutritional deterioration, and may allow early intervention in these high-risk patients. It has been reported that up to 45% of critically ill children are malnourished on admission.[4] Children with chronic diseases are at an even higher risk of malnutrition. An initial nutritional assessment should include a nutrition/growth history, medical history, anthropometric data, nutrition-focused physical examination, and review of laboratory data.[2] Growth charts should also be reviewed and utilized throughout admission.

Expert comment Growth charts

The World Health Organization (WHO) growth charts should be used for infants and children up to 2 years of age. These growth curves are international standards of growth potential for healthy, well-nourished, breastfed babies. The Centers for Disease Control (CDC) growth curves are a national reference for children aged 2–19 years. In addition, specialty growth curves should be utilized as a supplement for children with particular disorders, including Down syndrome and Turner syndrome. Anthropometry includes height/length, weight, and head circumference, as well as mid-upper arm circumferences (MUACs) and triceps skinfold (TSF) thicknesses. Weight/length (<2 years) and body mass index (BMI; >2 years) should be calculated. Standard deviations (SDs) are available for weight, height, BMI, head circumference, MUAC, and TSF. The z scores, defined as SDs from the mean, are used to compare children of various ages and sex.[2] The z scores can then be used in the classification of malnutrition.

During the dietitian's nutritional assessment, she obtained a detailed dietary history from Lilly's parents. Lilly had not been eating well for the past 3 weeks. She has been suffering pain while swallowing, resulting in her only taking small quantities of soft foods, such as yogurt, bananas, and juices. Her peak weight 4 weeks ago was 23 kg and is currently 20 kg on admission today. Her parents explain that she appears more emaciated than usual and is more tired throughout the day. On physical examination, Lilly has hair loss, dry mucous membranes, and blistered lips with some ulcerations. The dietitian plotted her height and weight on the growth chart. Her height was just above the 25th percentile for age and weight at the third percentile for age. The dietitian then measured her MUAC and TSF thickness, which were 17 cm and 7 cm, respectively.

> ⊕ **Clinical tip** Performing circumference and skin fold anthropometric measurements
>
> Anthropometric measurements such as MUAC and TSF can be used to assess fat mass and serve as indices of malnutrition.[1] MUAC is calculated as the circumference of the arm at the point between the acromion process of the scapula and the olecranon process of the elbow, with the patient's arm by their side and a 90-degree bend at the elbow. TSF is measured using a skinfold calliper at the point used for measuring MUAC. The clinician pulls skin and subcutaneous fat away from muscle and takes a reading between the calliper blades. Multiple readings (usually three) should be taken in both MUAC and TSF thickness values, and averages should be recorded.[2] Standardized tables can be used based on age and sex.[5] All anthropometric data should be taken into consideration when assessing nutrition status.

> ⊕ **Expert comment** Anthropometric measurements
>
> To ensure accuracy, anthropometric measurements should be performed by a trained clinician/ dietitian. TSF is a useful indicator of total body fat stores when compared to reference data for appropriate age groups. Caution should be taken in children who are acutely ill. For example, in oncological patients undergoing chemotherapy or haematopoietic stem cell transplantation, steroid therapy and fluid overload (with subcutaneous oedema) can make these measurements unreliable. However, recent studies have shown that anthropometric data can predict outcomes, such as length of mechanical ventilation, hospital-acquired infections, and mortality in critically ill children.[6–8]

As the dietitian completed her documentation of her nutritional assessment, she discussed with the medical team that Lilly is categorized as having 'severe malnutrition'. Her BMI is currently 12.8 kg/m^2, which is lower than –2 z scores, based on the CDC criteria She also has weight loss that exceeds 10% of her usual body weight. Her MUAC and TSF thickness are concerning for decreased fat stores. The dietitian asks the medical team to order additional laboratory testing, including a C-reactive protein, prealbumin and chemistry panel.

> ✪ **Learning point** Diagnosing paediatric malnutrition
>
> The American Society for Parenteral and Enteral Nutrition (ASPEN) has recently provided a practical definition for malnutrition and described the characteristics of paediatric malnutrition.[3,9] Historically, anthropometric data alone were used to categorize malnutrition as mild, moderate, and severe. However, these authors highlight the importance of considering other critical components when thinking about a child's nutritional state. Firstly, the authors categorize the aetiology of malnutrition into either illness related or non-illness related. Secondly, if related to the patient's illness, the length of malnutrition is considered acute (<3 months) or chronic (>3 months). Lastly, the mechanism of malnutrition should be considered. These factors, in addition to traditional anthropometric data, comprise a more comprehensive definition of paediatric nutrition. Upon admission to the PICU, children will have one or more variables to use to categorize the degree of malnutrition. When only a single data point is available, z scores for weight-for-length, BMI-for-age, length/height-for-age, and MUAC can be used. Children with z scores of –1 to –1.9 have mild malnutrition, –2 to –2.9 have moderate malnutrition, and –3 or less have severe malnutrition.[9] Becker et al. also described the categorization of nutrition if two or more indicators are available, based on WHO data for patients <2 years of age.[9]

Overnight, Lilly's condition continued to worsen. She developed worsening hypoxia requiring endotracheal intubation and mechanical ventilation. Repeat CXR showed evolving bilateral pulmonary infiltrates. She was diagnosed with acute respiratory distress syndrome, based on her clinical, radiographic, and laboratory findings. A central venous catheter and arterial line were placed for monitoring. She was started on a norepinephrine infusion for continued hypotension, with resulting improved stability. Her parents were updated regarding Lilly's critical condition.

> ⊘ **Evidence base** Enteral feeding and vasoactive infusions
>
> In a retrospective analysis of 339 patients, Panchal et al. compared children aged 1–18 years who were fed versus not fed while receiving vasoactive infusions during the first four days of ICU admission.[10] They reported no significant adverse GI outcomes, such as necrotizing enterocolitis or bowel perforation, in children receiving EN while on vasoactive agents. It is important to note that the authors classified children receiving any amount of EN to the fed group and therefore no conclusions can be drawn regarding an association with the amount of enteral feeding being delivered. Initiation and gradual advancement of enteral feeding in patients with haemodynamic stability on a single vasoactive infusion is deemed safe. Feedings may be advanced slowly with the caveat that the clinician must have high vigilance for any GI manifestation of poor perfusion or intolerance. In patients who require ongoing fluid boluses or those on double vasoactive or escalating vasoactive infusions, EN may be deferred until haemodynamic stability is achieved.

On morning rounds, the paediatric resident asked whether it would be appropriate to begin EN. The resident expressed his concern that Lilly had been on dextrose-containing IV fluids with normal saline but had not received any nutrition for the past 2 days. The dietitian stated on rounds that she agreed and would like to start providing some nutrition, although was concerned that given her severe malnutrition status, she might have electrolyte instability during the initiation of feeding.

> ✪ **Learning point** Refeeding syndrome
>
> Clinicians should anticipate refeeding syndrome in high-risk patients. Early awareness can prevent significant clinical deterioration. Refeeding syndrome is defined as clinical and biochemical changes that occur to accommodate cellular processes in response to nutritional repletion in a malnourished child.[11,12] Risk factors for refeeding syndrome in children include, but are not limited to, anorexia nervosa; failure to thrive; prolonged fasting (>5 days); children with complex health needs; and oncological, inflammatory, GI, and cardiac diseases. During starvation, the body becomes deplete of electrolytes. Fats and proteins are broken down during gluconeogenesis by the liver for energy. Shifts in electrolytes occur in response to fluid shifts to maintain homeostasis. Upon restoration of nutrition, intracellular shifts in electrolytes accelerates owing to an increase in metabolic demand as the liver converts to an anabolic state to produce protein and glycogen. This often results in hypophosphataemia, hypokalaemia, and hypomagnesaemia. Hyperglycaemia also occurs as a result of a lack of inadequate insulin supply, and thiamine deficiency can a occur as a result of an acute increase in carbohydrate and glucose load.[12] Clinical symptoms of refeeding syndrome include cardiovascular, respiratory, haematological, and musculoskeletal complications that are often a manifestation of hypophosphataemia. Cardiac complications can include ventricular dysrhythmias and cardiac systolic dysfunction, which can often be worsened by fluid retention in refeeding syndrome.[12] Weakness from hypophosphataemia can result in respiratory failure secondary to respiratory muscle weakness. Paraesthesia, tetany, and seizures are neurological complications of refeeding syndrome. Musculoskeletal symptoms can include myopathy and rhabdomyolysis.[12-14] These life-threatening manifestations highlight the importance of vigilant surveillance and recognition of patients at high risk for refeeding syndrome. Electrolytes should be promptly replaced in cases of derangement and re-checked frequently. Refeeding syndrome may be prevented by careful attention to those at risk and by very careful and gradual introduction of EN with strict vigilance and frequent checking of electrolyte levels.

⊕ **Clinical tip** When to use parenteral nutrition

Although EN is the preferred route of nutrition delivery, some children are unable to tolerate feeding their GI tract. Children with surgical GI disorders, short bowel syndrome, motility disorders, congenital heart disease, and hypermetabolic states such as trauma or burns may not be able to receive EN. A careful discussion should begin early. The multidisciplinary medical team will need to balance the risks and benefits of starting parenteral therapy. EN remains the primary target for feeding if the GI tract is working properly. Risks of parenteral nutrition (PN) include thrombotic occlusions, infectious complications, metabolic derangements and liver dysfunction, especially during long term use. Once PN is initiated, continued discussions should occur daily to consider when a patient can be transitioned to EN.

⊘ **Evidence base** Timing of parenteral nutrition

A multicentre, randomized controlled trial by Fivez et al., published in 2016, investigated early initiation of PN (day 1 of admission) versus late initiation of PN (7 days after admission).[15] Three centres enrolled 1440 infants and children were randomized to one of two arms in the study. The investigators reported an absolute risk reduction in new infections and a decreased time to ICU discharge readiness in the late PN group. This large trial in children provides evidence in practice where it is currently lacking; however, applicability and generalizability to patients should be done with caution. Many children in the late PN group were discharged before they received PN and most children in the study were not moderately or severely malnourished.

⑥ **Expert comment** Enteral nutrition

Clinicians must decide between providing EN versus PN when beginning to provide nutrition therapy in the severely malnourished child at risk for refeeding syndrome. EN is preferred. If tolerated, EN by mouth, nasogastric tube, or surgically placed feeding route should begin as early as possible. Contraindications would include obstructive GI physiology, malabsorption, or intolerance of feedings. Electrolyte abnormalities should be corrected before nutrition therapy commences. Clinicians should begin feedings slowly to determine clinical and electrolyte stability. As a general guideline, patients should begin receiving approximately 25% of estimated resting energy expenditure (REE; based on predictive equations) or based on patient/family dietary recall when starting feedings. Feeds should be advanced slowly by increasing caloric intake by 10%–25% per day over the course of a week. If the patient's actual caloric intake is less than estimated REE, the patient's caloric intake should serve as the starting point for feeding. Protein should not be restricted to allow for rebuilding muscle mass. Advancement of feedings should always be at clinician discretion based on patient tolerance and stability. Serum chemistries should be monitored frequently. Daily weights should be obtained to ensure appropriate fluid balance.

⊘ **Evidence base** Gastric versus postpyloric feeding

According to ASPEN Pediatric Nutrition Support Guideline Recommendations, there is currently insufficient evidence to recommend gastric versus postpyloric feeding as a uniform strategy in critically ill children.[16] Gastric feeding is thought to be more physiological. Postpyloric feeding may be considered in patients at high risk for aspiration or in patients in whom gastric feeding has been unsuccessful. Initiation of feeding should not be delayed if there is difficulty or inexperience in placing a postpyloric feeding tube.

⑥ **Expert comment** Energy requirement

Total energy requirements for children include REE, physical activity-associated energy requirements, diet-induced thermogenesis, and energy necessary for growth. However, during illness, metabolic needs in children are altered. In acute stress, the body transitions to catabolism, resulting in the breakdown of endogenous protein, carbohydrate, and fat stores to provide energy. This response is thought to be driven by a higher energy requirement. However, children treated in the ICU have various factors that will lower energy requirements, such as temperature regulation, sedation, assisted ventilation, and decreased activity level. Mechanical ventilator support with sedation may also decrease energy expended for respiratory effort and lower insensible energy losses due to warmed, humidified air. Therefore, calories provided based on equations that were developed in healthy children often overestimate the energy requirement and may result in overfeeding. Overfeeding may increase the CO_2 burden in such patients (secondary to caloric excess) and this may be poorly tolerated in patients with respiratory insufficiency or failure.

Monitoring a child's growth over time is the best indicator of appropriate nutrition status during their stay in the ICU. It is therefore important to document serial weight and height/length measurements during the ICU stay. These measurements can help guide nutrition, fluid balance status, medication delivery, and mechanical ventilator therapy. It is essential to raise awareness of the importance of at least weekly weights, if not more frequently, during discussion on multidisciplinary rounds.

Indirect calorimetry (IC) allows accurate measurement of REE. However, in the absence of IC, estimated basal metabolic energy expenditure can be calculated. One commonly used predictive method is the Schofield weight equation. It is important to note that all predictive equations usually overestimate energy needs but can be used as a guide when determining a patient's energy prescription.

✚ Clinical tip Protein requirements

Protein requirements vary depending on the age of the child and may be calculated using the handy guide shown in Table 18.1.

Table 18.1 Protein requirements (ASPEN Clinical Guidelines for critically ill children)

Age (years)	Protein (g/kg/day)
0–2	2–3
2–13	1.5–2
13–18	1.5

Source: Data from *J Parenter Enteral Nutr*, 33(3), Mehta NM, Compher C, A.S.P.E.N. Clinical Guidelines: nutrition support of the critically ill child, pp. 260–76, Copyright (2009), The American Society for Parenteral and Enteral Nutrition.

★ Learning point Enteral nutrition in the critically ill child

EN remains the preferred route of nutrition delivery in critically ill children. The benefits of enteral feeding, as well as enteral feeding early in critical illness, has been well described. Studies have demonstrated improved mortality and decreased length of ICU stay in children receiving early EN. However, it is essential to consider the timing, route, potential tolerance, and barriers to providing EN for each individual child. The benefits of EN in a population of children who are often in a catabolic state with significant physiological stress and inflammation may seem intuitive. Providing optimal nutrition does not reduce protein breakdown, but might improve protein synthesis, reduce nutrient deficits, and improve GI tolerance. As always, risks should also be weighed when deciding to provide EN. These risks include aspiration of gastric contents into an unprotected airway, GI dysmotility, and GI perforation. Once feeding begins, interruptions are very common in the ICU owing to procedures and clinician perception of intolerance based on abdominal distention and gastric residual volume measurements. Standardized unit feeding algorithms have shown evidence in minimizing these interruptions. Algorithms have also been shown to help children reach an adequate volume of nutrition early in their hospitalization.[18]

Over the course of the next week, Lilly continued to require mechanical ventilation for respiratory failure. Despite receiving EN, Lilly had not gained weight. The decision was made to perform IC, given her oncological diagnosis and her inability to wean from mechanical ventilation over the past week. She completed IC after she achieved a steady state on the mechanical ventilator. Based on these findings, her nutrition prescription was adjusted to meet her metabolic needs.

✚ Clinical tip Estimating resting energy expenditure

The Schofield weight equation can be used to calculate estimated REE, in kilocalories (kcal), based on age, weight, and sex for children. For example, the patient in this case is an 8-year-old female who weighs 20 kg. The corresponding Schofield equation to calculate her estimated REE is 22.5 × (kg) + 499.[17] This would equal 949 kcal.

★ Learning point Indirect calorimetry

IC is a method used in the PICU to measure REE in mechanically ventilated patients. Advances in technology have allowed for a portable metabolic cart brought to the bedside, measuring breath-to-breath oxygen (VO_2) and carbon dioxide (VCO_2) production. During aerobic metabolism, heat is produced, as oxygen consumed as a substrate, and carbon dioxide is released as a byproduct. Using the modified Weir equation, measurement of VO_2 and VCO_2 can be used to determine REE.[19] Short measurements of gas exchange may be used to predict 24-hour REE values, but these measurements must meet criteria for steady state (minimum fluctuation in VCO_2 and VO_2 values) for at least 5 minutes. Owing to limited resources in most PICUs, a targeted approach to IC has been suggested to apply this method in those at highest risk of metabolic derangement (Table 18.2).[19] Limitations that prevent accurate IC include ventilator circuit or endotracheal tube leak, chest tube air leak, fraction of inspired oxygen requirement >60%, or patients receiving high-frequency oscillatory ventilation.

Table 18.2 Suggested criteria for indirect calorimetry in the Paediatric Intensive Care Unit

1. Underweight (BMI <5th percentile for age), at risk of overweight (BMI >85th percentile for age), or overweight (BMI >95th percentile for age)
2. >10% weight gain or loss during medical–surgical Intensive Care Unit stay
3. Failure to consistently meet prescribed caloric goals
4. Failure to wean or escalation in respiratory support
5. Need for muscle relaxants for >7 days
6. Neurological trauma (traumatic, hypoxic, and/or ischaemic) with evidence of dysautonomia
7. Oncological diagnoses (including stem cell or bone marrow transplantation)
8. Need for mechanical support >7 days
9. Suspicion of severe hypermetabolism (status epilepticus, hyperthermia, systemic inflammatory response syndrome, dysautonomic storms) or hypometabolism (hypothermia, hypothyroidism, drug-induced coma)
10. Intensive Care Unit length of stay >4 weeks

BMI, body mass index.
Source: Adapted from *J Parenter Enteral Nutr*, 33(3), Mehta NM, Bechard LJ, Leavitt K, et al., Cumulative energy imbalance in the pediatric intensive care unit: role of targeted indirect calorimetry, pp. 336–44, Copyright (2009), with permission from The American Society for Parenteral and Enteral Nutrition.

Lilly began to improve, gradually weaning off mechanical ventilation and tolerating full nasogastric feedings. She was made nil-per-mouth in preparation for extubation. Once Lilly was extubated successfully and demonstrated respiratory stability, the team restarted enteral feeing. With her nasogastric feeding tube still in place, they resumed feeds that night. Over the next several days, she also began to take small sips of water and juice by mouth after a formal speech and swallow assessment. The clinical team monitored her weight and nutritional status routinely to monitor her progress. In discussion with oncology, a pain regimen was discussed to treat the discomfort caused by her mucositis. Owing to her improving trajectory, discussions began regarding transfer of care back to the oncology unit for continued treatment of her ALL.

Discussion

Nutrient delivery in critical illness may be overlooked in the complex management of a critically ill child. Yet, this remains one of the key components to a child's healing and recovery. The heterogeneous population in the PICU, with varying ages, diagnosis, severity of illness, and degree of malnourishment, complicates this further. Each patient requires an individual plan, taking into consideration their medical history, current problem area, and barriers to adequate nutrition. To accomplish this, a structured nutritional assessment is the first step in this process. This allows the medical team to obtain a baseline risk assessment and starting point. Once nutrition is initiated, ongoing re-evaluation, including frequent weight checks, must be obtained to monitor progress closely.

A final word from the expert

The prevalence of malnutrition in critically ill children remains high. Heightened awareness and screening for malnourished individuals is an important initial task on admission. Studies have shown that a malnourished state and decreased nutritional intake is associated with increased morbidity and mortality in this population. A nutritional assessment, with an individualized plan for macronutrient and micronutrient intake for each patient is essential. Energy requirements in critically ill children can be variable, and equations used to estimate energy expenditure are often inaccurate. In the absence of indirect calorimetry to measure accurate energy expenditure, clinicians must be vigilant for either underfeeding or overfeeding calories. Protein requirements are probably higher in critically ill children and may impact outcomes. Once nutritional needs are determined, a careful approach to select the best route, timing, and method of nutrient delivery must be selected. Patients must be monitored for intolerance to EN and risk of refeeding syndrome with dyselectrolytaemia. A dedicated PICU dietitian, use of an algorithmic stepwise nutrition guideline, increased awareness of the role of nutrition, and its impact on outcomes are factors that have been shown to promote optimal and safe nutrition in the PICU setting. As evidence continues to emerge, clinical guidelines will continue to be revised to provide guidance on the best evidence-based practice.

References

1. Mehta NM, Goday PS. *Pediatric Critical Care Nutrition.* New York: McGraw-Hill; 2015.
2. Green Corkins K, Teague EE. Pediatric nutrition assessment. *Nutr. Clin. Pract.* 2017;32:40–51.
3. Mehta NM, Corkins MR, Lyman B, et al. Defining pediatric malnutrition: a paradigm shift toward etiology-related definitions. *JPEN J. Parenter. Enteral Nutr.* 2013;37:460–81.
4. de Souza Menezes F, Leite HP, Koch Nogueira PC. Malnutrition as an independent predictor of clinical outcome in critically ill children. *Nutrition* 2012;28:267–70.
5. Abdel-Rahman SM, Bi C, Thaete K. Construction of lambda, mu, sigma values for determining mid-upper arm circumference z scores in U.S. children aged 2 months through 18 years. *Nutr. Clin. Pract.* 2017;32:68–76.
6. Grippa RB, Silva PS, Barbosa E, Bresolin NL, Mehta NM, Moreno YMF. Nutritional status as a predictor of duration of mechanical ventilation in critically ill children. *Nutrition* 2017;33:91–5.
7. Bechard LJ, Duggan C, Touger-Decker R, et al. Nutritional status based on body mass index is associated with morbidity and mortality in mechanically ventilated critically ill children in the PICU. *Crit. Care Med.* 2016;44:1530–7.
8. de Souza Menezes F, Leite HP, Koch Nogueira PC. Malnutrition as an independent predictor of clinical outcome in critically ill children. *Nutrition* 2012;28:267–70.
9. Becker P, Carney LN, Corkins MR, et al. Consensus statement of the Academy of Nutrition and Dietetics/American Society for Parenteral and Enteral Nutrition: indicators recommended for the identification and documentation of pediatric malnutrition (undernutrition). *Nutr. Clin. Pract.* 2015;30:147–61.
10. Panchal AK, Manzi J, Connolly S, et al. Safety of enteral feedings in critically ill children receiving vasoactive agents. *JPEN J. Parenter. Enteral Nutr.* 2016;40:236–41.
11. Pulcini CD, Zettle S, Srinath A. Refeeding syndrome. *Pediatr. Rev.* 2016;37:516–23.
12. Marinella MA. Refeeding syndrome in cancer patients. *Int. J. Clin. Pract.* 2008;62:460–5.
13. Marinella MA. Refeeding syndrome and hypophosphatemia. *J. Intensive Care Med.* 2005;20:155–9.

14. Fuentebella J, Kerner JA. Refeeding syndrome. *Pediatr. Clin. North Am.* 2009;56:1201–10.
15. Fivez T, Kerklaan D, Mesotten D, et al. Early versus late parenteral nutrition in critically ill children. *N. Engl. J. Med.* 2016;374:1111–22.
16. Mehta NM, Compher C. A.S.P.E.N. Clinical Guidelines: nutrition support of the critically ill child. *JPEN J. Parenter. Enteral Nutr.* 2009;33:260–76.
17. Schofield WN. Predicting basal metabolic rate, new standards and review of previous work. *Hum. Nutr. Clin. Nutr.* 1985;39(Suppl. 1):5–41.
18. Hamilton S, McAleer DM, Ariagno K, et al. A stepwise enteral nutrition algorithm for critically ill children helps achieve nutrient delivery goals. *Pediatr. Crit. Care Med.* 2014;15:583–9.
19. Mehta NM, Bechard LJ, Leavitt K, Duggan C. Cumulative energy imbalance in the pediatric intensive care unit: role of targeted indirect calorimetry. *JPEN J. Parenter. Enteral Nutr.* 2009;33:336–44.

INDEX

Notes

Abbreviations found in the index can be found in the List of Abbreviations

Tables and figures are indicated by *t* and *f* following the page number